Fluids, Electrolytes, and Acid-Base Disorders Handbook

SECOND EDITION

EDITORS

Jeffrey J. Bruno, PharmD, BCPS, BCNSP, BCCCP, FCCM

Nicki L. Canada, MS, RD, LD, CNSC

Todd W. Canada, PharmD, BCNSP, BCCCP, FASPEN

Anne M. Tucker, PharmD, BCNSP

Joseph V. Ybarra, PharmD, BCNSP

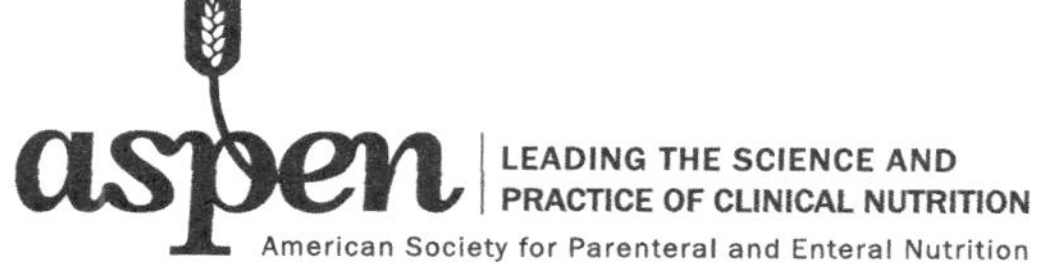

About ASPEN

The American Society for Parenteral and Enteral Nutrition (ASPEN) is a scientific society whose members are health care professionals; physicians, dietitians, nurses, pharmacists, other allied health professionals, and researchers; that envisions an environment in which every patient receives safe, efficacious, and high-quality patient care.

ASPEN's mission is to improve patient care by advancing the science and practice of clinical nutrition and metabolism.

Print ISBN 978-1-889622-43-9
eBook ISBN 978-1-889622-44-6

Suggested citation: Bruno J, Canada N, Canada T, Tucker AM, Ybarra JV, eds. ASPEN Fluids, Electrolytes, and Acid-Base Disorders Handbook, Second Edition. Silver Spring, MD: American Society for Parenteral and Enteral Nutrition; 2020.

3 4 5 6 7 8 9 10

Printed in the United States of America.

Contents

Foreword

I am delighted to write the foreword to *ASPEN Fluids, Electrolytes, and Acid-Base Disorders Handbook, Second Edition*. The management of fluids, electrolytes, and acid-base problems is of vital importance. However, the task of managing these issues if often left to many of the more inexperienced members of a medical team. Without thorough training, patients may be at risk for numerous complications. Maintaining a patient's hydration and electrolyte balance is complex and requires an in-depth foundation. Further, managing adults or children who have developed fluid and/or electrolyte disorders can be some of the most challenging aspects of clinical medicine. Such disorders may lead to significant hemodynamic, cardiovascular, respiratory, and neurologic complications, and if not appropriately corrected may lead to death.

Under the editorial guidance of Jeff Bruno, Nicki Canada, Todd Canada, Anne Tucker, and Joe Ybarra, this handbook will serve as a wonderful compendium for healthcare professionals who manage the nutrition care of their patients. The handbook will also provide an excellent reference for routine medical care beyond that centered on nutrition. The handbook is nicely laid out in a sequential order from normal physiologic needs of the patient to defined approaches to disorders in hydration, electrolytes, and acid-base disturbances. The handbook offers stepwise approaches to correct the most important of such disorders, and then has separate sections on common clinical scenarios (Chapter 5) and the medical approach to their care. Of key importance is a strong chapter on pediatric considerations (Chapter 6). Each chapter is replete with critical tables and formulas to guide the reader and provide them with a practical approach to patient care.

Key experts in each area have contributed to the six core chapters presented herein. This handbook serves as the perfect companion to other ASPEN resources, including *The ASPEN Adult Nutrition Support Core Curriculum, Third Edition* and ASPEN's evidence-based clinical guidelines and standards documents.

ASPEN believes that the reader will find the easy-to-read format and comprehensive tables and figures to be an excellent guide for bedside clinical use.

Lingtak-Neander Chan, PharmD, BCNSP
President, ASPEN
Professor of Pharmacy, University of Washington School of Pharmacy
Seattle, Washington

Preface

Appropriate treatment of fluid and electrolyte disorders is imperative in clinical practice to provide quality patient care and ensure positive outcomes. Clinicians and trainees encounter situations daily that require the ability to recognize such disorders, determine their etiology, and provide management recommendations regardless of clinical practice environment. The updated 2nd edition of the *ASPEN Fluids, Electrolytes, and Acid-Base Disorders Handbook* was designed to be a comprehensive bedside handbook on fluids, electrolytes, and acid-base disorders and how each relates to patient care, including appropriate identification and treatment strategies.

The handbook offers something for everyone, from novice to the advanced practitioner irrespective of health care background. Experts in the field of fluids, electrolytes, and acid-base disorders were sought to provide the most up-to-date, evidenced-based recommendations. This handbook serves as the perfect pocket companion to the ASPEN adult and pediatric core curriculums, evidence-based guidelines, and standards documents. Its easy-to-read format consisting of tables, figures, bullet point statements, and step-by-step guides make it ideal for bedside use. We hope that this handbook quickly becomes your go-to pocket guide for management of fluids, electrolytes, and acid-base disorders.

The *ASPEN Fluids, Electrolytes, and Acid-Base Disorders Handbook, Second Edition* is organized into six chapters. Chapter 1 lays the foundation for the reader by providing an overview of water regulation and electrolyte balance. Chapters 2 through 4 provide detailed overviews of disorders related to water, individual electrolytes, and acid-base homeostasis. Clinical scenarios presented in chapters 1 through 4 allow users to better grasp concepts and further develop clinical skills. Chapter 5 focuses on common clinical situations in which in-depth understanding of fluids, electrolytes and acid-base balance is required. While the handbook primarily focuses on adult patients, chapter 6 provides insight into pediatric considerations related to fluids, electrolytes, and acid-base homeostasis and management. To ensure completeness, nutrition support principles and strategies have been incorporated where appropriate.

In closing, we would like to acknowledge that this publication would not have been possible without the countless hours of dedication from our contributors and support from the ASPEN Board of Directors and publications staff. We would like to specifically thank Kassie Stovell, ASPEN Director, Publications for her patience and dedication in bringing this publication to print. Her attention to detail and insights into medical publishing will certainly add to the future success of this handbook. It definitely takes a village to bring a book to print.

ASPEN Fluids, Electrolytes, and Acid-Base Disorders Handbook, Second Edition Editors

Editors

Jeffrey J. Bruno, PharmD, BCPS, BCNSP, BCCCP, FCCM
Director, PGY2 Critical Care Pharmacy Residency
Clinical Pharmacy Specialist – Critical Care / Nutrition Support
The University of Texas MD Anderson Cancer Center
Houston, TX

Nicki L. Canada, MS, RD, LD, CNSC
Assistant Director, Clinical Nutrition
Texas Children's Hospital
Houston, TX

Todd W. Canada, PharmD, BCNSP, BCCCP, FASHP, FTSHP, FASPEN
Nutrition Support Clinical Pharmacy Specialist
The University of Texas MD Anderson Cancer Center
Houston, TX

Anne M. Tucker, PharmD, BCNSP
Clinical Pharmacy Specialist – Critical Care/Nutrition Support
The University of Texas MD Anderson Cancer Center
Houston, Texas

Joseph V. Ybarra, PharmD, BCNSP
Director of Corporate Clinical Pharmacy
Division of Clinical Excellence, CHRISTUS Health
Irving, TX

CHAPTER 1

Regulation of Water and Electrolyte Balance

Composition of Body Fluids[1,2]

1. Water

- Water is the major constituent of the human body, accounting for 50% and 60% of body weight in females and males, respectively (Figure 1-1). Accordingly, total body water (TBW) can be calculated as follows:
  - Women: TBW (L) = weight (kg) × 0.5 (L/kg)
  - Men: TBW (L) = weight (kg) × 0.6 (L/kg)
- Water is associated with lean body mass. Muscle contains approximately 75% water, while adipose tissue contains only 10% water. Factors such as percentage of body fat, age, and sex affect the percentage of TBW (Table 1-1).
- In obese patients (ie, body mass index [BMI] ≥ 30 kg/m^2 or >125% ideal body weight), lean body weight (LBW) can be used to determine TBW.

  LBW (women) = [1.07 × weight (kg)] – 148 × [weight (kg)/height (cm)]^2

  LBW (men) = [1.1 × weight (kg)] – 128 × [weight (kg)/height (cm)]^2

Figure 1-1. Body Fluid Composition.

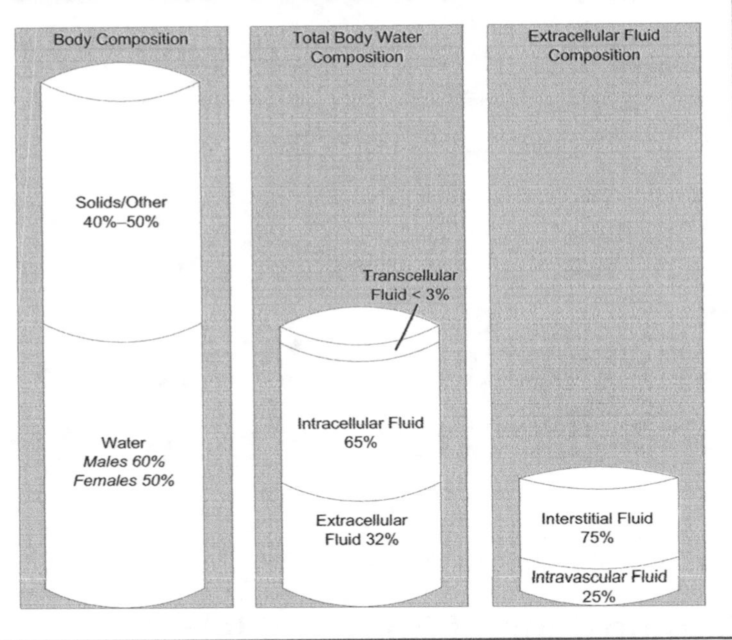

- Alternatively, equations that consider the above factors, such as the Watson formula, can be utilized to calculate TBW.

Women: TBW (L) = –2.097 + [0.1069 × height (cm)] + [0.2466 × weight (kg)]

Men: TBW (L) = 2.447 – [0.09156 × age (y)] + [0.1074 × height (cm)] + 0.3362 × weight (kg)]

Table 1-1. Factors That Affect Total Body Water.

Factor	Description
Fat	Fat contains little water. TBW decreases with increasing body fat.
Age	Muscle mass declines and the proportion of fat increases with age; thus, TBW decreases with increasing age.
Sex	Women have proportionately higher body fat than men; thus, women have less TBW.

TBW, total body water.

2. Solutes

- Solutes that are normally present in body fluids can be divided into 2 general categories: electrolytes and nonelectrolytes.
- Electrolytes are substances that dissociate in solution and carry a charge (eg, sodium, chloride, potassium, phosphorus, bicarbonate).
- Nonelectrolytes are substances that do not dissociate in solution (eg, creatinine, urea, bilirubin, glucose).

Fluid Compartments[1,3]

1. TBW is distributed among 3 main compartments: the intracellular (ICF), extracellular (ECF), and transcellular fluid (TCF) compartments (Figure 1-1).
2. ICF accounts for approximately 65% of TBW.
    - ICF stability is vital to normal cell function and is protected from variations by the cell membrane and the ECF compartment.
3. ECF accounts for approximately 32% of TBW.
    - ECF includes both the interstitial and intravascular spaces.
    - The interstitial space accounts for approximately 75% of the ECF. It includes fluid within the lymphatic system and the fluid surrounding individual cells.
    - The intravascular space accounts for approximately 25% of the ECF. It includes fluid within the blood vessels.
4. TCF accounts for less than 3% of TBW.
    - It includes specialized fluids such as cerebrospinal fluid, aqueous humor of the eye, and secretions of the gastrointestinal tract, among others.

Movement of Water and Solutes[4,5]

Semipermeable membranes separate the fluid compartments of the body. Several processes control the movement of water and solutes between these compartments.

1. Active transport involves the use of energy (typically adenosine triphosphate, ATP) to move solutes across cell membranes against a

concentration gradient (ie, from areas of lower concentration to those of higher concentration). An example is the sodium-potassium-ATPase pump, which pumps potassium into cells in exchange for sodium in order to maintain ICF potassium concentrations of ~150 mEq/L despite ECF concentrations of only 3.5–5 mEq/L.

2. Passive transport does not require energy and entails the movement of solutes across cell membranes along a gradient (eg, concentration, pressure). Gas exchange in the lungs is an example of passive transport, with a net flow of carbon dioxide out of cells and oxygen into cells.

3. Osmosis is the passive movement of water between the ECF and ICF compartments in response to osmotic gradients. Water moves from areas of lower osmolality to areas of higher osmolality in order to maintain homeostasis.

   - The concentration of effective osmoles (solutes that cannot passively cross cell membranes) is responsible for generating osmotic gradients. The osmotic pressure in each fluid compartment is primarily dependent on 1–2 solutes.

   - ECF osmolality is primarily dependent on sodium.

   - ICF osmolality is primarily dependent on potassium and phosphate.

Serum Osmolality[5]

1. Under normal conditions, the serum osmolality (ie, osmolality of the intravascular space) is 275–290 mOsm/kg H_2O.

   - Serum osmolality can be determined by laboratory analysis (ie, measured via blood draw) or estimated with the following equation:

     Serum osmolality (mOsm/kg H_2O) = 2 × serum sodium (mEq/L) + [serum glucose (mg/dL)/18] + [blood urea nitrogen (mg/dL)/2.8]

   - As reflected in the equation, serum osmolality is primarily dependent on the serum sodium concentration, but it can also be affected by large changes in serum glucose (eg, hyperglycemic hyperosmolar state) and/or azotemia (eg, acute kidney injury [AKI]).

   - In addition, the introduction of large amounts of effective osmoles that are not normally present in the body (eg, propylene glycol) can result in an elevated measured serum osmolality. (Note that such elevations will not be captured with the above equation.)

2. Alterations in serum osmolality elicit compensatory mechanisms to re-establish sodium and water homeostasis in the ECF.

Regulation of ECF[4,6-10]

The ECF is the most clinically important compartment because it contains both the intravascular and interstitial compartments. Volume, composition, and concentration of the ECF are regulated by a complex interplay of renal, metabolic, and neurohormonal processes.

Intravascular Volume and Concentration[7]

Effective blood volume (EBV) is defined as the volume of circulating intravascular fluid available for tissue perfusion. Typically, systolic blood pressure is used as a surrogate marker for EBV. Decreases in the EBV (or systolic blood pressure) trigger compensatory mechanisms to help maintain adequate tissue perfusion. Increases in the EBV (or systolic blood pressure) trigger mechanisms to help the body eliminate excess fluids (Figure 1-2).

1. Stimulation of the sympathetic nervous system triggers the release of catecholamines (epinephrine, norepinephrine, dopamine), which provide an initial, short-term response to compensate for a decrease in EBV. Catecholamines increase cardiac contractility and heart rate, thus increasing cardiac output. They also cause vasoconstriction leading to increased blood pressure.

2. Activation of the renin-angiotensin-aldosterone system results in an increase in both blood pressure (mediated by angiotensin II) and intravascular volume (mediated by aldosterone), providing a subsequent rise in EBV (Figure 1-3). See Table 1-2 for other factors that influence aldosterone secretion.

3. Natriuretic peptides are secreted in response to elevated cardiac pressures or increases in intravascular volume. Three types of natriuretic peptides exist, all of which cause increased sodium excretion, vasodilation, and suppression of the renin-angiotensin-aldosterone system, ultimately decreasing intravascular volume.

   - Atrial natriuretic peptide is produced by the atrial myocardium.
   - Brain natriuretic peptide is produced by the ventricular myocardium.
   - C-type natriuretic peptide is produced by the vascular endothelium.

Figure 1-2. Regulation of Effective Blood Volume and Systolic Blood Pressure.

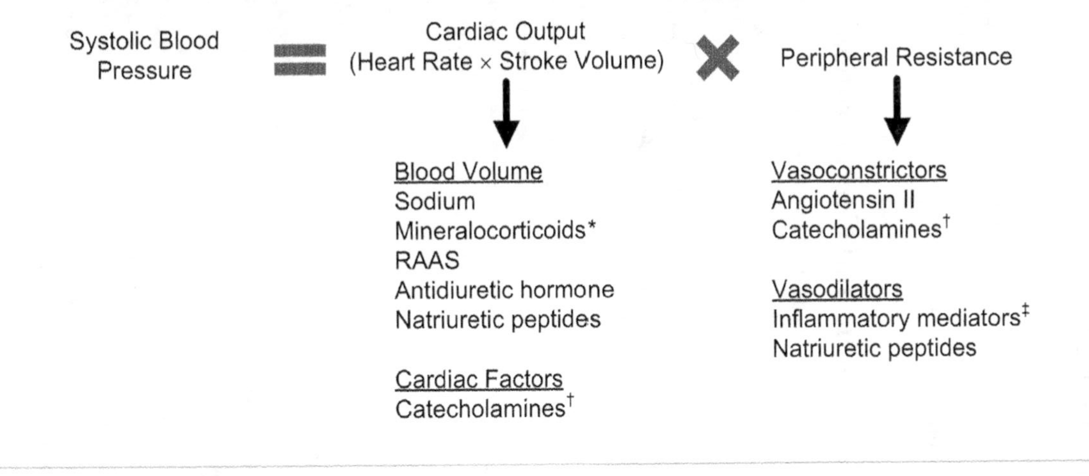

RAAS = renin-angiotensin-aldosterone system
* eg, aldosterone
† Catecholamines—epinephrine, norepinephrine, dopamine
‡ Inflammatory mediators—histamine, serotonin, bradykinin, complement component 3a and 5a, prostaglandins, prostacyclins

Figure 1-3. The Renin-Angiotensin-Aldosterone System.

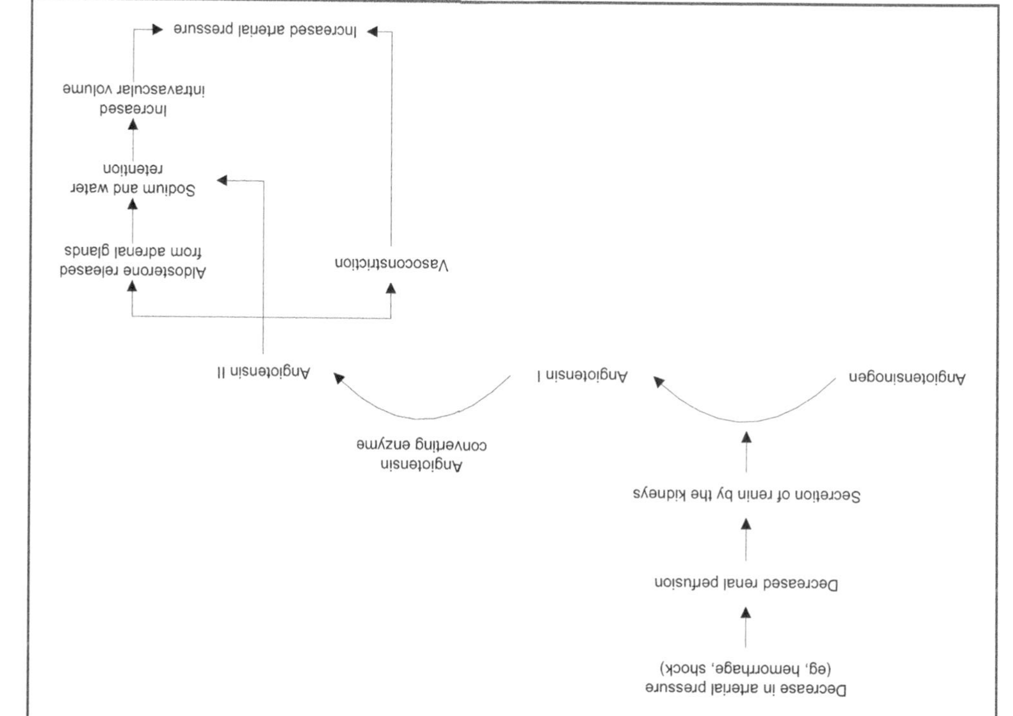

Table 1-2. Factors That Influence the Secretion of Aldosterone.

Decrease secretion	Increase secretion
Hypokalemia	Hyperkalemia
Atrial natriuretic peptide	Angiotensin II
Hypernatremia	Hyponatremia
	Adrenocorticotropic hormone

4. Arginine vasopressin (also referred to as antidiuretic hormone, ADH) is produced by the hypothalamus and secreted by the posterior pituitary gland in response to changes in serum osmolality. ADH acts on the distal tubules and collecting ducts in nephrons to increase water reabsorption and concentrate urine.

    - An elevation in serum osmolality will result in an increased release of ADH, leading to increased water reabsorption.
    - Elevations in serum osmolality also activate the hypothalamus-stimulated thirst mechanism, prompting the intake of fluids by mouth (if feasible) and complementing the effects of ADH in relation to water retention.
    - A reduction in serum osmolality will result in the opposite effects (ie, decreased release of ADH and cessation of the thirst mechanism).

Role of the Kidneys[8–10]

The kidneys help maintain homeostasis of the ECF compartment by eliminating waste products (urea, creatinine, and uric acid) and adjusting urinary excretion of water and electrolytes to match exogenous intake and endogenous production (Table 1-3). Approximately every 30 minutes, the kidneys filter the entire plasma volume, resulting in 135–180 L of filtered fluid per day in a normal adult.

1. Urine output can be characterized by volume in milliliters per kilogram per hour.

    - Normal urinary output ranges from 0.5 to 2 mL/kg/h.
    - Oliguria is defined as a urine output < 0.5 mL/kg/h (or < 400 mL/d).
    - Anuria is < 50–100 mL of urine output in 24 hours.
    - Polyuria is > 2 mL/kg/h.

2. A reduction in urine output could be representative of AKI.

Table 1-3. Major Functions of the Nephron.

Component	Major functions
Glomerulus	Filters electrolytes, amino acids, glucose, urea, and other solutes from the blood to form a plasma ultrafiltrate Should not filter visceral proteins (albumin) or red blood cells; the presence of these colloids in urine may indicate injury or damage to the glomerulus.
Proximal tubule	Reabsorbs 65%–70% of sodium and water Reabsorbs 90% of filtered bicarbonate Reabsorbs nearly all glucose and amino acids Reabsorbs potassium, phosphorus, calcium, magnesium, urea, and uric acid Secretes many organic bound drugs[a]
Loop of Henle	Reabsorbs 15%–25% of sodium Is a major site of active regulation of magnesium excretion
Distal tubule	Is a major site of active regulation of calcium excretion Reabsorbs sodium and chloride and secretes potassium under the influence of aldosterone Reabsorbs water in the presence of ADH
Collecting ducts	Reabsorb water and urea relative to concentrations of ADH present (dilution or concentration of urine) Secrete hydrogen and ammonia to final urine pH (can be as low as 4.5–5)

ADH, antidiuretic hormone.

[a]Penicillin, probenecid, indomethacin, methotrexate, furosemide, chlorothiazide, hydrochlorothiazide, amiloride, dopamine, morphine, quinine, triamterene, acetazolamide, salicylates, atropine, procainamide, and chlorpromazine.

3. AKI can be characterized into prerenal, intrinsic, or postrenal.

- Prerenal AKI occurs as a result of intravascular depletion (ie, hypovolemia) or an inability to perfuse the kidneys (eg, cardiogenic shock)
- Intrinsic AKI occurs as a result of a direct nephrotoxic insult (eg, administration of foscarnet or cidofovir), and may also be a secondary consequence of persistent prerenal injury (eg, cardiogenic shock-induced ischemia).
- Postrenal AKI occurs as a result of factors downstream from the actual kidney (eg, bladder outlet obstruction, extrinsic ureteral compression due to malignancy, urinary catheter obstruction), leading to obstruction of urinary flow.
- For a full discussion of renal injury or failure, please see Chapter 5.

4. Acute oliguria is often the first sign of AKI or impairment because rises in blood urea nitrogen (ie, azotemia) and serum creatinine may lag behind the injury by several days. A thorough evaluation of the oliguric patient can be helpful in identifying the underlying problem and providing timely treatment.

   - The fractional excretion of sodium (FE_{Na}), which characterizes the amount of filtered sodium that is reabsorbed by the tubules, can be used to help differentiate prerenal from other types of AKI (ie, intrinsic or postrenal).
   - Figure 1-4, describes use of FE_{Na} in the evaluation of acute azotemia and/or oliguria. Urine sodium, serum sodium, urine creatinine, and serum creatinine should be obtained simultaneously (or as close in time as possible for accuracy).
     - Recent administration of diuretics and/or hypertonic saline can influence urine sodium measurements and subsequently impair the interpretation of FE_{Na} calculation results.

Figure 1-4. Interpretation of the Fractional Excretion of Sodium (FE_{Na}).

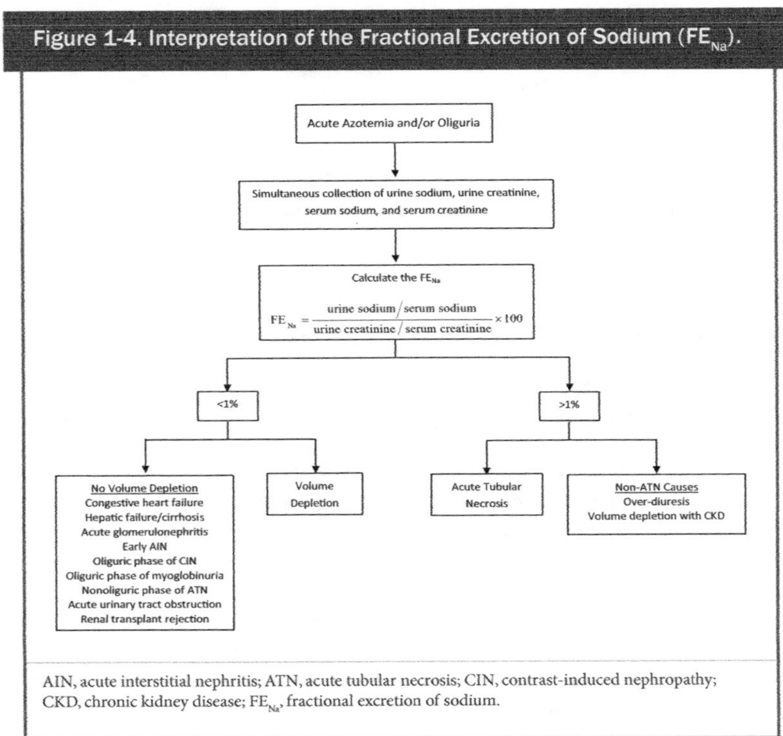

AIN, acute interstitial nephritis; ATN, acute tubular necrosis; CIN, contrast-induced nephropathy; CKD, chronic kidney disease; FE_{Na}, fractional excretion of sodium.

- FE_{Na} < 1% with azotemia usually indicates a low urine sodium concentration and favors a diagnosis of intravascular volume depletion from fluid loss or third-spacing; however, a FE_{Na} < 1% does not guarantee prerenal azotemia. In addition, a FE_{Na} < 1% may also be seen in nonazotemic patients (ie, without AKI) in the setting of moderate salt intake.

- FE_{Na} results around 1% are nonspecific and should be interpreted with caution because fluctuations in sodium intake or excretion (due to diuretics) can bias calculations.

- FE_{Na} > 1% with azotemia usually indicates a higher urine sodium concentration and is suggestive of acute tubular necrosis (from intrinsic renal damage). It can also occur with volume depletion secondary to diuretic use or in the setting of chronic renal failure. In nonazotemic patients (ie, without AKI), a FE_{Na} > 1% may also be seen due to excessive sodium intake.

Fluid Balance and Provision[1,6,11–14]

To maintain a proper fluid balance, fluid gains (intake) should be in equilibrium with fluid losses (output). On average, a healthy adult requires a fluid intake of 30–40 mL/kg per day. Table 1-4 summarizes the total fluid intake (ie, from drinking water or other beverages and eating food) considered adequate for individuals living in the United States.

1. Daily fluid requirements are affected by many variables.
   - As expected, total daily fluid requirements increase with age from infancy to childhood to adulthood; however, infants and children require more fluid per kilogram than adults.
   - Men require more fluid per day than women to maintain adequate hydration.
   - Active adults require more fluid per day than sedentary adults.
   - Active adults living in warm, dry climates may need upwards of 6 L/d to maintain fluid balance.
2. Fluid intake is mainly derived from dietary intake (including the generation of water from the oxidation of carbohydrates, proteins, and fats).
   - Solid foods contain varying amounts of water. The water content of fruits and vegetables can be as high as 80%–95%, while lean raw

Table 1-4. Adequate Total Water Intake for Individuals Living in the United States.

Sex	Age, y/Life Stage Group	Adequate Intake, L/d
Female	9–13	2.1
	14–18	2.3
	19–30	2.7
	31–50	2.7
	50–70	2.7
	>70	2.7
	Pregnancy	3
	Lactation	3.8
Male	9–13	2.4
	14–18	3.3
	19–30	3.7
	31–50	3.7
	50–70	3.7
	>70	3.7

meats are approximately 60% water and nuts and grains are as little as 5% water.

- Oxidative metabolism of food provides approximately 300 mL of water per day.
- Oral fluids, intravenous (IV) fluids (Table 1-5), and enteral fluids all contribute to total intake.
- Figure 1-5 reflects the distribution of 3 different IV fluids within the body, inclusive of the impact on intravascular fluid volume.
    - Following administration of dextrose 5% in water, the carbohydrate (ie, glucose) content is metabolized, resulting in the availability of only free water. Hence, fluid distribution resembles that of TBW (ie, approximately two-thirds intracellular and one-third extracellular).
    - Hypotonic fluids, such as dextrose 5% in water or 0.45% sodium chloride, can be utilized to correct TBW deficits given the provision of more free water compared to effective osmoles.
    - With 0.9% sodium chloride, given an osmolality of 308 mOsmol/L (approximating normal serum osmolality) derived from sodium

Table 1-5. Composition of Select Intravenous Fluids.

	Solution	Dextrose, g/L	Osmolality, mOsm/L	Tonicity	Electrolytes, mEq/L				
					Na^+	Cl^-	K^+	Mg^{2+}	Ca^{2+}
Crystalloids	D5W (5% dextrose)	50	252	Hypotonic	–	–	–	–	–
	0.225% NaCl (¼ normal saline)	–	77	Hypotonic	38.5	38.5	–	–	–
	0.45% NaCl (½ normal saline)	–	154	Hypotonic	77	77	–	–	–
	0.9% NaCl (normal saline)	–	308	Isotonic	154	154	–	–	–
	3% NaCl (hypertonic saline)	–	1026	Hypertonic	513	513	–	–	–
	Ringers lactate	–	275	Isotonic	130	109	4	–	3
	PlasmaLyte[a]	–	294	Isotonic	140	98	5	3	–
	Normosol-R	–	294	Isotonic	140	98	5	3	
Colloids	Hetastarch 6%[b]								
	• Hespan		309	Isotonic	154	154	–	–	–
	• Hextend		307	Isotonic	143	124	3	0.9	5
	Albumin in 0.9% NaCl[c]	–	See footnote	See footnote	130–160	130–160	–	≤1	–
	Mannitol[d]	–	See footnote	See footnote	–	–	–	–	–

[a]PlasmaLyte A and PlasmaLyte 148 are 2 separate products that differ only in pH (7.4 vs 5.5, respectively).
[b]Hetastarch 6% is available in 0.9% sodium chloride (Hespan) or Lactated Electrolyte injection (Hextend). Note the differences in the electrolyte content of each product.
[c]Albumin is available in 5% and 25% concentrations. Albumin 5% solution is osmotically equivalent to plasma. Albumin 25% is hypertonic, with each 100 mL osmotically equivalent to 500 mL of normal plasma.
[d]Mannitol is available in various concentrations ranging from 5% to 25%. The 5% mannitol has an osmolality of 275 mOsm/L and is an isotonic colloid. All other concentrations of mannitol are hypertonic colloids.

Figure 1-5. Theoretical Distribution of 3 Different Intravenous Fluids.

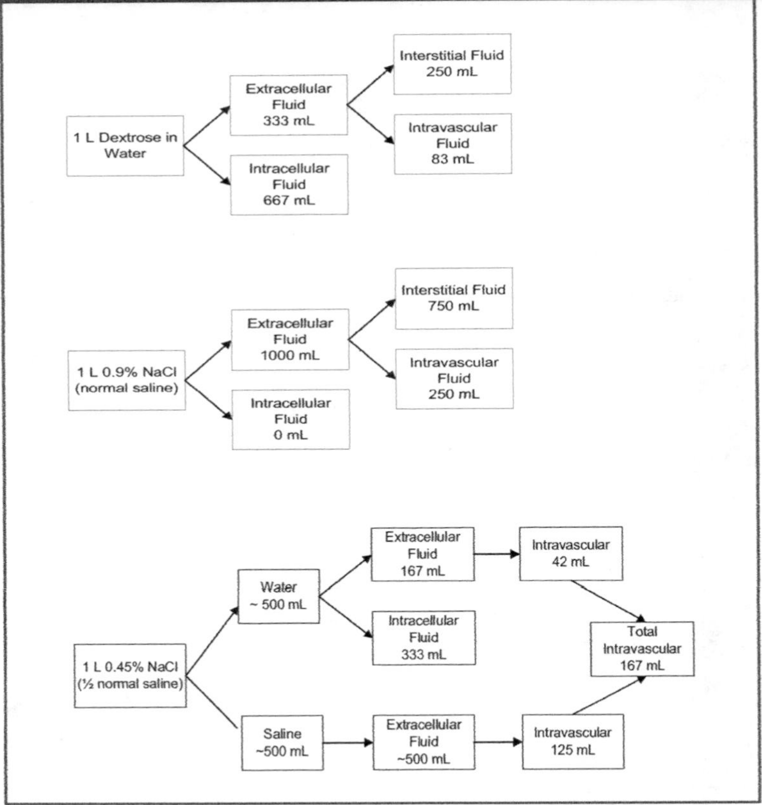

and chloride (effective osmoles), the entire administered volume should in theory remain in the ECF compartment, with subsequent distribution into the interstitial and intravascular spaces.

- Isotonic fluids, such as 0.9% sodium chloride, Ringer's lactate, or PlasmaLyte, can be utilized as a replacement fluid to correct intravascular volume deficits. Intravascular volume is a determinant of blood pressure.

3. Output is any fluid loss from the body (Table 1-6), and it can be due to sensible or insensible losses.

   - Sensible losses refer to fluid output that can be measured directly and quantified (eg, urine, emesis, and output from nasogastric or gastrostomy tubes, ostomies, surgical drains). Fluid provision to account for sensible losses should be tailored to include both an appropriate volume as well as an appropriate electrolyte content.

Table 1-6. Volume and Average Electrolyte Content of Gastrointestinal Secretions.

Source/ Type of Secretion	Volume, L/d	Electrolyte Content, mEq/L			
		Na^+	K^+	Cl^-	HCO_3^-
Saliva	1.5	10	26	10	30
Stomach	1.5	60	10	130	0
Duodenum	Variable	140	5	80	0
Ileum	3	140	5	104	30
Colon	Variable	60	30	40	0
Pancreas	Variable	140	5	75	115
Bile	Variable	145	5	100	35

Adapted with permission from Whitmire SJ. Fluids and electrolytes. In Matarese LE, Gottschlich MM, eds. *Contemporary Nutrition Support Practice: A Clinical Guide*. 1st ed. Philadelphia, PA: Saunders; 1998:130.

- Insensible losses refer to fluid output that cannot be directly measured (eg, losses from the skin or respiratory tract) and *typically account for 10 mL/kg of fluid loss per day.* Elevated body temperatures, higher ambient temperatures, and faster respiratory rates can all increase insensible losses. Insensible losses are increased by 25% (ie, approximately 2.5 mL/kg/d) for each 1°C increase in temperature above 37°C.

4. In lieu of pre-existing fluid disorders, fluid intake (oral and intravenous) should be adjusted accordingly to keep a net zero balance while maintaining adequate hydration.

   - Fluid intake and output and daily weight should be closely monitored. Each liter of fluid retained will result in approximately 1 kg of weight gain.

   - Weight gains or losses that occur over a short period of time may indicate fluid gains and losses, respectively, and can be used in conjunction with physical examination to help determine overall fluid balance.

Patient Scenario 1

James is a 27-year-old man who reports to the emergency center with a 3-day history of nausea and vomiting attributed to a "stomach bug." His wife states that over the past 24 hours he has become progressively more confused and lethargic. He has been vomiting multiple times throughout the day and has not been able to tolerate any solid food or fluids. His blood pressure is 82/53, and he has difficulty following conversations and is unsteady on his feet. Laboratory tests are done, and toxicology laboratory results are all negative. The abnormal laboratory values are listed below. What IV fluid would be the most appropriate for James?

Sodium, 147 mEq/L
Potassium, 3.2 mEq/L
Chloride, 98 mEq/L
Carbon dioxide, 34 mEq/L
Blood urea nitrogen, 28 mg/dL
Creatinine, 1.6 mg/dL

James is experiencing dehydration from vomiting and an inability to take in oral fluids. He is symptomatically hypotensive and requires immediate fluid resuscitation with an isotonic fluid.

1. Choose an appropriate IV resuscitation fluid—isotonic fluids.

- Crystalloid vs colloid
    - Crystalloids are the most widely used resuscitation fluids and are appropriate for most patients presenting with hypovolemia.
    - Colloids contribute to oncotic pressure and may be helpful in patients with significant third-spacing of fluids or in the setting of hypoalbuminemia.
- Hypertonic vs isotonic vs hypotonic
    - Hypertonic fluids, such as 3% sodium chloride and mannitol, are reserved for specific indications and do not have a role in fluid resuscitation. These agents will be discussed in subsequent chapters.
    - Isotonic fluids will distribute more into the intravascular compartment than hypotonic fluids, helping to restore intravascular volume and increase EBV, thus raising blood pressure.

2. Consider treatment options.

- Fluid resuscitation with an IV isotonic crystalloid fluid is the most appropriate intervention for the patient at this time (in addition to suppressing nausea and vomiting, determining the etiology of his illness, and providing supportive care and treatment as needed).

- Any isotonic crystalloid solution would be appropriate in this patient, and no compelling evidence supports choosing one over another.
- Note that Ringer's lactate, PlasmaLyte, and Normosol-R solutions contain small amounts of electrolytes, including potassium; therefore, serum electrolytes should be monitored routinely given this patient's elevated serum creatinine.

Patient Scenario 2

Amy is a 43-year-old woman living in Phoenix, Arizona, who runs approximately 20 miles per week. She has 3 children, aged 9 years, 4 years, and 7 months, and currently breastfeeds the youngest. On average, Amy drinks about 4 L of fluids per day (water and other beverages) and consumes a normal diet of 3 meals per day. Recently her breast milk production has significantly declined. Amy inquires about her fluid intake and how it may affect her breast milk production.

1. Assess Amy's fluid needs.
   - According to Table 1-4, Amy should consume at least 3.8 L of fluids per day.
   - Due to her active lifestyle, Amy's fluid needs will be higher than average.
   - The warm, dry climate of Phoenix will also dehydrate Amy more quickly than a temperate, humid climate, thus increasing her daily fluid needs.
2. Assess Amy's intake.
   - Currently, Amy drinks about 4 L of fluid per day.
   - Oxidative metabolism from oral intake will contribute approximately 300 mL/d.
3. Consider possible recommendations.
   - Several factors are contributing to Amy's increased fluid needs: lactation, active lifestyle, and the local climate.
   - Amy should increase her fluid intake by 1–2 L/d to maintain adequate hydration and help increase and maintain breast milk production.

Patient Scenario 3

Elaine is a 68-year-old woman (65 kg) who has been admitted to the hospital for shortness of breath. A computed tomographic scan of the chest with IV contrast was ordered to rule out pulmonary embolism. The next day, Elaine's urine output dropped from 60 to 20 mL/h. Past medical history is significant for only gastric reflux and hypertension, both of which are controlled with diet and lifestyle modifications. She does not takes any medications. She appears well hydrated on physical exam. Laboratory tests and urine studies are ordered. What is Elaine's FE_{Na}, and how might it be interpreted?

Sodium, 138 mEq/L
Potassium, 3.8 mEq/L
Chloride, 102 mEq/L
Carbon dioxide, 26 mEq/L
Blood urea nitrogen, 22 mg/dL
Creatinine, 1.2 mg/dL
Urine sodium, 15 mEq/L
Urine creatinine, 45 mg/dL

1. Assess Elaine's urine output and calculate FE_{Na}.

    - Elaine's weight is 65 kg, and her current urine output is 20 mL/h. This output translates to only 0.3 mL/kg per hour, which is consistent with oliguria.
    - FE_{Na} calculations yield 0.3%. Given the absence of any history of renal, cardiac, or liver disease as well as the absence of hypovolemia, the most likely cause of Elaine's oliguria is contrast-induced nephropathy (recent exposure to IV contrast).
    - Although her serum creatinine is not yet elevated, a slight elevation over the next several days should be expected. The level will likely peak 3–5 days after the administration of IV contrast before gradually returning to normal.

2. Provide supportive care to prevent any further injury, including avoiding nephrotoxic agents and maintaining adequate hydration for renal perfusion.

References

1. Rose BD, Post TW. *Clinical Physiology of Acid-Base and Electrolyte Disorders*. 5th ed. New York, NY: McGraw-Hill; 2001.
2. Watson PE, Watson ID, Batt RD. Total body water volumes for adult males and females estimated from simple anthropometric measurements. *Am J Clin Nutr*. 1980;33(1):27–39.
3. Canada TW, Boullata JI. Fluid and electrolytes. In: Rolandelli RH, Bankhead R, Boullata JI, Compher CW, eds. *Enteral and Tube Feeding*. 4th ed. Philadelphia, PA: Elsevier Saunders; 2005:95–109.
4. Moukarzel A. Understanding and managing fluid and electrolyte abnormalities. In: A.S.P.E.N. 22nd Clinical Congress Course Syllabus. 1999:247–254.
5. Bruno JJ, Canada TW. Electrolyte disorders in the critically ill population. In: Erstad B, ed. *Critical Care Pharmacotherapy*. 1st ed. Lenexa, KS: American College of Clinical Pharmacy; 2016:58–97.
6. Whitmire SJ. Fluids and electrolytes. In: Matarese LE, Gottschlich MM, eds. *Contemporary Nutrition Support Practice: A Clinical Guide*. 1st ed. Philadelphia, PA: Saunders; 1998:127–144.
7. McDonough AA. Mechanisms of proximal tubule sodium transport regulation that link extracellular fluid volume and blood pressure. *Am J Physiol Regul Integr Comp Physiol*. 2010;298(4):R851–861.
8. George AL Jr, Neilson EG. Chapter 303. Cellular and molecular biology of the kidney. In: Jameson JL, Fauci AS, Kasper DL, Hauser SL, Longo DL, Loscalzo J, eds. *Harrison's Principles of Internal Medicine*. 20th ed. New York, NY: McGraw-Hill; 2018. https://accessmedicine.mhmedical.com/content.aspx?bookid=2129§ionid=181950772. Accessed November 13, 2019.
9. Waikar SS, Bonventre JV. Chapter 304. Acute kidney injury. In: Jameson JL, Fauci AS, Kasper DL, Hauser SL, Longo DL, Loscalzo J, eds. *Harrison's Principles of Internal Medicine*. 20th ed. New York, NY: McGraw-Hill; 2018. https://accessmedicine.mhmedical.com/content.aspx?bookid=2129§ionid=186950567#1157019088. Accessed November 13, 2019.
10. Steiner RW. Interpreting the fractional excretion of sodium. *Am J Med*. 1984;77(4):699–702.
11. Mirtallo J, Canada T, Johnson D, et al. Safe practices for parenteral nutrition [published correction appears in *JPEN J Parenter Enteral Nutr*. 2006;30(2):177]. *JPEN J Parenter Enteral Nutr*. 2004;28:S39–S70.
12. Sawka MN, Cheuvront SN, Carter R 3rd. Human water needs. *Nutr Rev*. 2005;63(6 Pt 2): S30–S39.
13. National Research Council. *Dietary Reference Intakes for Water, Potassium, Sodium, Chloride, and Sulfate*. Washington, DC: The National Academies Press; 2005.
14. Cox P. Insensible water loss and its assessment in adult patients: a review. *Acta Anesthesiol Scand*. 1987;31(8):771–776.

CHAPTER 2

Fluid Disorders

Fluid Balance[1]

As introduced in Chapter 1, regulation of fluid balance involves an interplay of the gastrointestinal (GI), endocrine, and renal systems. Under normal conditions, these systems work in harmony to help avoid fluid disorders.

1. GI tract
   - The fluid and electrolyte concentration of GI secretions vary depending on the specific location along the GI tract (see Table 1-6 in Chapter 1).
   - Collectively, the GI tract produces nearly 7 L of fluid each day, almost all of which is reabsorbed under normal conditions.
   - Approximately 100–200 mL of fluid is lost in feces.
2. Endocrine system
   - The renin-angiotensin-aldosterone system (RAAS) regulates sodium excretion by the kidney and affects blood pressure (see Figure 1-3 in Chapter 1).

Table 2-1. Primary Changes Responsible for Fluid and Electrolyte Disorders.

Change	Outcome
Loss or gain of water and sodium from the ECF	Hypovolemia, hypervolemia
Loss or gain of TBW	Dehydration, overhydration
Loss or gain of electrolytes	Electrolyte disorders[a] (eg, hypokalemia vs hyperkalemia, hypophosphatemia vs hyperphosphatemia)

ECF, extracellular fluid; TBW, total body water

[a]Disorders of sodium are predominantly a result of alterations in TBW.

- The hypothalamus produces antidiuretic hormone (ADH) (subsequently released by the posterior pituitary gland) in response to alterations in serum osmolality, influencing water reabsorption in the kidneys.
- In addition, the hypothalamus regulates the thirst mechanism, influencing oral fluid intake.

3. Kidneys

- Sodium and water are filtered and reabsorbed by the kidneys to maintain homeostasis.
- In addition to their response to RAAS activation and ADH, the kidneys also respond to changes in effective blood volume (EBV) by adjusting urine output and electrolyte content, particularly sodium.

If dysfunction occurs in any of these key systems, fluid and electrolyte disorders may develop (Table 2-1). Of note, this chapter will focus solely on fluid disorders; for electrolyte disorders, please see Chapter 3.

Fluid Disorders[2,3]

Fluid disorders can be divided into 2 main categories: those related to the loss or gain of fluid in the extracellular fluid (ECF) compartment (hypovolemia vs hypervolemia, respectively) and those related to the loss or gain of total body water (TBW) (dehydration vs over-hydration, respectively).

1. Gain or loss of fluid in the ECF compartment

- Hypervolemia indicates ECF volume overload.
- Hypovolemia indicates ECF volume depletion.

- As discussed in Chapter 1, sodium is the primary effective osmole for the ECF compartment. Hence, hypovolemia and hypervolemia also indicate a loss or gain in total body sodium, respectively.

2. Gain or loss of TBW

   - Gain or loss of TBW results in cellular over-hydration (ie, water intoxication) or dehydration, respectively.
   - Water intoxication is rare but can occur in patients with low body mass, high-intensity athletes who consume large amounts of fluids, patients with psychiatric polydipsia, and patients who receive excessive amounts of hypotonic intravenous fluids (eg, dextrose 5% in water).
   - Dehydration can occur in patients with prolonged nausea, vomiting, or diarrhea (ie, sensible losses) or those with excessive and unconsidered insensible losses (eg, through the skin as sweat, through the lungs from respirations), accompanied by insufficient fluid intake or provision.
   - A change in TBW is reflected by a change in serum sodium concentration and serum osmolality. When TBW is in excess of sodium content, hyponatremia ensues. Alternatively, hypernatremia reflects a deficit of TBW relative to total body sodium content. In most cases, patients will maintain EBV. For further discussion, see sodium disorders in Chapter 3.

Proper diagnosis of fluid disorders depends on knowledge of normal body fluid composition (as discussed in Chapter 1), thorough physical examination, work-up/identification of possible etiologies (Table 2-2), and evaluation of electrolyte disorders (as discussed in Chapter 3).

Hypovolemia[4,5]

Hypovolemia, also known as volume depletion, is characterized by a reduction in the volume of the ECF compartment relative to its capacity. Hypovolemia can be characterized as absolute or relative.

- Absolute hypovolemia refers to a reduction in total circulating blood volume due to the loss of sodium and water (ie, a net reduction in ECF volume).
- Relative hypovolemia refers to the presence of insufficient volume, particularly intravascular volume, in the setting of an expanded size of the ECF compartment.

Table 2-2. Examination of Patients With Fluid Disorders.

Type of Examination	Examination Elements
Physical examination	• Pulse rate • Postural blood pressure • Jugular venous pressure • Skin turgor
Other parameters associated with volume status	• Intake/output records for fluid balance • Urine color • Central venous pressure (if available) • Pulmonary capillary wedge pressure (if available)
Review of medical record for predisposing comorbidities/ consideration of potential new diagnosis(es)	• Heart failure • Cirrhosis • Nephrotic syndrome • Addison's disease or Cushing's disease • Hypopituitarism or Hyperpituitarism • Hypothyroidism
Laboratory and radiologic examinations	• Albumin • Hematocrit • Serum sodium • Urine sodium • Serum glucose • Serum triglycerides • Renal function (BUN/SCr) • Thyroid function (TSH, T_4, T_3) • Serum and urine osmolality • Chest x-ray • Echocardiogram

BUN, blood urea nitrogen; SCr, serum creatinine; T_3, triiodothyronine; T_4, thyroxine; TSH, thyrotropin.

Pathophysiology[5]

1. Absolute hypovolemia

- Extrarenal
    - The most frequent extrarenal cause of absolute hypovolemia is massive bleeding; however, many other causes are possible, including GI losses (Table 2-3).

Table 2-3. Causes of Absolute and Relative Hypovolemia.

Type of Hypovolemia	Extrarenal Losses	Renal Losses
Absolute	Hemorrhage (eg, gastrointestinal or trauma) Fluid loss from the gastrointestinal tract (eg, vomiting, diarrhea, nasogastric suctioning, fistula drainage, ostomy drainage) Skin losses (eg, excessive sweating or burns) Wound drainage Respiratory losses Dialysis	Diuretics (particularly loop and thiazide diuretics) Enhanced diuresis (eg, osmotic diuresis from hyperglycemia, excessive protein administration) Salt-wasting disease (eg, Fanconi's syndrome, interstitial nephritis, medullary cystic disease, urinary tract obstruction, polycystic kidney disease, cerebral salt-wasting) Adrenal insufficiency/ hypo-aldosteronism
Relative	Edematous states (eg, heart failure, cirrhosis) Generalized vasodilation (eg, sepsis, pregnancy) Third-space loss (eg, pancreatitis, peritonitis, rhabdomyolysis, small bowel obstruction)	Nephrotic syndrome

   - When the reduction in ECF is isotonic (ie, the loss of sodium and water is of a concentration that resembles a normal serum sodium concentration), plasma sodium and osmolality remain within normal range, resulting in a shift of fluid from the interstitial space to the intravascular space in attempt to maintain EBV and tissue perfusion.
   - If the reduction in ECF is not isotonic, plasma sodium and osmolality will change, resulting in hypernatremia or hyponatremia (see Chapter 3 for more detail).
- Renal
   - The kidneys regulate filtration and reabsorption of sodium. When renal mechanisms are compromised or modified (eg, via use of diuretics), the amount of sodium and water present in the urine can increase, resulting in absolute volume depletion.

2. Relative hypovolemia

- Extrarenal
  - Extrarenal causes of relative hypovolemia include vasodilation, third-space loss, or edematous states.
  - Arterial vasodilation can be an appropriate physiologic response (as seen with pregnancy and sepsis) or exogenously induced via medications (eg, hydralazine).
  - Third-space loss (also known as third-space sequestration) occurs when fluid accumulates extracellularly in spaces that normally have minimal to no fluid. Such accumulation can be seen with burns, pancreatitis, and GI obstruction, among other conditions.
    - Other potential areas of third-space fluid accumulation include between the pleura, in the pericardial sac, or within the peritoneal cavity.
  - Edematous states (ie, fluid accumulation in the interstitial space) are considered states of relative hypovolemia (as well as secondary hypervolemia) and will be addressed separately later in this chapter.
  - Remember, volume status is dictated predominantly by fluid contained in the intravascular space. Fluid contained in the interstitial space, or third-space, has no effect on EBV, resulting in relative hypovolemia.
- Renal
  - Relative hypovolemia can occur with nephrotic syndrome (Table 2-4), defined as damage to the renal glomerulus with subsequent proteinuria, hypoalbuminemia, and often, hyperlipidemia.

Table 2-4. Causes of Nephrotic Syndrome.

Primary Causes	Secondary Causes
Glomerulonephritis	Diabetes mellitus
IgA nephropathy	Amyloidosis
Membranous nephropathy	Infection
Minimal-change nephropathy	Sjögren's syndrome
	Systemic lupus erythematosus
	Sarcoidosis
	Cancer (solid and hematologic)
	Drugs (lithium, NSAIDs, interferon α)

IgA, immunoglobulin A; NSAIDs, nonsteroidal anti-inflammatory drugs.

- With hypoalbuminemia, intravascular oncotic pressure is compromised, resulting in capillary leak. Fluid from the intravascular space consequently moves to the interstitial space, leading to relative hypovolemia.

Clinical Manifestations and Physical Assessment[5]

1. Clinical findings of hypovolemia depend on the total volume, rate, and time course of the volume loss and the patient's ability to compensate.

2. Signs and symptoms are typically apparent in physical examination when ECF volume is decreased by 5%–15% and are related to tissue hypoperfusion (Table 2-5).

3. Circulatory collapse is likely to occur when volume depletion exceeds 10%–20%.

Table 2-5. Clinical Presentation and Diagnosis of Hypovolemia.

Signs and Symptoms	Laboratory Assessment
• Dizziness	• Random urine sodium < 15 mEq/L
• Mental status changes	• FE_{Na} < 1%
• Reduced tears	• Random urine osmolality > 450 mOsm/kg H_2O
• Cool, clammy skin	• BUN/SCr > 20:1
• Dry mucous membranes	• Hematocrit increased
• Decreased skin turgor	• Serum albumin increased
• Reduced CVP	
• Tachycardia (HR > 100 beats/min)[a]	
• Hypotension (SBP < 90 mm Hg)[a]	
• Orthostatic changes in HR and/or SBP	
• Reduced urine output (< 0.5 mL/kg/h)	
• Improvement in HR and SBP after administering a fluid challenge	
• Improvement in HR and SBP with passive leg raise	
• Weight loss	

BUN, blood urea nitrogen; CVP, central venous pressure; FE_{Na}, fractional excretion of sodium; HR, heart rate; SBP, systolic blood pressure; SCr, serum creatinine

[a]Relative to a patient's baseline values, milder increases in heart rate and/or decreases in blood pressure may also be clinically relevant

Diagnosis[5–7]

The diagnosis of hypovolemia is based on signs/symptoms and correlation with laboratory assessment (Table 2-5). The typical laboratory findings detailed below arise from activation of compensatory mechanisms (ie, RAAS, release of ADH) to restore homeostasis.

1. Urine sodium < 15 mEq/L
    - Low urine sodium occurs as sodium reabsorption by the kidneys is increased in an attempt to maintain EBV.
    - A spot urine sample is sufficient for evaluating the urine sodium level.
2. Fractional excretion of sodium (FE_{Na}) < 1%
    - FE_{Na} refers to the calculated percentage of filtered sodium excreted in the urine (refer to Chapter 1, Figure 1-4).
    - A FE_{Na} < 1% typically accompanies the azotemia/oliguria seen with hypovolemia.
3. Urine osmolality > 450 mOsm/kg H_2O
    - With normally functioning kidneys, urine should be concentrated in hypovolemic states secondary to compensatory mechanisms that result in increased water reabsorption.
4. Blood urea nitrogen (BUN)/serum creatinine (SCr) ratio > 20:1
    - Volume depletion frequently increases the BUN secondary to a decline in glomerular filtration rate and an increase in urea recycling.
5. Hematocrit and albumin
    - Unless the etiology is hemorrhage, hematocrit and albumin levels often increase in the setting of hypovolemia secondary to hemoconcentration. However, these values can be difficult to interpret and assessment is not always reliable because the patient's baseline values must be known in order to make clinical judgment.

Treatment[5,8,9]

The goals of treatment are to restore intravascular volume, prevent organ/tissue hypoperfusion, and promote hemodynamic stability. Volume repletion to restore normovolemia should be based on the patient's volume deficit; however, this value usually cannot be calculated precisely. The adequacy of volume repletion should be assessed through frequent physical examination and repeat laboratory data analysis.

1. Mild to moderate hypovolemia

- Increasing dietary sodium and water intake may be sufficient to correct mild volume depletion.
- Oral fluid administration should only be considered in patients who are conscious and have a functioning GI tract. In patients who are unconscious or unable to drink by mouth due to other reasons, enteral (ie, per feeding tube) administration of fluids should be pursued.
- Oral rehydration solutions should contain at least 2% glucose and 50–90 mEq/L of sodium to take advantage of the sodium/glucose cotransport in the GI tract by promoting small intestinal sodium reabsorption (coupled transport of sodium and glucose at this site). Recommended oral rehydration solutions, including a specific formula from the World Health Organization, are listed in Table 2-6.
- If patients are unable to tolerate and/or absorb enough sodium and water via the oral/enteral route, intravenous (IV) fluids may be necessary.

Table 2-6. Oral Rehydration Solutions.

ORS[a]	Sodium, mEq/L	Potassium, mEq/L	Carbohydrate, g/L	Osmolarity, mOsm/L
WHO Reduced Osmolarity formula	70	20	27	245
CeraLyte 70	70	20	41	235
TRIORAL	75	20	13.5	245
Gatorade G2 (ready to drink) + 1/2 teaspoon of salt[b]	70	3.2	22.5	256
Pedialyte	45	20	25	270

ORS, oral rehydration solution; WHO, World Health Organization.

[a]Visit The Oley Foundation for ORS recipes (http://www.oley.org).

[b]Gatorade® G2 (ready to drink) contains ~18.5 mEq of sodium per 32 ounces (946 mL). Addition of ½ teaspoon of salt to 32 ounces results in a sodium concentration of ~70 mEq/L. Potassium levels are well below the recommended amount for an ORS.

2. Moderate to severe hypovolemia

- With more severe hypovolemia, IV fluids are often required.
- The clinical situation (including factors such as the patient's hemodynamic status, etiology of hypovolemia, and laboratory findings) will determine which fluid is the most suitable in a given situation (refer to Table 1-5 and Figure 1-5 in Chapter 1).
- In patients with hemodynamic instability or compromise, isotonic fluids (eg, 0.9% sodium chloride, Ringer's lactate, PlasmaLyte) should be given.
    - A 20–30 mL/kg bolus of fluid is recommended in most adults to acutely expand the intravascular space, followed by a continuous infusion of the same IV fluid. The infusion should be maintained at a rate greater than the total fluid output (including urine output, insensible losses, and any other losses present) until normovolemia is achieved.
    - Albumin solutions (or other colloid-containing solutions) may be useful in patients with protein-losing states or those with increased interstitial volume.
- In the majority of patients without hemodynamic instability, isotonic IV fluids (as mentioned above) or 0.45% sodium chloride can be used.
    - The plasma sodium concentration can help dictate which solution should be used. For example, if a patient has hypernatremia (ie, a greater deficit of water than solute), 0.45% sodium chloride should be administered. Of note, in patients with concomitant hypoglycemia, dextrose can be added to the above IV fluids (eg, dextrose 5%-sodium chloride 0.45%, commonly referred to as D5-1/2NS).
    - It is not recommended to use 0.225% sodium chloride for management of hypovolemia because the low tonicity of this solution can lead to a shift of water from the ECF to the ICF compartment, with risk of hemolysis.
    - Hypertonic saline (3% sodium chloride) should not be used for fluid resuscitation; use should be reserved for patients with severely symptomatic hyponatremia (see Chapter 3 for more detail).

3. Relative hypovolemia

- Treatment of relative hypovolemia depends on reversal of the underlying cause and relies less on volume replacement. See discussion of edematous states later in this chapter for specific treatment recommendations.

Hypervolemia[5]

Hypervolemia, or volume expansion, refers to the situation in which ECF volume exceeds compartment capacity and is a result of elevated total body sodium (ie, when renal sodium retention exceeds renal and extrarenal losses). Hypervolemia is classified as primary or secondary depending on if renal sodium retention is a result of a kidney or adrenal gland disorder or secondary to diseases of other organs (eg, heart failure), respectively. See Table 2-7 for a list of causes of primary and secondary hypervolemia.

Pathophysiology[5]

1. Primary hypervolemia

    - Most commonly, primary hypervolemia arises from direct injury to the kidney, resulting in disruption of normal filtration processes and excessive sodium retention. An increase in total body sodium leads to water retention and a subsequent expansion of the ECF.

    - Conditions associated with excessive mineralocorticoid activity (eg, Cushing's disease, adrenal tumors) can also lead to primary hypervolemia.

2. Secondary hypervolemia

    - Secondary hypervolemia is often associated with heart failure and/or cirrhosis.

        - Renal sodium retention occurs secondary to decreased EBV despite total ECF volume expansion because the majority of fluid is contained in the interstitial space.

Table 2-7. Causes of Primary and Secondary Hypervolemia.

Primary Hypervolemia	Secondary Hypervolemia
Anuric/oliguric acute kidney injury	Heart failure (with reduced ejection fraction)
Chronic kidney disease	Cirrhosis
Glomerular disease	Idiopathic edema
Bilateral renal artery stenosis	Iatrogenic (excessive IV fluids)
Mineralocorticoid excess (Cushing's disease, adrenal tumor)	

IV, intravenous.

- Volume depletion triggers the release of angiotensin II and norepinephrine. These hormones cause enhanced sodium reabsorption in the kidneys and reduced urinary sodium excretion.

Clinical Manifestations and Physical Assessment[5]

1. Signs and symptoms of hypervolemia (Table 2-8) depend on the relative distribution of fluid between the intravascular and interstitial spaces of the ECF compartment.

2. Distribution of fluid

   - If cardiac and hepatic function are normal, hydrostatic and oncotic forces remain intact and excess volume is distributed proportionately throughout the ECF compartments; however, if cardiac and/or hepatic function is altered, distribution of fluid is disproportionate.

     - Arterial overload: hypertension
     - Venous overload: elevated jugular venous pressure and central venous pressure
     - Interstitial fluid accumulation: peripheral edema, pleural effusions, ascites, and/or pulmonary edema

3. Patient assessment should consist of a thorough patient history, review of systems, and physical examination.

Table 2-8. Clinical Presentation and Diagnosis of Hypervolemia.

Signs	Symptoms	Laboratory Values
Hypertension	Dyspnea	Elevated BNP
Peripheral edema	Tachypnea	Low to normal serum sodium
Pleural effusions	Swelling of the extremities	Urine sodium < 15 mEq/L
Ascites	Abdominal distension	Low to normal urine osmolality
Pulmonary rales	Difficulty ambulating	Low to normal BUN
Elevated jugular venous pressure		Low hematocrit and albumin (dilutional effect)
Enlarged liver		
S_3 gallop heart sound		
Weight gain		

BNP, B-type natriuretic peptide; BUN, blood urea nitrogen; S_3, third heart sound.

Diagnosis[5]

Hypervolemia is usually evident from physical examination in conjunction with a review of the patient's past medical history (ie, comorbidities) and laboratory tests (Table 2-8 and Table 2-9).

1. Any combination of 2 or more of the following is diagnostic for hypervolemia: peripheral edema, raised jugular venous pressure, pulmonary symptoms, and pleural effusions.

Treatment[5,10,11]

1. Treat the underlying cause, which is paramount for reducing the probability of further occurrences of hypervolemia.

Table 2-9. Common Etiologies, Clinical Manifestations, and Diagnosis of Hypervolemic States.

Etiology	Clinical Findings	Diagnosis
Heart failure	Pitting edema Dyspnea on exertion Orthopnea Paroxysmal nocturnal dyspnea Lung crackles S_3 and S_4 gallop heart sounds Jugular venous distention Hepatojugular reflux	Echocardiogram Chest x-ray B-type natriuretic peptide Low serum sodium concentration (hypervolemic hyponatremia)
Nephrotic syndrome	Diffuse edema or anasarca Ascites Periorbital edema	24-h urine protein collection to check for protein loss Plasma protein assays Hypoalbuminemia
Cirrhosis	Chronic alcohol abuse Ascites Jaundice Easy bruising Testicular atrophy Gynecomastia	Elevated liver enzymes Hypoalbuminemia Elevated PT Increased total bilirubin

PT, prothrombin time; S_3, third heart sound; S_4, fourth heart sound.

2. Decrease ECF volume excess.

- Limit sodium and water intake (< 45–90 mEq/d or 2–4 g/d and 1–1.5 L/d, respectively). In hospitalized patients, total intake should include all potential sources, including IV fluids (eg, maintenance fluids, piggyback medications, parenteral nutrition), oral intake, and blood transfusions.
    - The use of concentrated enteral formulas or parenteral nutrition may be needed to minimize free water intake.
- Administer diuretics to alleviate sodium and water excess (see Table 2-10).
    - The choice of diuretic will depend on the underlying cause.
    - In heart failure, cirrhosis, and kidney failure, diuretics are given to enhance the renal excretion of sodium by blocking sites of sodium reabsorption along the nephron.

Table 2-10. Mechanism of Action of Diuretic Agents.

Agent	**Site of Action**	**Drug Target**	**Primary Effect**
Loop diuretics (furosemide, torsemide, bumetanide, ethacrynic acid)	Ascending limb of loop of Henle	Blocking of Na^+/K^+/$2Cl^-$ cotransporter	Inhibits reabsorption of sodium and chloride resulting in increased excretion of water, sodium, chloride, potassium, magnesium, and calcium. Potent diuresis (water loss > sodium loss).
Thiazide diuretics (hydrochlorothiazide, chlorothiazide)	Distal convoluted tubule	Blocking of Na^+/Cl^- cotransporters	Inhibits sodium reabsorption resulting in increased excretion of sodium, water, potassium, hydrogen ions. Moderate diuresis (sodium loss > water loss).
"Potassium-sparing" diuretics (spironolactone, eplerenone, triamterene, amiloride)	Collecting duct	Competes with aldosterone at receptor sites (spironolactone, eplerenone) or inhibits the Na^+/K^+ exchange mechanism in the distal renal tubule (triamterene, amiloride)	Potassium retention with mild increase in sodium and water excretion; diuretic/natriuretic effect is mild given site of action in the collecting duct.
Carbonic anhydrase inhibitors (acetazolamide)	Proximal renal tubule	Blocking of Na^+/H^+ exchange	Reduction of hydrogen ion excretion with increased excretion of sodium, potassium, bicarbonate, and water.

Edematous States[12]

In edematous states, EBV is decreased, but total ECF increases given expansion of the interstitial space. Thus, edematous states are commonly described as either relative hypovolemia or secondary hypervolemia, depending on the perspective. Heart failure, cirrhosis, and nephrotic syndrome are commonly associated with the development of edema.

Pathophysiology[13]

A relative decrease in cardiac output in heart failure or splanchnic vasodilation in cirrhosis results in a decrease in EBV and a subsequent activation of the neurohormonal system (eg, RAAS) with retention of sodium and water. Atrial and carotid baroreceptors stimulate ADH release, which then acts on the distal tubules and collecting ducts in the kidney to increase water reabsorption. Renal vasoconstriction diminishes perfusion and ultimately, the glomerular filtration rate.

All of the above leads to a compensatory increase in EBV, although it is physiologically inappropriate and counterproductive for the underlying condition(s). Ultimately, some of the retained fluid stays in the intravascular compartment, but altered capillary hemodynamics result in most of the fluid entering the interstitial space, eventually resulting in edema.

1. Heart failure

    - In patients with heart failure with reduced ejection fraction, the reduction in cardiac output correlates to a reduction in EBV.
    - The kidney works to restore EBV by retaining sodium and water; however, increased hydrostatic pressure results in fluid overload, primarily in the interstitial space.

2. Cirrhosis

    - In patients with cirrhosis, splanchnic arterial vasodilation leads to the development of portal hypertension, which facilitates accumulation of fluid in the abdominal cavity (ie, ascites).
    - Secondary hyperaldosteronism may also play a role in increased sodium and water retention in these patients.
    - In addition, severe hypoalbuminemia results in decreased oncotic pressure within the vasculature, subsequently resulting in edema.

3. Nephrotic syndrome

- Increased interstitial fluid results from primary sodium retention and excessive proteinuria secondary to kidney disease.
    - With increased proteinuria, hypoalbuminemia develops, which lowers serum oncotic pressure, creating a disorder of water distribution throughout the body.
    - The amount of water in the intravascular space decreases (lowering the EBV), whereas water content in the interstitial space increases, resulting in edema.
    - Sodium retention due to impaired renal excretion exacerbates the above fluid disorder.
    - Refer to Table 2-4 for common causes of nephrotic syndrome.

Clinical Manifestations and Physical Assessment

Edema on physical examination may manifest as systemic (eg, anasarca) or pulmonary venous congestion (eg, dyspnea, shortness of breath) depending on the etiology and severity (Table 2-9).

Diagnosis[14–16]

Upon recognition of edema, attention should turn to identifying the underlying etiology.

1. Heart failure

- To help distinguish between a primary cardiac or pulmonary disorder, an echocardiogram can be conducted along with measurement of B-type natriuretic peptide.
    - B-type natriuretic peptide is released by cardiac myocytes in response to volume overload, and it may be elevated in patients with hypervolemia secondary to heart failure.

2. Cirrhosis

- Abnormal accumulation of fluid within the peritoneal cavity (ie, ascites) can be directly visualized with imaging (eg, computed tomographic scan of the abdomen) or presumed if shifting dullness is identified upon percussion of the abdomen during physical examination.

- Cirrhosis is the cause for approximately 80% of all cases of ascites in the Western world.

3. Nephrotic syndrome

   - Protein excretion > 3.5 g/d with a 24-hour urine collection characterizes nephrotic proteinuria.

Treatment[14,17,18]

The management of edematous states centers on improving EBV by addressing the underlying etiology, facilitating sodium and water elimination, and restricting sodium and water intake. Goals of therapy include relief of edema symptoms, improvement of end organ function, and reduction of tissue edema.

1. Heart failure

   - Loop and thiazide diuretics are recommended in patients with edema and/or congestion associated with heart failure. Diuresis reduces cardiac filling pressure (ie, preload), resulting in improved symptoms and exercise tolerance as well as a potential reduction in the risk of hospitalization. Neither loop nor thiazide diuretics confer a mortality benefit.

   - Spironolactone and eplerenone, mineralocorticoid/aldosterone receptor antagonists, are recommended in heart failure patients with an ejection fraction less than or equal to 35% given the drugs' proven ability to reduce mortality and risk of hospitalization.

2. Cirrhosis

   - Spironolactone, an aldosterone receptor antagonist, is the preferred diuretic agent in cirrhosis due to its moderate diuretic effect (avoids compromising intravascular volume). In addition, hyperaldosteronism is thought to be a primary mediator of sodium and water retention in cirrhosis.

3. Nephrotic syndrome

   - In nephrotic syndrome, the diuretic response with loop diuretics is suboptimal, generally requiring greater than 200 mg/d of furosemide.

   - The addition of diuretics with alternate renal mechanisms of action (including thiazide diuretics, which act on the distal tubule) may help enhance sodium excretion.

Patient Scenario

A 67-year-old woman with chronic congestive heart failure (baseline left ventricular ejection fraction of 25%) is admitted to the hospital. On physical examination, she has distended neck veins and pedal edema, and she is exhibiting signs of pulmonary edema. What would be the appropriate treatment to alleviate this patient's symptoms?

1. Choose an appropriate treatment plan.

    - Limit sodium intake to 2 g/d and water intake to 1.5 L/d.
    - Choose an appropriate diuretic.
        - Loop diuretics are the most widely used diuretics in heart failure and are appropriate in this patient.
        - Thiazide diuretics work in the distal convoluted tubule where only 5%–10% of sodium is filtered and are thus relatively weak diuretics. However, they may be used in advanced/decompensated heart failure in combination with loop diuretics to promote more effective diuresis.

2. Avoid side effects and over-diuresis.

    - After the patient is started on diuretic therapy, she exhibits a 6-kg weight loss with marked clinical improvement. However, her BUN rises from 14 to 60 mg/dL and her serum creatinine increases from 1.1 to 2.6 mg/dL. What is the explanation for the rapid decline in renal function?
        - The patient is likely experiencing decreased tissue perfusion due to over-diuresis causing a reduction in EBV.
        - Reduction in edema must be carefully balanced with maintenance of sufficient EBV and cardiac output in patients with heart failure.
        - Patient assessment should be conducted daily (at a minimum) to evaluate for signs of under-diuresis vs over-diuresis in order to balance the risk-benefit profile of such therapy.

References

1. Verbalis JG. Disorders of body water homeostasis. *Best Pract Res Clin Endocrinol Metab.* 2003;17(4):471–503.
2. Andreoli TE. Water: normal balance, hyponatremia and hypernatremia. *Ren Fail.* 2000;22(6):711–735.
3. McGee S, Abernethy WB, Simel DL. Is this patient hypovolemic? *JAMA*. 1999;281(11): 1022–1029.
4. Mange K, Matsuura D, Cizman B, et al. Language guiding therapy: the case of dehydration versus volume depletion. *Ann Intern Med.* 1997;127(9):848–853.
5. Slotki IN, Skorecki K. Disorders of sodium balance. In: Yu AS, Chertow GM, Luyckx V, Marsden PA, Skorecki K, Taal MW, eds. *Brenner and Rector's The Kidney*. 11th ed. Philadelphia, PA: Elsevier;2019:389–442.
6. Andreoli TE, Safirstein RL. Fluid and electrolyte disorders. In: Andreoli TE, Benjamin I, Griggs RC, Wing EJ, eds. *Andreoli and Carpenter's Cecil Essentials of Medicine.* 8th ed. Philadelphia, PA: Saunders Elsevier; 2010: chapter 28.
7. Rose BD, Post TW. *Clinical Physiology of Acid-Base and Electrolyte Disorders.* 5th ed. New York, NY: McGraw-Hill; 2001:707–711.
8. Kelly DG, Nadeau J. Oral rehydration solution: a "low-tech" oft neglected therapy. *Pract Gastroenterol.* 2004;28(10):51–62.
9. The Oley Foundation. Oral rehydration solution (ORS) recipes. https://cdn.ymaws.com/oley.org/resource/resmgr/ors_recipes/ORS_recipes_handout.pdf. Accessed November 22, 2019.
10. Ellison DH. Edema and the clinical use of diuretics. In: Greenberg A, ed. *Primer on Kidney Diseases.* 4th ed. Philadelphia, PA: Saunders; 2005:136–148.
11. Lexi-Drugs Online. Lexicomp Online Web site. https://www.wolterskluwercdi.com/lexicomp-online/. Accessed November 22, 2019.
12. Schrier RW. Water and sodium retention in edematous disorders: role of vasopressin and aldosterone. *Am J Med.* 2006;119(7 suppl 1):S47–S53.
13. Schrier RW. Pathogenesis of sodium and water retention in high output and low-output cardiac failure, nephrotic syndrome, cirrhosis, and pregnancy. *N Engl J Med.* 1988;319(17):1127–1134.
14. Ponikowski P, Voors AV, Anker SD, et al. 2016 ESC guidelines for the diagnosis and treatment of acute and chronic heart failure. *Eur Heart J.* 2016;37(27):2129–2200.
15. European Association for the Study of Liver. EASL clinical practice guidelines for the management of patients with decompensated cirrhosis. *J Hepatol.* 2018;69(2):406–460.
16. Orth SR, Ritz E. The nephrotic syndrome. *N Engl J Med.* 1998;338(17):1202–1211.
17. Brater DC. Diuretic therapy. *N Engl J Med.* 1998;339(6):387–395.
18. Somberg JC, Molnar J. Therapeutic approaches to the treatment of edema and ascites: the use of diuretics. *Am J Ther.* 2009;16(1):98–101.

CHAPTER 3

Electrolyte Disorders

Electrolyte disorders are a common occurrence in clinical practice and are seen in all practice settings, from outpatient clinics to the intensive care unit (ICU). An understanding of electrolyte disorders is vital for all clinicians regardless of practice setting. This chapter discusses the appropriate diagnosis and management of electrolyte disorders related to sodium, potassium, magnesium, calcium, and phosphorus.

Sodium

Overview

Sodium disorders are the most common electrolyte disturbances encountered in clinical practice. Although many cases are mild and asymptomatic, understanding the etiologies, treatments, and management strategies of sodium disorders is clinically important because the disorders and the treatments are associated with significant morbidity and mortality if not recognized early and managed appropriately.

1. Homeostasis and physiological function[1,2]

- The normal sodium range is 135–145 mEq/L (1 mEq/L = 1 mmol/L).

- Sodium is the most abundant extracellular cation and acts as a functionally impermeable solute (ie, an effective osmole because sodium cannot move passively across cell membranes).

- Sodium is the major osmotically active substance in the extracellular fluid (ECF) and maintains the concentration, volume, and osmolality of the ECF compartment.

- The conduction of action potential in nerves and muscle tissue is dependent on sodium concentration.

2. Dietary intake

   - One gram of sodium chloride is equal to 17 mEq of sodium and 17 mEq of chloride.

   - Adequate sodium intake for adults is 20–26 mEq (1200–1500 mg) per day depending on age and comorbidities.

   - The typical Western diet contains 100–250 mEq (6–15 g) of sodium per day.

3. Excretion

   - Sodium intake and urinary sodium excretion are balanced in healthy patients, with excess sodium excreted in the urine to maintain homeostasis. The range for urine sodium excretion varies widely and is dependent on diet. Typically, the average patient will excrete 40–200 mEq of sodium per day in the urine.

   - In the setting of inadequate sodium intake, the kidneys compensate by increasing the amount of sodium reabsorbed; when necessary, urinary excretion can be as little as < 1% of all filtered sodium.

   - Extrarenal sodium losses via gastrointestinal (GI) fluids and sweat are outlined in Chapter 1.

Hyponatremia

Prevalence and Mortality[3,4]

1. Hyponatremia is the most common electrolyte disturbance encountered in clinical practice.

2. An estimated 30%–45% of hospitalized patients will have hyponatremia (serum sodium < 135 mEq/L) and 2%–6% will have a serum sodium < 125 mEq/L.

- Approximately 30% of critically ill patients experience hyponatremia.
- Ambulatory care patients, who have not been extensively studied, have an estimated prevalence of hyponatremia of 7%–21%.
- Hyponatremia will develop in 18% of nursing home patients.

3. Mortality depends on the acuity and severity of hyponatremia.

- Whether the increase in mortality among hyponatremic patients is due to the underlying illness causing hyponatremia, the hyponatremia itself, or the treatment of hyponatremia is unknown.
- A serum sodium level < 130 mEq/L is associated with a mortality rate of 11.2%, and this rate dramatically increases to 25% when the serum sodium level falls below 120 mEq/L.

Risk Factors[3,5,6]

1. Increasing age (> 30 years old) is associated with an increased risk of both hyponatremia at hospital admission and hospital-acquired hyponatremia.

- Older individuals have a decreased ability to adapt to environmental, disease-related, drug-related, and other iatrogenic changes in sodium and water balance due to reductions in total body water, decrease in thirst sensation, decrease in renal responsiveness to antidiuretic hormone (ADH), and a decrease in glomerular filtration rate (GFR).

2. Lower body weight is associated with an increased risk of developing hyponatremia.

3. Administration of hypotonic intravenous (IV) fluids (see Chapter 1) can lead to iatrogenic hyponatremia.

4. Thiazide and thiazide-like diuretics (chlorthalidone, chlorothiazide, hydrochlorothiazide, indapamide, metolazone) frequently cause hyponatremia by increasing the renal excretion of sodium.

5. Hyponatremia can be seen in the postoperative period due to a combination of nonosmotic ADH release (in response to pain or stress

despite a normal serum osmolality) and administration of hypotonic intravenous fluids (eg, 0.45% sodium chloride).

Etiology[7]

Hyponatremia has various causes that are discussed in more detail under the diagnostic approach to hyponatremia section. A general description of hyponatremia is an imbalance of extracellular water and sodium wherein water is in excess relative to sodium.

1. Alterations in intake and output of water from the body can lead to hyponatremia. The major mechanisms for regulating water intake are thirst and secretion of ADH from the pituitary gland and its effect on the kidneys.

2. Osmoregulation and baroregulation of the release of ADH from the pituitary gland depends on the osmolality of the serum. Injury or damage to the pituitary gland can lead to inappropriate secretion of ADH regardless of serum osmolality or effective blood volume (EBV), leading to increased reabsorption of water in the kidney tubules.

3. Third-spacing of fluids in certain conditions (eg, bowel obstruction, pancreatitis, sepsis, and trauma) may cause capillary leak resulting in reduced EBV. A reduction in EBV will signal ADH release from the pituitary gland.

4. The kidneys play a major role in sodium and water regulation in the body because they are primarily responsible for reabsorption or excretion of sodium and water based on signals from various endocrine hormones.

    - Adrenal insufficiency causes hypoaldosteronism, which results in renal sodium wasting (see the adrenal insufficiency section in Chapter 5).

    - Heart failure may result in hyperaldosteronism causing sodium retention, thus leading to water retention and volume overload. Hyponatremia can result from retention of more water relative to sodium (ie, hypotonic hypervolemic hyponatremia).

    - Injury or damage to the kidneys may impair the reabsorption of sodium, thus causing sodium wasting in the urine.

Clinical Presentation[7-9]

1. Neurological symptoms are the primary clinical manifestation of hyponatremia and can range from mild symptoms, such as gait disturbances, concentration deficits, nausea, and headaches, to severe symptoms like psychosis, seizures, and coma (Table 3-1).

Table 3-1. Classification of Symptoms Associated With Hyponatremia.[2,7-9]

Severity	Serum Sodium Level, mEq/L	Clinical Manifestations
Mild		Commonly asymptomatic[a]
Moderately Severe	125-129	Nausea Headache Confusion
Severe	< 125	Vomiting Agitation Psychosis Seizures Abnormal/deep somnolence Coma (GCS ≤ 8)

GCS = Glasgow Coma Score

[a]Symptoms depend on the patient's baseline serum sodium level and the rate of decline. Patients with mild chronic hyponatremia may experience subclinical symptoms such as slight cognitive deficits and gait disturbances that are not easily recognized as symptoms of hyponatremia.

2. The severity of symptoms due to hyponatremia is generally related to the acuity of onset (ie, how fast hyponatremia develops) and the patient's baseline serum sodium level prior to the onset (ie, the absolute decrease in serum sodium).

   - Acute hyponatremia (onset < 48 hours) is associated with symptoms more commonly than chronic hyponatremia. Oftentimes, patients with acute hyponatremia present with more severe neurological symptoms than patients with chronic hyponatremia.

   - Chronic hyponatremia (onset > 48 hours) that occurs over days or weeks is often considered "asymptomatic," but it commonly causes subtle clinical abnormalities. Clinical signs include gait disturbances, falls, and concentration and cognitive deficits. The cognitive deficits or motor disturbances due to hyponatremia may not be clinically overt or apparent to the patient and/or family members. Additionally, chronic hyponatremia directly contributes to osteoporosis, increasing the potential for bone fractures from falls.

Diagnosis/Diagnostic Tests[10]

1. In addition to diagnostic studies, a comprehensive patient history, physical assessment, and evaluation of current medications are vital to help confirm the etiology of hyponatremia.

2. Serum sodium should be closely monitored (ie, every 4–6 hours).

3. Serum osmolality (normal range 275–290 mOsm/kg) will aid in diagnosing the type of hyponatremia and potential causes.

- Osmolality vs osmolarity
  - Osmolality is a measurement of concentration per weight (mOsm/kg).
  - Osmolarity is a measurement of concentration per volume (mOsm/L).
  - Since 1 L of H_2O weighs 1 kg, the numerical values of these 2 concentration measurements are equal when solutes are dissolved in water. Oftentimes the terms serum osmolality and serum osmolarity are used interchangeably.
- As described in Chapter 1, serum osmolality may be directly measured via blood sample or estimated (ie, calculated) using Equation 1.

Equation 1: Calculated serum osmolality

$$\text{Serum osmolality (mOsm/kg)} = [2 \times \text{serum sodium (mEq/L)}] + \left[\frac{\text{serum glucose (mg/dL)}}{18}\right] + \left[\frac{\text{blood urea nitrogen (BUN, mg/dL)}}{2.8}\right]$$

- An evaluation of serum osmolality (ie, hypotonic, hypertonic, or isotonic) in the context of hyponatremia can aid in determining the underlying etiology (as discussed later in the sodium section).
- Practitioners should calculate the serum osmol gap, which is defined as the difference between the measured and calculated serum osmolality (normal osmol gap is < 10 mOsm/kg).
  - An osmol gap > 10 mOsm/kg may indicate pseudohyponatremia or toxic ingestion of an osmotically active substance (eg, ethylene glycol, propylene glycol, methanol).

4. Evaluation of the urine sodium concentration will help the clinician determine if the kidneys are wasting or conserving sodium.

- A 24-hour urine sodium collection is the most accurate method to obtain a urine sodium concentration. The normal range is 40–200 mEq per 24 hours, but it varies with sodium intake.
- A one-time (ie, spot-check) urine sodium concentration is less nursing intensive but is also less accurate. The normal value should

be > 20 mEq/L, but it varies with sodium intake. No reference range exists for one-time urine sodium levels because many variables may alter sodium excretion throughout the day (eg, dietary sodium intake, diuretics and other medications, acid-base status). Results should be interpreted cautiously and samples should not be taken within 24 hours of diuretic use.

5. Urine osmolality (normal range 300–850 mOsm/kg) may help determine if the kidneys are appropriately concentrating the urine.

6. Physical examination should take place with particular emphasis on volume status of the patient and signs/symptoms of hyponatremia.

7. Determine if hyponatremia is acute or chronic, if possible. If the duration or onset of hyponatremia is unknown, assume it is a chronic condition.

Goals of Therapy[2,7-9,11]

1. The goal of therapy for hyponatremia is to increase serum sodium levels to the point that the patient is no longer symptomatic.

   - Regardless of the severity of symptoms due to hyponatremia, the rate and magnitude of sodium correction should reverse clinical manifestations of hyponatremia without posing a risk to the patient.

   - The rate at which the sodium level should be corrected and the sodium correction thresholds depend on the rate of onset of hyponatremia.

     - Acute hyponatremia (duration of several minutes to hours): Correction can occur at the same rate of onset of hyponatremia (ie, no daily sodium correction threshold). Oftentimes these patients are symptomatic and require rapid correction (see Management section).

     - Acute hyponatremia (duration of 24–48 hours): Rate of correction should not exceed 10 mEq/L in 24 hours.

     - Chronic hyponatremia (duration > 48 hours): Slow correction is necessary because these patients have adapted to having lower serum sodium levels. The rate of sodium correction should not exceed 8 mEq/L in 24 hours. An increase in serum sodium of 4 to 8 mEq/L should be targeted to minimize the risk of osmotic demyelination syndrome (ODS).

2. Recommended serum sodium correction thresholds are based on avoidance of ODS.

- ODS is a neurological condition characterized by damage (ie, demyelination) of nerve cells in the brain and can occur if serum sodium is corrected too rapidly. The typical onset of ODS is 3–5 days after sodium correction. Clinical manifestations include paraparesis or quadriparesis, difficulty swallowing or speaking, diplopia, and/or locked-in syndrome. Frequent neurological monitoring (eg, every 6 hours) can help detect early manifestations of ODS. Magnetic resonance imaging can be useful in detecting ODS, even in asymptomatic patients.
- A review of 51 patients with hyponatremia revealed no cases of ODS among those who experienced a serum sodium correction of < 12 mEq/L/d (n = 13); however, among the 38 patients whose serum sodium was corrected by > 12 mEq/L/d, 37% developed ODS.
- ODS is predominantly a concern in patients with chronic hyponatremia; however, caution must still be exercised when managing patients with acute hyponatremia.
- Factors that place patients at a higher risk of developing ODS include:
    - Serum sodium ≤ 105 mEq/L
    - Hypokalemia
    - Alcoholism
    - Malnutrition
    - Advanced liver disease

3. Ultimately, the goal of serum sodium correction is to end symptoms (typically serum sodium levels of 125–130 mEq/L), not to correct sodium to normal levels in all patients.

- Patients with acute onset of hyponatremia will likely tolerate sodium levels within normal range if this was their baseline sodium level.
- Patients with chronic hyponatremia merely need to be corrected to a stable baseline sodium level at which they are asymptomatic.

Management

The method of management of hyponatremia will depend on the severity of symptoms and the acuity of onset. Severe symptoms should be treated aggressively to safely correct serum sodium levels and resolve symptoms. Less severe symptoms may not require any direct interventions to increase serum sodium levels, but only require correcting the underlying disorder or removing an offending agent to allow sodium levels to correct over time.

Hyponatremia With Severe Symptoms[2,7,12,13]

- Hyponatremia *with severe symptoms,* such as vomiting, confusion, obtundation, seizures, and/or coma is a life-threatening emergency and should be treated promptly. Development of such symptoms can be indicative of increased intracranial pressure, which may result in brain herniation. An acute rise in serum sodium of 4–6 mEq/L may be needed to halt neurological symptoms, such as seizures, and hopefully, prevent impending brain herniation.
  - For acute hyponatremia, a 4–6 mEq/L increase in serum sodium within the initial 1–4 hours of symptoms onset can be targeted.
  - For chronic hyponatremia, serum sodium should be increased by the lowest amount needed for symptom resolution, with a maximum rise of 4–6 mEq/L within the initial 6 hours (maximum correction 6–8 mEq/L in 24 hours; 12–14 mEq/L in 48 hours; 14–16 mEq/L in 72 hours).
- Intravenous 3% NaCl (513 mEq of sodium/L) is considered the standard of care for severely symptomatic hyponatremia. This therapy can be administered as small intermittent boluses, as a continuous infusion, or as a combination of these 2 methods.
  - *Bolus infusion*
    - Small volume (ie, 100–150 mL) bolus dose administration of 3% NaCl can be considered. The 2014 European clinical practice guidelines for the diagnosis and treatment of hyponatremia recommend a 150-mL fixed dose (or 2 mL/kg, whichever is less) administered over 20 minutes, with repeat bolus dosing twice as needed until symptoms subside or the serum sodium level has increased by 5 mEq/L (whichever occurs first). Serum sodium levels should be monitored 20 minutes after each bolus dose is completed.

- In the absence of free water loss in the urine, each 1 mL/kg of 3% NaCl should increase the serum sodium level by 1 mEq/kg. Hence, intermittent bolus dose administration with repeat laboratory work theoretically allows for a controlled and immediate rise in serum sodium levels to halt neurologic injury.

- Continuous IV infusion
  - Administration of 3% NaCl via continuous infusion can also be considered for management of severely symptomatic hyponatremia.
  - In contrast to bolus dose administration, there is no standard approach, with "protocol" dosing varying widely in available literature (eg, initial infusion rates of 20–83 mL/h, including potential adjustments to the infusion rate based on follow-up serum sodium levels).
  - As an alternative to protocol-based dosing (ie, one size fits all), the initial 3% NaCl infusion rate can also be calculated using the formula in Table 3-2. Essentially, given a patient's serum sodium level, the change in serum sodium expected following administration of 1 L of 3% NaCl is determined.
    - For example, if a 70-kg male patient presented with a serum sodium of 120 mEq/L, each liter of 3% NaCl would be expected to result in a rise in serum sodium of approximately 9 mEq/L.

Table 3-2. Infusate Characteristics and Expected Change in Serum Sodium.[8]

$$\text{Change in serum sodium (mEq/L)} = \frac{\text{Infusate sodium (mEq/L)} - \text{Serum sodium (mEq/L)}}{\text{Total body water (L)} + 1}$$

Solution	Tonicity	Na^+, mEq/L	ECF distribution, %
3% NaCl (hypertonic saline)	Hypertonic	513	100[a]
0.9% NaCl (normal saline)	Isotonic	154	100
Lactated Ringer's[b]	Isotonic	130	97
PlasmaLyte[b,c]	Isotonic	140	98
Normosol-R[b]	Isotonic	140	98

ECF, extracellular fluid.

Please refer to Chapter 1 for calculation of total body water.

[a]In addition to its complete distribution to the ECF compartment, this infusate induces osmotic removal of water from the intracellular compartment.

[b]Also contains other electrolytes (see Table 1-5 for more information).

[c]PlasmaLyte A and PlasmaLyte 148 are 2 separately labeled products that differ only in pH (7.4 vs 5.5, respectively).

- If the desired change in serum sodium is 5 mEq/L, this would entail approximately 555 mL of 3% NaCl. If this change is desired in the first 6 hours, then the initial infusion rate of 3% NaCl should be 93 mL/h.
- It should be emphasized that that the formula in Table 3-2 is only intended to guide the initial IV infusion rate. The formula provides an estimate of need, and the infusion rate should be adjusted/ guided by serial sodium monitoring conducted every 2–6 hours.

- Following acute correction of the serum sodium, subsequent management may include continuous IV infusion of 3% NaCl or 0.9% NaCl (as dictated by the clinical situation) until the etiology of hyponatremia is determined and targeted interventions are initiated.
- Serum sodium monitoring should occur every 4 hours when 3% NaCl is being administered. Once the serum sodium level has stabilized and symptoms have resolved, the frequency of monitoring can be reduced to every 6–12 hours and then daily.
- Logistical considerations with 3% NaCl
  - Central line administration is preferred given that the solution is hypertonic (osmolality of 1026 mOsm/L) and has the potential to cause phlebitis; however, the lack of central line access should not delay administration in symptomatic patients. In addition, recent literature reveals a "low" incidence of infusion-related adverse events in patients administered 3% sodium chloride via peripheral vein.
  - As noted above, serum sodium monitoring should occur every 4 hours when administering 3% NaCl, allowing for detection and prompt intervention for excessive elevations.
  - Lastly, it is recommended that institutions develop policies guiding use of 3% NaCl (ie, prescribing and administration specifics).

Hyponatremia With Moderately Severe Symptoms[2,7,12–15]

1. In the management of patients with moderately severe symptoms from hyponatremia, the goal is to prevent symptom progression.
   - A single bolus dose of 3% NaCl 150 mL intravenously over 20 minutes is recommended (see bolus infusion section above), with a target rise in serum sodium of 5 mEq/L in 24 hours.
   - Discontinue any offending medications (see Figure 3-1 and Table 3-3) or fluids that may contribute to hyponatremia. Practitioners should

Figure 3-1. Assessment of Serum Osmolality in Hyponatremia.[2]

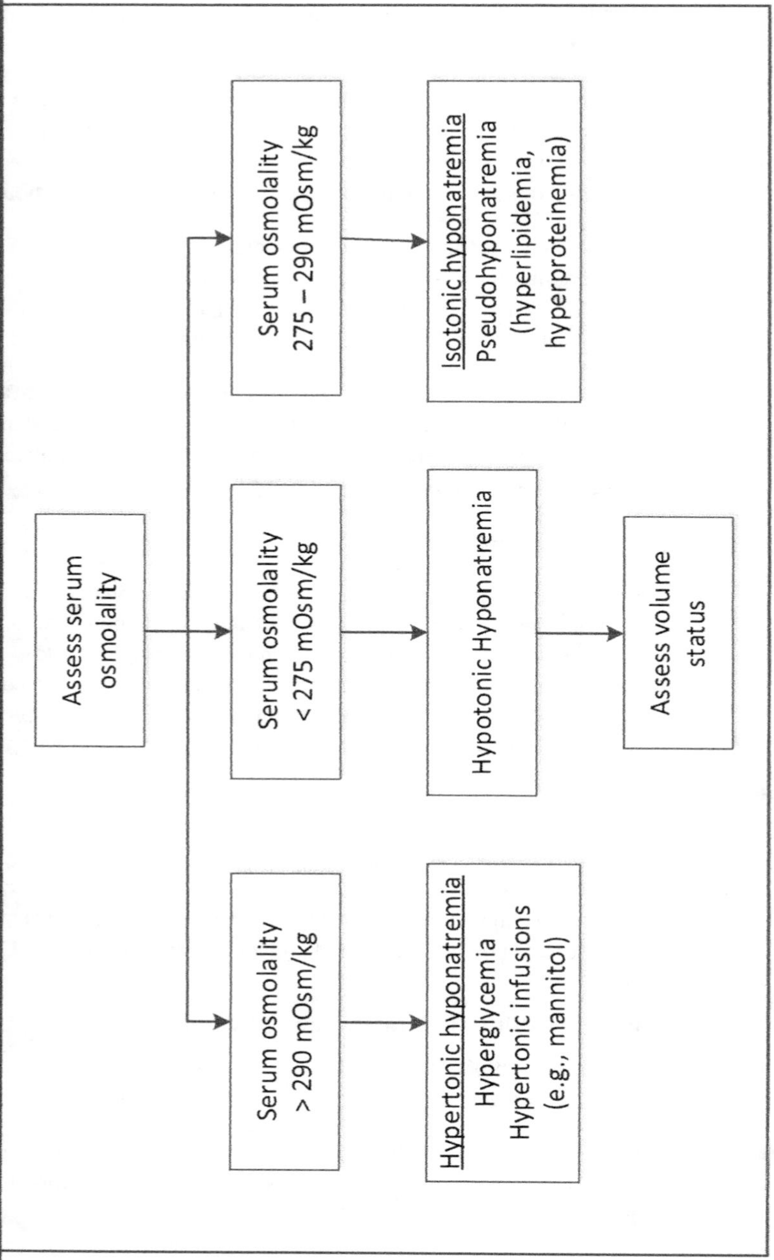

Table 3-3. Causes of Syndrome of Inappropriate Antidiuresis.[1,7,14,15]

Cause	Examples
Malignancy	• Central nervous system • Ewing's sarcoma • Gastrointestinal (stomach, duodenum, pancreas) • Genitourinary/gynecologic (ureter, bladder, prostate, endometrium) • Lung • Lymphomas • Mesothelioma
Pulmonary disorders	• Aspergillosis • Asthma • Cystic fibrosis • Pneumonia • Tuberculosis
Drugs/medications[a]	• Amitriptyline • Carbamazepine • Chemotherapy (cyclophosphamide, ifosfamide, vincristine) • Chlorpropamide • Clofibrate • Desmopressin • Haloperidol • Lamotrigine • MDMA (ecstasy or molly) • Opiates (eg, fentanyl, morphine, hydromorphone) • Nicotine • Nonsteroidal anti-inflammatory drugs (eg, aspirin, celecoxib, diclofenac, etodolac, ibuprofen, indomethacin, ketoprofen, naproxen, meloxicam, piroxicam, sulindac) • Oxcarbazepine • Oxytocin • Selective serotonin reuptake inhibitors (eg, citalopram, escitalopram, fluoxetine, paroxetine, sertraline) • Valproic acid • Vasopressin

Continued on next page

Table 3-3. *Continued.*

Cause	Examples
Central nervous system disorders	• AIDS • Cerebrovascular accident • Delirium tremens • Guillain-Barré syndrome • Head trauma (subarachnoid hemorrhage, subdural hematoma) • Hydrocephalus • Hypopituitarism • Infections (eg, CNS abscess, encephalitis, meningitis, Rocky Mountain spotted fever, malaria) • Multiple sclerosis
Other	• Hereditary disorders • Idiopathic • Transient (endurance exercise, general anesthesia, nausea, pain, stress)

AIDS, acquired immunodeficiency syndrome; CNS, central nervous system; MDMA, 3,4-methylenedioxymethamphetamine

[a]Act by increasing the secretion of antidiuretic hormone (ADH) from the pituitary and/or potentiating the effect of ADH.

be cognizant of the potential use of hypotonic diluents (eg, 0.45% NaCl or 5% dextrose in water) for IV piggyback medications, such as antimicrobials, and request a change to 0.9% NaCl if compatible. Conduct a risk vs benefit analysis of all offending medications, considering alternatives as feasible.

- Initiate a prompt diagnostic assessment.

Asymptomatic Hyponatremia[2,7,12–15]

1. Asymptomatic hyponatremia can be treated conservatively, particularly in patients with chronic hyponatremia.

   - As noted above, discontinue any offending medications or fluids that may contribute to hyponatremia and initiate a prompt diagnostic assessment.

   - Assess the urine osmolality and serum osmolality.

     - Concentrated urine (urine osmolality greater than serum osmolality) may indicate a reduced EBV and is treated with infusion of isotonic saline (Table 3-2).

- Dilute urine (urine osmolality less than serum osmolality) may indicate fluid overload and is treated with water restriction and close observation.

- If the onset of hyponatremia is acute and the decrease in serum sodium exceeds 10 mEq/L, consider a single IV infusion of 3% NaCl 150 mL over 20 minutes (see bolus infusion section below).

Diagnostic Approach to Hyponatremia[1]

Once the patient is acutely stabilized, attention can shift to determining the underlying etiology of hyponatremia using the diagnostic methods discussed earlier (see Diagnosis/Diagnostic Tests section). Identification of the etiology will allow the clinician to determine the most appropriate management strategies to facilitate resolution, and hopefully, avoid recurrence.

1. First, assess serum osmolality (Figure 3-1).

   - *Hypertonic hyponatremia*: serum osmolality > 290 mOsm/kg.

     - *Osmotically active substances other than sodium contribute to* increased serum osmolality, causing water to move from the intracellular fluid (ICF) to the ECF in order to equilibrate osmolality. This movement will cause sodium dilution in the ECF, leading to hyponatremia.

     - Common causes of hypertonic hyponatremia include hyperglycemia and infusion of hypertonic fluids (with no or little sodium) or medications (mannitol).

     - Treatment centers on correcting the underlying cause (eg, providing insulin or reducing dextrose load for hyperglycemia) or discontinuing the offending agents.

       - Traditionally, for each 100 mg/dL increase in blood glucose above 100 mg/dL, serum sodium is expected to fall by 1.6 mEq/L. Equation 2 can be used to calculate the corrected serum sodium level in the presence of hyperglycemia.

Equation 2: Corrected serum sodium for hyperglycemia

Corrected serum sodium (mEq/L) =

serum sodium (mEq/L) + [0.016 [serum glucose (mg/dL) − 100]]

- *Isotonic hyponatremia*: serum osmolality 275–290 mOsm/kg.
  - Isotonic hyponatremia occurs with an increase in the nonaqueous portion of the serum; however, the sodium concentration in the aqueous portion of the serum remains normal.
  - It is historically related to older, less accurate laboratory methodologies for measuring serum sodium levels.
  - Common causes include hyperlipidemia and hyperproteinemia (seen in certain hematologic malignancies).
  - Treatment focuses on correction or treatment of the underlying cause. Since the sodium level of the aqueous portion of the serum is normal, clinicians should not attempt to correct the serum sodium.

- *Hypotonic hyponatremia*: serum osmolality < 275 mOsm/kg (Figure 3-2).
  - Hypotonic hyponatremia is the most common and most clinically relevant type of hyponatremia.
  - Depending on the fluid status of the patient, hypotonic hyponatremia can be classified as hypovolemic, euvolemic, or hypervolemia.

2. Assess the patient's volume status.

- Hypovolemia signs and symptoms include dry mouth/tongue, increased thirst, sunken eyes, decreased skin turgor, tachycardia, decreased blood pressure, decreased urine output, and/or dark urine color in the absence of jaundice (indicating concentrated urine).
  - Fluid losses such as vomiting, diarrhea, high output drain or ostomy, hemorrhage or bleeding, and high nasogastric tube output can all contribute to hypovolemia. See Table 1-6 for a description of the electrolyte content for specific sites of GI fluid loss.
- Hypervolemia signs and symptoms include ascites, pleural effusions on chest x-ray, extremity swelling or edema, anasarca, increased blood pressure, and/or increased brain natriuretic peptide > 300 pg/mL.
- *Hypovolemic hypotonic hyponatremia* reflects a deficit of both sodium and water, but sodium losses exceed water losses.
  - A one-time or spot-check urine sodium level should be assessed.

Figure 3-2. Assessment of Volume status in Hypotonic Hyponatremia.

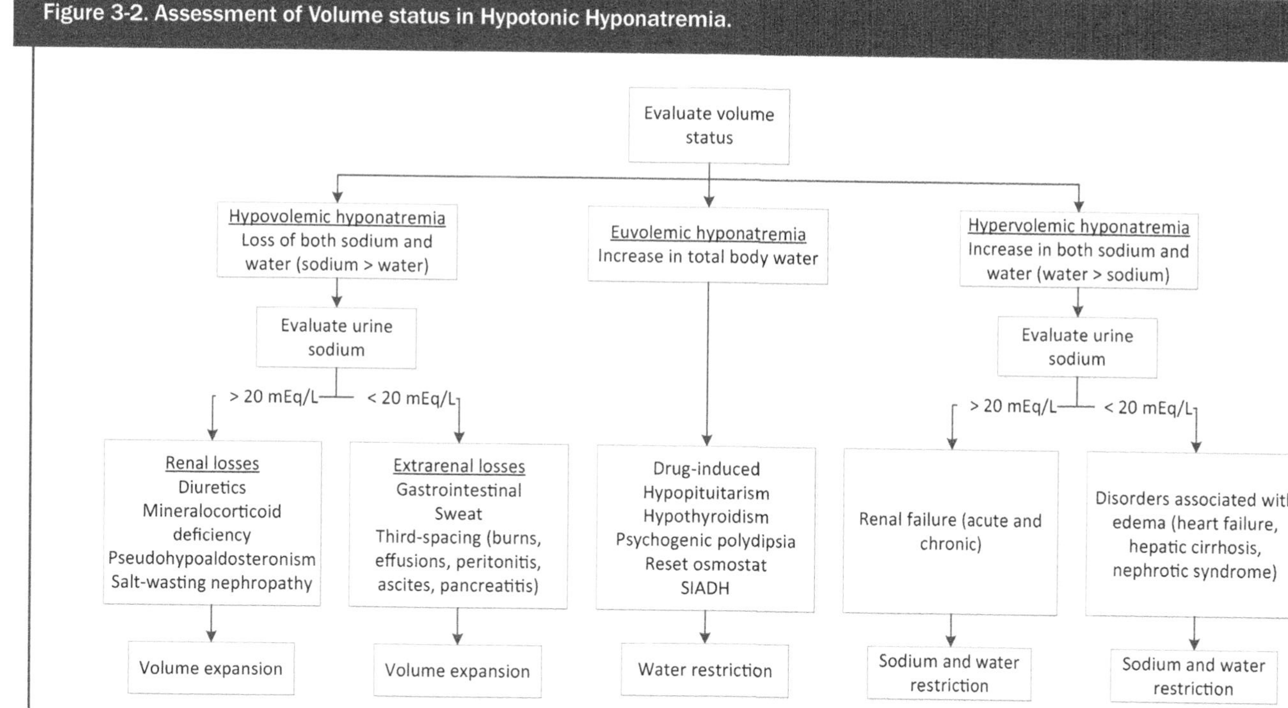

SIADH, syndrome of inappropriate antidiuretic hormone.

- A common cause is fluid loss, which can be categorized as renal or extrarenal.
  - Renal losses (urine sodium > 20 mEq/L) include fluid loss from the use of diuretics, mineralocorticoid deficiency, pseudohypoaldosteronism, solute diuresis, salt-wasting nephropathy, and/or cerebral salt wasting.
    - Diuretics can lead to increased fluid loss through renal excretion. Thiazide and thiazide-like diuretics (chlorthalidone, chlorothiazide, hydrochlorothiazide, indapamide, metolazone) are more commonly associated with hyponatremia. These agents act solely on the distal tubules, causing sodium wasting, and do not interfere with the kidney's ability to concentrate urine (resulting in more water resorption compared with other classes of diuretics). They also do not interfere with the ability of ADH to cause water resorption. Hence, with thiazide diuretic use, sodium losses in the urine are relatively greater than water losses.
      - Loop diuretics (budesonide, ethacrynic acid, furosemide, torsemide) are rarely associated with hyponatremia because they impair the urine-concentrating mechanisms of the kidney (ie, water losses in the urine are relatively greater than sodium losses, which can result in hypernatremia due to creation of a total body water deficit).
    - Mineralocorticoid deficiency is primarily a deficiency in aldosterone, which impairs reabsorption of sodium in the distal convoluted tubule, leading to sodium wasting.
    - Pseudohypoaldosteronism is caused by genetic disorders that induce aldosterone resistance or by medications that antagonize aldosterone (eg, eplerenone, spironolactone).
    - Solute diuresis is induced by elevated BUN, hyperglycemia, and/or mannitol. Patients will waste both sodium and water; however, more sodium losses may occur due to the presence of other osmotically active solutes (eg, glucose, mannitol, urea).
    - Salt-wasting nephropathy is a tubular and interstitial injury caused by nephrotoxic medications or inherited disorders.
    - Cerebral salt wasting can be seen following injury (eg, trauma) to the brain and is characterized by excessive sodium losses in the urine despite "normal" kidney function; the precise mechanism of action remains unknown.

- Extrarenal losses (urine sodium < 20 mEq/L) include fluid loss from excessive sweating, GI loss, or third-spacing (also known as sequestration), which is commonly seen with burns, effusions, peritonitis, pancreatitis, and ascites.

  - Treatment is to provide volume expansion with isotonic fluids (Table 3-2); in the setting of severe symptoms, hypertonic saline (3% NaCl) should be administered (as previously discussed).

- *Euvolemic hypotonic hyponatremia* reflects an increase in total body water while total body sodium remains the same.
  - Common causes are related to disorders associated with increased water retention.
    - Syndrome of inappropriate antidiuretic hormone (SIADH) is an excess of ADH secretion resulting in water retention. ADH is secreted mainly from the pituitary gland; however, small amounts are secreted in lung tissue as well.
      - In hyponatremia, SIADH is an overarching term describing a pathological condition in which the pituitary and/or other cells secrete ADH independent of serum osmolality or EBV. Water permeability of the renal collecting ducts can be affected by both genetic and pharmacological factors regardless of ADH secretion. For the purpose of accuracy, the phrase syndrome of inappropriate antidiuresis (SIAD) will be used throughout the text to describe any condition that results in increased water permeability in the renal collecting ducts.
      - Causes of SIAD are listed in Table 3-3.
    - Psychogenic polydipsia results in increased water intake secondary to excessive thirst due to psychosis or dry mouth from antipsychotic medications.
    - Hypothyroidism, mainly in patients with primary hypothyroidism and myxedema, can cause euvolemic hyponatremia. The mechanism is not completely understood, but it may be related to a diminished ability of the kidneys to excrete water. Some patients may have reduced cardiac output, which can lead to the release of ADH via the carotid sinus baroreceptors; however, not all hypothyroid patients have increased levels of ADH.
    - Cortisol deficiency can also lead to euvolemic hyponatremia. This outcome may be in part due to the reduction in systemic blood

    pressure and cardiac output, with subsequent stimulation of baroreceptors due to a decrease in EBV.

    - Reset osmostat occurs when the threshold for ADH release is reduced, resulting in plasma sodium levels below normal but stable (120–130 mEq/L).

  - Treatment includes treating the underlying disorder and restricting fluids to < 1–1.5 L of fluid per day.

  - Oral NaCl tablets may also be considered for sodium supplementation. Each 1 g tablet of NaCl provides approximately 18 mEq of sodium.

  - Refractory SIAD may require administration of vasopressin-2 receptor antagonists. Currently, 2 agents are approved by the US Food and Drug Administration, conivaptan (available for intravenous use) and tolvaptan (available as an oral tablet). These agents cause an aquaresis (excretion of free water).

- *Hypervolemic hypotonic hyponatremia* reflects an increase in total body water and sodium, but water gains are greater than sodium gains.

  - One-time or spot-check urine sodium level should be assessed.

  - Common causes are mainly due to activation of the renin-angiotensin-aldosterone system (RAAS). See Figure 1-3.

    - Renal failure (urine sodium > 20 mEq/L), both acute and chronic, can lead to both sodium and water retention.

    - Disorders associated with fluid retention and edema (urine sodium < 20 mEq/L), such as heart failure or hepatic cirrhosis, can cause both sodium and water retention.

  - Treatment is sodium and fluid restriction; loop diuretics in addition to aldosterone receptor antagonists (spironolactone, eplerenone) should be considered in patients with heart failure; aldosterone receptor antagonists are preferred in patients with cirrhosis.

Monitoring[6]

1. The degree of monitoring should reflect the severity of hyponatremia and ensure an appropriate rate of sodium correction without posing a risk to the patient.

2. Asymptomatic patients treated conservatively may require daily or twice daily sodium level assessments to ensure the serum sodium is not being overcorrected or corrected too rapidly, thus putting the patient at risk for ODS.

3. Symptomatic patients who are being aggressively treated with continuous infusion hypertonic saline (ie, 3% NaCl) should have serum sodium levels monitored at least every 2–4 hours to ensure a safe sodium correction rate. Patients treated with bolus doses of 3% NaCl should have sodium levels monitored 20 minutes after each bolus and then at 6 and 12 hours once sodium levels have stabilized.

4. Patients at risk for hyponatremia should have regular follow-up (eg, every 3–6 months) with their managing clinician to monitor sodium levels, especially in the presence of medications or comorbidities that may precipitate hyponatremia.

Hypernatremia

Prevalence and Mortality[12,16,17]

1. An estimated 1%–3% of all hospitalized patients will have hypernatremia (serum sodium > 145 mEq/L); however, it occurs more commonly in critically ill patients (9%).

2. The mortality of patients with hypernatremia ranges from 42% to 60%.

   - Mortality increases to over 75% when serum sodium levels are > 160 mEq/L.

   - The mortality associated with chronic hypernatremia is lower than with acute hypernatremia.

   - Mortality associated with hypernatremia is often due to underlying disease processes and not directly attributable to hypernatremia alone.

Risk Factors[12,16]

1. The risk of hypernatremia is highest when the ability to recognize thirst and/or gain access to water is impaired.

2. Infants, the elderly, patients with underlying cognitive dysfunction or altered mental status, and mechanically ventilated patients have the highest risk for hypernatremia.

Etiology[16,18]

Hypernatremia has various causes that are discussed in more detail under the diagnostic approach to hypernatremia section. A general description of hypernatremia is an imbalance of extracellular water and sodium wherein sodium is in excess relative to water.

1. Alterations in the intake and output of fluids from the body can lead to hypernatremia. The major mechanisms for regulating water intake are thirst and secretion of ADH from the pituitary gland and its effect on the kidneys.

2. Fluid loss via the kidneys, GI tract or through sweating may result in loss of more water relative to sodium, resulting in hypernatremia. Even though sodium is lost via the above-mentioned routes, relatively more water is lost.

3. Insufficient secretion of ADH or ineffective action of ADH on the kidneys may result in an inability of the kidneys to reabsorb water. This is known as diabetes insipidus (DI).

4. Hypernatremia can arise from iatrogenic causes. Many medications can lead to water loss (Figure 3-3), and overadministration of sodium-containing isotonic (eg, 0.9% NaCl) or hypertonic (eg, 3% NaCl) fluids can contribute to hypernatremia.

Clinical Presentation[9,16]

1. The clinical manifestations of hypernatremia are primarily neurological (Table 3-4).

2. Infants typically present with symptoms associated with mild or moderate hypernatremia; however, elderly patients are commonly asymptomatic until sodium levels exceed 160 mEq/L.

3. The severity of symptoms depends on the rate of onset of hypernatremia.

   - Acute increases in sodium (< 48 hours) are more commonly associated with symptoms compared to chronic sodium changes.

   - Chronic hypernatremia (onset > 48 hours) that occurs over days or weeks is often asymptomatic.

4. Thirst response may be present initially, but it may dissipate as hypernatremia progresses.

Figure 3-3. Medications Associated with Hypernatremia.[16,18]

Hyponatremia[a]	**Hypernatremia**
Carbamazepine	Induce nephrogenic DI
Cisplatin	• Amphotericin B
Cyclophosphamide	• Demeclocycline
Nicotine	• Foscarnet
Opiate derivatives	• Methoxyflurane
SSRIs	• Lithium
• Citalopram, escitalopram, fluoxetine, paroxetine, sertraline	Cause excessive water loss
Thiazide diuretics/thiazide-like diuretics	• Conivaptan, tolvaptan (aquaresis via vasopressin-2 receptor antagonism)
• Chlorthalidone, chlorothiazide, hydrochlorothiazide, indapamide, metolazone	• Loop diuretics (furosemide, bumetanide, torsemide)
	• Lactulose (osmotic cathartic)
Tricyclic antidepressants	• Mannitol (acts as osmotic diuretic)
• Amitriptyline, clomipramine, desipramine, doxepin, nortriptyline	• Tube feeds > 1.5 kcal/mL (osmotic catharic)
Vincristine	Iatragenic
	• Hypertonic sodium infusion (3% NaCl)

ADH, antidiuretic hormone; DI, diabetes insipidus; SSRIs, selective serotonin reuptake inhibitors.

[a]Acts by increasing the secretion of ADH from the pituitary and/or potentiating the effect of ADH.

Diagnosis/Diagnostic Tests[9,16 10,19]

1. In addition to diagnostic studies, a comprehensive patient history, physical assessment, and evaluation of current medications are vital to help confirm the etiology of hypernatremia.

2. Serum sodium should be closely monitored (eg, every 6–12 hours) depending upon the severity of symptoms and/or aggressiveness of management.

3. Serum osmolality (normal range, 275–290 mOsm/kg) is of little use in hypernatremia because hypernatremia is always associated with hypertonicity.

Table 3-4. Clinical Manifestations of Hypernatremia.

Severity of Hypernatremia	Serum Sodium Level, mEq/L	Symptoms
Mild	145–150	Commonly asymptomatic[a] Thirst
Moderate	151–160	Anorexia Excessive thirst Insomnia Lethargy Muscle twitching/weakness
Severe	> 160	Weakness Altered mental status Irritability Lethargy Seizures Stupor Coma

[a]Symptoms depend on the patient's baseline serum sodium level and the rate of increase.

4. One-time or spot-check urine sodium (normal values are > 20 mEq/L) will aid in determining if decreased renal sodium excretion or increased free water loss is present.

5. Urine osmolality (normal range, 300–850 mOsm/kg) will help to determine if the kidneys are appropriately concentrating urine. In hypernatremia, urine osmolality < 850 mOsm/kg indicates a defect in the secretion or effect of ADH or the presence of an osmotic diuresis.

6. Urine output (normal output is 0.5–2 mL/kg/h) will aid in determining if excessive fluid losses are occurring.

7. Physical examination should take place with particular emphasis on volume status and signs/symptoms of hypernatremia.

8. Determining if hypernatremia is acute or chronic should be performed if possible. If the duration or onset of hyponatremia is unknown, assume it is a chronic condition.

Goals of Therapy[16]

1. The goal of therapy for hypernatremia, similar to that of hyponatremia, is to correct serum sodium levels to the point that the patient is no longer symptomatic. The rate of sodium correction should be tightly controlled and not exceed the recommended rate of correction to avoid adverse effects, primarily cerebral edema.

2. Regardless of the severity of symptoms due to hypernatremia, the rate and magnitude of sodium correction should reverse clinical manifestations of hypernatremia without posing a risk to the patient.

    - The rate at which the sodium level is corrected is dependent on the rate of onset of hypernatremia.

        - Acute hypernatremia: Sodium correction can occur at the same rate of onset of hypernatremia. Oftentimes these patients are symptomatic and require rapid correction.

        - Chronic hypernatremia: Slow correction is necessary because these patients have adapted to having higher serum sodium levels.

    - No true consensus exists on the rate of correction; however, for the safety of the patient, the rate should not exceed 8–10 mEq/L in 24 hours or 18 mEq/L in 48 hours.

        - Cerebral edema and swelling can occur if serum sodium levels are corrected too rapidly. Clinical manifestations of cerebral edema include seizures, permanent brain injury, and death.

    - The goal of serum sodium correction is to end symptoms and gradually correct the water deficit without posing a risk to the patient.

Management

The management of hypernatremia depends on the severity of symptoms and the acuity of onset of hypernatremia. Treat severe symptoms aggressively to safely correct serum sodium levels and resolve symptoms. Less severe symptoms may not require any direct interventions to correct serum sodium levels; correcting the underlying disorder or removing an offending agent may be sufficient to allow sodium levels to correct over time.

Symptomatic Hypernatremia[16]

1. Mild symptoms such as thirst should be treated conservatively.

   - Administration of hypotonic fluids (eg, 0.45% NaCl or 5% dextrose in water) can slowly decrease sodium levels and alleviate mild symptoms. Restrict exogenous sodium administration as much as possible.

     - Calculate the water deficit and administer fluids based on the rate of correction for the chosen infusate (Table 3-5).

     - If possible, allow the patient to drink water as tolerated to help correct hypernatremia. This approach may allow for correction of hypernatremia without the use of IV fluids. Oral rehydration solutions can also be utilized because they typically contain ≤ 75 mEq Na/L, but practitioners should be cognizant of the differing sodium content within each product (see Table 2-6). Soup broth should be avoided given a typical sodium content of ≥ 80 mEq/L.

2. Moderate to severe symptoms including muscle twitching, lethargy, stupor, seizures, and coma should be treated aggressively and considered a life-threatening emergency.

   - Provide rapid correction with hypotonic IV fluids (Table 3-5).

     - Serum sodium may be corrected as rapidly as 0.5–1 mEq/L/h until symptoms resolve.

     - Rate of correction should not exceed 8–10 mEq/L in 24 hours or 18 mEq/L in 48 hours to prevent the development of cerebral edema and convulsions.

Table 3-5. Formulas for the Management of Hypernatremia.[12,16]

Water deficit (L) = Total body water (L) × [(Serum sodium (mEq/L)/140) − 1]

$$\text{Change in serum sodium (mEq/L)} = \frac{\text{Infusate sodium (mEq/L)} - \text{Serum sodium (mEq/L)}}{\text{Total body water (L)} + 1}$$

Solution	Tonicity	Na^+, mEq/L	Free water per liter, mL
0.9% NaCl (normal saline)	Isotonic	154	0
0.45% NaCl (½ normal saline)	Hypotonic	77	500
Lactated Ringer's	Isotonic	130	0
5% dextrose	Hypotonic	–	1000

Please refer to Chapter 1 for calculation of total body water.

Diagnostic Approach to Hypernatremia[1]

A standard, systematic approach to diagnose hypernatremia is extremely helpful to the bedside clinician. Once the etiology of hypernatremia is established, the clinician can determine exactly how to manage hypernatremia.

1. Assess the patient's volume status (Figure 3-4).

    - Carefully examine fluid intake and output.
    - Hypovolemia signs and symptoms include dry mouth/tongue, increased thirst, sunken eyes, decreased skin turgor, tachycardia, decreased blood pressure, decreased urine output, and/or dark urine color in the absence of jaundice.
        - Excessive fluid losses can be caused by vomiting, diarrhea, high output drain or ostomy, hemorrhage or bleeding, and/or high nasogastric tube output.
    - Hypervolemia signs and symptoms include ascites, pleural effusions on chest x-ray, extremity swelling or edema, anasarca, increased blood pressure, and/or increased brain natriuretic peptide > 300 pg/mL.
    - *Hypovolemic hypernatremia* reflects a deficit of both sodium and water, but water losses exceed sodium losses.
        - Assess a one-time or spot-check urine sodium level if oliguria is present (urine output < 0.5 mL/kg/h).
        - Common causes are renal or extrarenal fluid loss.
            - Renal losses (urine sodium > 20 mEq/L) can be attributed to acute kidney injury (AKI) or chronic kidney disease (CKD; patients are not able to appropriately concentrate urine and lose excess water), diuretics, solute diuresis (induced by elevated BUN, hyperglycemia, mannitol), and/or urinary obstruction.
            - Extrarenal losses (urine sodium < 20 mEq/L) can be attributed to excessive sweating, GI losses, and/or respiratory losses.
        - Treatment is volume expansion through the provision of fluids.
            - If the patient is symptomatically hypovolemic (ie, hypotensive), provide volume expansion with isotonic IV fluids (eg, Ringer's lactate, PlasmaLyte, 0.9% NaCl) until blood pressure stabilizes.

Figure 3-4. Diagnostic Approach to Hypernatremia.

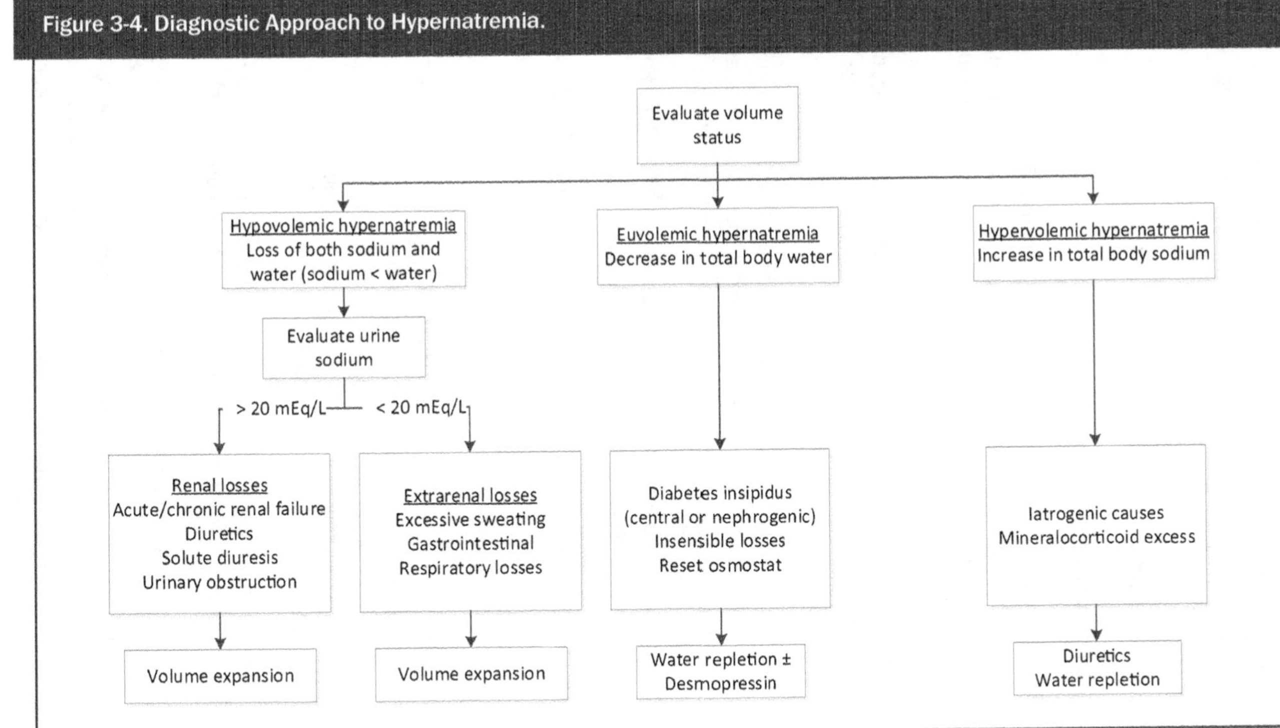

- Once the blood pressure stabilizes or if the patient is not hypotensive, use hypotonic fluids to correct water deficit.
    - Calculate the water deficit (Table 3-5).
    - Correct no more than half the water deficit in the first 24 hours. Correct the remainder of the water deficit over the next 48 hours.
    - The water deficit can be corrected orally, enterally, or parenterally.

- *Euvolemic hypernatremia* reflects a decrease in total body water, but total body sodium remains normal.
    - Common causes include pure water loss.
        - DI causes excessive water excretion via the kidneys. Potential causes are listed in Figure 3-5.
            - Central DI, also called neurohypophyseal or neurogenic DI, is a deficiency in the secretion of ADH from the pituitary.

Figure 3-5. Causes of Diabetes Insipidus.

Nephrogenic	Central
Advanced renal disease	Central nervous system infection
Drugs	Central nervous system malignancy
• Amphotericin B, aminoglycosides (amikacin, gentamicin, tobramycin), cidofovir, demeclocycline, didanosine, foscarnet, ifosfamide, mannitol, vasopressin V2-receptor antagonists	Cerebral hemorrhage Cerebrovascular accident (involving pituitary) Head trauma Hypoxic encephalopathy
Hypercalcemia	Neurosurgery (pituitary)
Hypokalemia	Idiopathic
Lithium toxicity	
Polycystic kidney disease	
Familial	
• Inherited aquaporin-2 defect	
• Inherited vasopressin V2-receptor defect	

It can be caused by autoimmune injury to the ADH-secreting cells, trauma, pituitary surgery, or hypoxic or ischemic encephalopathy.

  - Nephrogenic DI is due to the kidney's inability to respond to endogenous ADH. Circulating levels of ADH are normal, but the kidney has varying degrees of resistance to the water reabsorption effects of ADH. Nephrogenic DI may be hereditary, associated with medications (Figure 3-5) or hypercalcemia, or transiently observed in the latter stages of pregnancy.
  - Urinary water loss exceeds sodium loss resulting in dilute urine (urine will not be maximally concentrated).
- Insensible fluid losses may occur that cannot be quantified. Examples include fluid losses through sweating and breathing and via the skin secondary to fever or thermal injury.
- Reset osmostat occurs when the body has a higher threshold for ADH secretion in response to hyperosmolarity. Thus, the body excretes fluids renally despite the presence of hypernatremia.

- Euvolemic hypernatremia may be treated by replacing water deficit and removing and/or treating the underlying cause.
  - A desmopressin challenge may be used to determine if DI is central or nephrogenic (Table 3-6).
    - A desmopressin test dose (0.1 mg orally or 1 mcg subcutaneously or intravenously or 10 mcg intranasally) may

Table 3-6. Urine Osmolality and Response to ADH in Hypernatremia.

Urine osmolality	Response to ADH?	Diagnosis
Low (< 300 mOsm/kg)	Yes	Central DI
	No	Nephrogenic DI
Normal (300–850 mOsm/kg)	Yes	Central DI (usually with volume depletion)
	No	Nephrogenic DI
	No	Osmotic diuresis
High (> 850 mOsm/kg)	No	Water loss/dehydration
	No	Impaired thirst and/or no access to water
	No	Intake of excess exogenous sodium

ADH, antidiuretic hormone; DI, diabetes insipidus.

be administered. If the patient's serum sodium responds to desmopressin (drastic decrease in urine output), the DI is likely central. If no response occurs, the DI is likely nephrogenic.

    - Desmopressin may be used to treat central DI with initial starting doses indicated below for various routes of administration. All are titrated based on the patient's response.
        - Desmopressin 0.05 mg orally twice a day.
        - Desmopressin 10 mcg intranasally in the evening.
        - Desmopressin 1–2 mcg subcutaneously or intravenously every 12 hours.
        - For nephrogenic DI, correct the underlying cause. Consider treatment using a dietary sodium restriction and a thiazide diuretic (eg, hydrochlorothiazide) to produce a mild ECF deficit. This approach should produce increased proximal tubule water reabsorption, decreased volume of filtrate presented to the distal nephron, and decreased urine output.

- *Hypervolemic hypernatremia* reflects an increase in total body sodium and total body water may be normal or increased.
    - Common causes are iatrogenic (due to overadministration of sodium-containing IV fluids) and mineralocorticoid excess (Cushing's syndrome, adrenal hyperplasia).
    - Treat by correcting underlying disorder, administering loop diuretics (eg, furosemide), and replacing water deficit.

Monitoring

1. The degree of monitoring should reflect the severity of hypernatremia and ensure an appropriate rate of sodium correction without posing a risk to the patient.

2. Asymptomatic patients treated conservatively may require daily or twice daily sodium level assessments to ensure the serum sodium is not being overcorrected too quickly, putting them at risk for cerebral edema.

3. Symptomatic patients who are being aggressively treated with hypotonic fluids should have serum sodium levels monitored at least every 4 hours to ensure safe sodium correction rates. Hypotonic fluids should be

discontinued if sodium levels reflect a correction rate that exceeds the recommended rate (8–10 mEq/L in 24 hours or 18 mEq/L in 48 hours).

4. Patients at risk for hypernatremia should have regular follow-up (eg, every 3–6 months) with their clinician to monitor sodium levels, especially in the presence of medications or comorbidities that may precipitate hypernatremia.

Patient/Family Counseling

1. The patient and caregivers should be educated and aware of the daily fluid intake necessary to maintain hydration. Any fluid restrictions should be clearly explained to the patient and/or caregiver.

2. Strict intake and output monitoring may be necessary in patients with high-output drains or ostomies. Patients may need to record and replace fluid losses daily to maintain adequate hydration.

3. All medications should be screened for their ability to potentially cause or exacerbate sodium disorders. Medications should be carefully reviewed by the clinician for medical necessity. The risks and benefits of continuing or discontinuing such medications should be discussed with the patient and/or caregiver.

4. Any excessive fluid losses, abnormal behavior, or signs or symptoms of sodium disorders should be reported to the patient's clinician immediately.

5. Diet intake should be adjusted to include or exclude products high in sodium based on the patient's underlying sodium disorder. The patient and caregivers should be instructed on how to properly read a nutrition label and interpret the sodium content. Always verify the patient's daily sodium allowance with the managing clinician.

Foods High in Sodium

1. Canned meats, vegetables, soups

2. Potato chips

3. Vegetable juice

4. Lunch meats

5. Cheese

6. Frozen meals

7. Processed foods have a higher likelihood of high sodium content.

Medications That May Contribute to Sodium Disorders

Many medications can predispose patients to sodium disorders. The patient's medication profile should be carefully screened and the patient counseled on those medications associated with sodium disorders. Some medications may need to be discontinued, while others may only need to have the dosage adjusted to manage the sodium disorders. Other medications may not require any intervention or may not be able to be discontinued due to necessity. In this instance, discussions with involved healthcare providers, the patient, and caregivers to weigh the risks and benefits of continuing the medication need to occur. See Figures 3-3 and 3-5 and Table 3-3 for medications commonly associated with sodium disorders.

Clinical Application

Patient Scenario 1

A 47-year-old man (70 kg) with small cell lung carcinoma presents to the emergency department (ED) with a 2-day history of confusion and lethargy. His vital signs are normal (heart rate 72 beats per minute, blood pressure 128/85 mm Hg, respiratory rate 16 breaths per minute, afebrile) on presentation, and he denies any fevers or chills. The patient's family denies any medications other than acetaminophen in the past 48 hours and reports that his diet and fluid intake have not changed recently. Review of systems and physical examination are negative except for the patient's altered mental status. Past medical history is significant only for small cell lung carcinoma. His laboratory results are as follows:

- Serum sodium, 112 mEq/L
- Serum creatinine, 0.8 mg/dL
- BUN, 15 mg/dL
- Glucose, 145 mg/dL
- Serum osmolality, 242 mOsm/kg

- Urine sodium (spot-check), 120 mEq/L
- Urine osmolality, 720 mOsm/kg

1. Assess the serum osmolality—*Hypotonic hyponatremia*
   - Measured serum osmolality, 242 mOsm/kg
     - Calculated serum osmolality, 237 mOsm/kg
2. Assess the patient's volume status—*Euvolemic hypotonic hyponatremia*
   - Vital signs are normal and do not represent a patient who is hypovolemic. The patient is not tachycardic or hypotensive, skin turgor on physical examination is normal, and there is no history of nausea, vomiting or other fluid loss.
   - Physical examination does not reveal signs of hypervolemia (edema, ascites, hypertension).
3. Differential diagnosis includes psychogenic polydipsia, SIAD, hypothyroidism, or reset osmostat.
   - The patient had no changes in fluid intake (which rules out psychogenic polydipsia) and has no history of hypothyroidism or hypopituitarism.
   - Urine is concentrated (urine osmolality, 720 mOsm/kg) with a urine sodium of 120 mEq/L, which indicates the kidneys are inappropriately concentrating urine in the setting of hypotonic hyponatremia.
   - The most likely cause is SIAD secondary to small cell lung cancer.
4. Treatment options include the following:
   - Correction of serum sodium to alleviate symptoms of hyponatremia. Cautious correction is warranted because the symptoms are not severe and the time of onset of hyponatremia is unknown (likely chronic, given the presumed etiology of SIAD).
   - Fluid restriction, predominantly by way of a free water restriction of less than 1–1.5 L/d, should be the primary treatment modality in this patient, with follow-up serum sodium measurement every 6 to 12 hours in conjunction with symptom monitoring. Sodium chloride tablets can be considered (eg, 2 g, 3 times a day); however, since this patient is confused, oral administration may not be feasible or safe. All hypotonic IV fluids should be discontinued, and medications given via IV piggyback should be mixed in 0.9% NaCl, if compatible.

- Target serum sodium elevation should be no more than 6–8 mEq/L in 24 hours and 12–14 mEq/L in 48 hours to minimize the risk of ODS.
- If symptoms worsen or the serum sodium continues to decline despite the above interventions, use of 3% NaCl would be warranted.
  - A one-time 150-mL bolus over 20 minutes can be administered, with follow-up serum sodium levels 20 minutes post infusion (and potential repeat dosing depending on symptom severity and serum sodium response).
  - Alternatively, a maintenance 3% NaCl infusion rate could be calculated using the formula provided in Table 3-2.
    - Each liter of 3% NaCl is expected to increase this patient's serum sodium by approximately 10 mEq/L, which is the maximum 24-hour elevation in the setting of presumed chronic hyponatremia. Therefore, the initial 3% NaCl infusion rate would be 40 mL/h and subsequently adjusted based on serial sodium monitoring every 4 hours (a higher initial infusion rate could be used to target a more rapid sodium rise of 5 mEq/L within 6 hours, depending on symptom severity at the time of prescribing).
- Ultimately, the underlying etiology of his hyponatremia needs to be addressed, which would entail treatment of his lung cancer.

Patient Scenario 2

A 78-year-old woman (60 kg) with a history of uncontrolled hypertension presents to her local physician with a 5-day history of severe nausea and vomiting, fever of 39.1 °C (102.4 °F) and worsening fatigue. Her vital signs reveal a blood pressure of 112/72 mm Hg, heart rate of 106 beats per minute, and a respiratory rate of 18 breaths per minute. She reports not being able to keep any food or liquids down. Her physical examination is notable for decreased skin turgor and dry mucous membranes. Laboratory tests reveal a serum sodium level of 165 mEq/L, BUN of 26 mg/dL, and serum creatinine of 0.86 mg/dL. Urine sodium is < 5 mEq/L. All other laboratory values are within normal limits. She currently takes no medications at home.

1. Assess the volume status.

   - Vital signs reflect hypovolemia as evidenced by decreased blood pressure (she is baseline hypertensive), increased heart rate, decreased skin turgor, and dry mucous membranes.

2. Assess urine sodium.

- Urine sodium levels in this patient are consistent with sodium conservation and hypovolemia.

3. Differential diagnosis includes extrarenal losses.

- These losses are likely due to history of vomiting and high fevers.

4. Treatment options include the following:

- Correction of water deficit slowly over a period of at least several days because the hypernatremia is likely chronic based on the onset of vomiting.
    - Calculate the water deficit. The patient has a free water deficit of 5.3 L.
    - Administer hypotonic fluids intravenously to correct half of the water deficit (2.65 L) in the first 24 hours.
        - 0.45% NaCl: 1 L only contributes 500 mL towards the water deficit so approximately 5.3 L will be needed in the first 24 hours.
        - Dextrose 5% in water: 1 L contributes 1000 mL towards the water deficit so approximately 2.65 L will be needed in the first 24 hours.
    - Administer the remainder of the water deficit using hypotonic fluids intravenously over the next 48 hours.
    - Rate of correction should not exceed 8–10 mEq/L in 24 hours or 18 mEq/L in 48 hours to prevent the development of cerebral edema and convulsions.

Potassium

Overview

Potassium disorders are one of the more common electrolyte disorders in hospitalized patients. Abnormalities of potassium are oftentimes mild and asymptomatic; however, understanding the etiology, treatment, and management is clinically important. Lack of early recognition of the disorders and the treatments themselves are both associated with significant morbidity and mortality if not managed appropriately. Potassium disorders are encountered frequently and are applicable to any practice setting.

1. Homeostasis and physiological function[20,21]

   - Normal potassium range is 3.5–5 mEq/L (1 mEq/L = 1 mmol/L).
   - Potassium is the second most abundant cation in the body and is the major intracellular cation.
   - Potassium concentrations are regulated by the sodium-potassium-adenosine triphosphatase pump, which maintains higher levels of potassium in the intracellular space compared to the extracellular space.
   - Potassium is essential for cellular metabolism, glycogen and protein synthesis, and regulation of electrical activity across cell membranes, especially in the myocardium.

2. Dietary intake[21,22]

   - One gram of potassium is equal to 25 mEq of potassium.
   - Adequate potassium intake for adults is 40–50 mEq (1600–2000 mg) per day depending on age and comorbidities.
   - The typical Western diet contains 25–62.5 mEq (1000–2500 mg) of potassium per day, and approximately 90% is absorbed in the upper GI tract.

3. Excretion[21]

   - The kidneys are the predominate organ for potassium regulation, and disorders can occur secondary to excessive losses of potassium through the kidneys or retention of potassium due to loss of the excretory function of the kidneys.
   - Extrarenal potassium losses via GI fluids and sweat account for 15% of excreted potassium.
   - Distal regulation of potassium secretion is determined by the amount of sodium in the distal and collecting tubules of the kidney, flow of urine, and aldosterone activity.

Hypokalemia

Prevalence and Mortality[20,21,23,24]

1. An estimated 15%–20% of hospitalized patients will have hypokalemia (serum potassium < 3.5 mEq/L), and 3%–6% will have a serum potassium < 3 mEq/L.

2. Mortality is dependent on the acuity and severity of hypokalemia.

   - Mortality during the first week of hospitalization has been shown to increase by 11% with each 0.1 mEq/L decline in serum potassium below 3.4 mEq/L.

   - Mortality significantly increases when serum potassium levels fall below 2.9 mEq/L.

Risk Factors[24-26]

1. Increasing age (> 65 years old) and higher comorbidity scores are associated with an increased risk of hypokalemia during a hospital admission.

2. Females are more likely to experience hypokalemia and have an increased risk of mortality compared with males.

3. Patients who have a history of alcohol abuse are more likely to experience hypokalemia.

4. Diuretics frequently cause hypokalemia by increasing the renal excretion of potassium.

5. A high-sodium diet can result in excessive urinary potassium loss.

Etiology[20-22,27]

1. Medications are the most common cause of hypokalemia (Figure 3-6).

2. Hypokalemia can result from an acute shift of potassium from the extracellular compartment to the intracellular compartment.

3. Abnormal loss of potassium can result secondary to loss through the kidneys induced by metabolic alkalosis or loss in stool induced by diarrhea (Figure 3-7).

Figure 3-6. Medications Commonly Associated with Potassium Disorders.[28-30]

Hypokalemia	Hyperkalemia

Transcellular (intracellular) shift
• β_2-adrenergic agonists
  ◦ Epinephrine
  ◦ Decongestants (pseudoephedrine, phenylpropanolamine)
  ◦ Bronchodilators (albuterol, terbutaline, ephedrine, isoproterenol)
• Theophylline
• Caffeine
• Verapamil intoxication
• Insulin overdose
	Transcellular (extracellular) shift
	• Nonselective β-blockers
	  ◦ Carvedilol, labetalol, nadolol, propranolol, sotalol, timolol
	• Succinylcholine
	• Digoxin
	• Mannitol
	• Intravenous amino acids:
	  ◦ Arginine, lysine, epsilon-aminocaproic acid
	• Herbal medications
	  ◦ Toad skin, chan su, oleander, foxglove, yew berry, lily of the valley, dogbane, Siberian ginseng, red squill

Increased renal excretion
• Diuretics
  ◦ Acetazolamide, hydrochlorothiazide, chlorothiazide, chlorthalidone, metolazone, bumetanide, ethacrynic acid, furosemide, torsemide
• Mineralocorticoids or effects of mineralocorticoids
  ◦ Fludrocortisone, hydrocortisone, licorice
• High-dose glucocorticoids
  ◦ Prednisone, methylprednisolone, dexamethasone, prednisolone, hydrocortisone
• High-dose antibiotics
  ◦ Penicillin, nafcillin, ampicillin
• Magnesium depleting drugs
  ◦ Aminoglycosides, cisplatin, oxaliplatin, carboplatin, foscarnet, amphotericin B, cetuximab
	Decreased renal excretion
	Alterations of renin-angiotensin-aldosterone system
	• ACE inhibitor
	  ◦ Benazepril, captopril, enalapril, fosinopril, lisinopril, quinapril, ramipril
	• Angiotensin receptor blocker
	  ◦ Azilsartan, candesartan, eposartan, irbesartan, losartan, olmesartan, telmisartan, valsartan
	• Aldosterone antagonist
	  ◦ Spironolactone, eplerenone
	• Nonsteroidal anti-inflammatory agents
	  ◦ Ibuprofen, naproxen, ketorolac
	• Calcineurin inhibitors
	  ◦ Tacrolimus, cyclosporine
	• Heparin
	• Lithium
	Blockade of sodium channels impairing renal tubular secretion
	• Triamterene
	• Amiloride
	• Trimethoprim
	• Pentamidine

Increased loss in stool • Sodium polystyrene sulfonate • Patiromer • Sodium zirconium cyclosilicate	Increased load • Potassium chloride or other potassium salts • Potassium penicillin G • Herbal medications ◦ Noni juice, alfalfa, dandelion, horsetail, nettle, milkweed, hawthorn berries

CHAPTER 3

Electrolyte Disorders

Figure 3-7. Nonmedication Causes of Hypokalemia.[23]

Loss in Stool	Loss in Urine
Infectious diarrhea • *Cholera*, *Salmonella*, *Strongyloides*, *Yersinia*, diarrhea associated with AIDS Tumors • Vipoma, villous adenoma of the colon, Zollinger-Ellison syndrome Jejunoileal bypass Enteric fistula Malabsorption Intestinal ion-transport defects • Congenital chloride diarrhea Cancer therapy • Chemotherapy, radiation enteropathy Geophagia	*Mineralocorticoid excess* Primary hyperaldosteronism • Adrenal adenoma, adrenal carcinoma, bilateral adrenal hyperplasia Congenital adrenal hyperplasia[a] • 11β-Hydroxylase deficiency, 17α-hydroxylase deficiency Renin-secreting tumors Ectopic corticotropin syndrome Cushing's syndrome • Adrenal, pituitary Glucocorticoid-responsive aldosteronism[a] Renovascular hypertension Malignant hypertension Vasculitis *Apparent mineralocorticoid excess* Liddle's syndrome[a] 11β-Hydroxysteroid dehydrogenase deficiency[a] *Impaired chloride-associated sodium transport* Bartter's syndrome[a] Gitelman's syndrome[a]

AIDS, acquired immunodeficiency syndrome.

[a]The disease is hereditary.

4. Patients experiencing refeeding syndrome can have depletion of serum phosphorus, potassium, and magnesium due to initiation of feeding after a period of starvation.

5. Inadequate dietary intake (< 1 g/d) is rarely the cause of hypokalemia unless the renal excretion of potassium fails to decrease promptly.

Clinical Presentation[12,26,28,31]

1. Patients with hypokalemia are commonly asymptomatic especially in mild disorders. In more severe cases, patients present with nonspecific symptoms such as nausea, vomiting, generalized weakness, lassitude, and constipation (Table 3-7).

2. Acute drops in potassium (< 48 hours) are more commonly associated with symptoms compared with chronic (≥ 48 hours) potassium changes.

3. Patients with underlying hypertension, heart failure, and cardiac arrhythmias are more likely to develop ventricular arrhythmias with mild to moderate hypokalemia.

Diagnosis/Diagnostic Tests[12,32-34]

1. Monitor serum potassium level frequently as hypokalemia is rarely suspected on the basis of clinical presentation.

2. Assess the patient's past medical and surgical history, as well as the medication and dietary supplement history; laboratory parameters (eg, serum magnesium level) should be evaluated for causes of hypokalemia.

Table 3-7. Clinical Manifestations of Hypokalemia.[12,28]

Severity of Hypokalemia	Serum Potassium Level, mEq/L	Symptoms
Mild	3-3.5	Commonly asymptomatic[a]
Moderate	2.5-2.9	Nausea Vomiting Lassitude Constipation Generalized weakness Cardiac arrhythmias
Severe	< 2.5	Rhabdomyolysis Paralysis leading to respiratory compromise Cardiac arrhythmias Death

[a]Symptoms depend on the patient's baseline serum potassium level and the rate of decline.

3. Conduct initial laboratory tests, including a basic metabolic profile, serum magnesium, serum calcium, BUN, serum creatinine, serum phosphorus, complete blood count, and serum glucose.
   - Concomitant hypomagnesemia often occurs with alcoholism, and it is a common feature in patients treated with diuretics and those with malabsorption disorders, as well as patients receiving cisplatin or gentamicin therapy.
   - Magnesium plays a vital role in the regulation of intracellular potassium and reduces renal potassium excretion.
   - Magnesium repletion is essential to ensure correction of potassium is not delayed.
4. Assess functional manifestations of hypokalemia.
   - A muscle strength evaluation should be completed to determine if a patient is experiencing muscle weakness associated with severe hypokalemia.
   - An electrocardiogram (ECG) should be obtained to assess cardiac abnormalities associated with hypokalemia such as a prolonged QT-interval or the presence of an arrhythmia.
5. Estimate the total body potassium deficit.
   - For every 0.3 mEq/L decrease in serum potassium concentration from normal, the total body potassium deficit is approximately 100 mEq (total body potassium content is approximately 50 mEq/kg body weight).
6. Obtain a urine potassium concentration.
   - A 24-hour urine potassium collection is the most accurate method to measure urinary potassium excretion (normal range, 22–160 mEq per 24 hours); however, it is not commonly used in routine practice.
   - In critically ill patients with severe hypokalemia, a one-time or spot-check urine potassium concentration may be beneficial, but it is also less accurate unless combined with a transtubular potassium concentration gradient (TTKG) or urine potassium-to creatinine ratio.
     - TTKG is a semiquantitative index because it adjusts for the gradient of potassium secretion and water reabsorption in the renal medullary collecting ducts.

$$\text{TTKG (\%)} = \frac{\text{Urine potassium (mEq/L)/serum potassium (mEq/L)}}{\text{Urine osmolality (mOsm/kg)/serum osmolality (mOsm/kg)}}$$

- TTKG is inaccurate if the urine osmolality is lower than the serum osmolality because it will underestimate potassium secretion.
- The urine sodium must be > 25 mEq/L to avoid underestimation of the potassium secretion.
- A value > 3 indicates a high renal potassium excretion rate.

- Urine potassium: creatinine ratio is an alternative method to determine potassium excretion and corrects for variations in urine volume.

$$\text{Urine potassium: creatinine ratio} = \frac{\text{Urine potassium (mEq/L)}}{\text{Urine creatinine (g)}}$$

  - The ratio is independent of the urine osmolality.
  - A value > 17.3 mEq/g indicates a high renal potassium excretion rate.
  - A value < 13 mEq/g suggests poor dietary potassium intake, GI losses, or an intracellular shift of potassium.
  - This method is inaccurate with reduced muscle mass because creatinine is lower in these patients and leads to falsely elevated ratios.

7. Assess acid-base balance if the source of hypokalemia is unknown.

- Low rate of urinary potassium excretion
  - Metabolic acidosis, asymptomatic patient
    - Common causes are GI losses secondary to laxative use or a villous adenoma.
- High rate of urinary potassium excretion (see TTKG and urine potassium: creatinine ratio above)
  - Metabolic acidosis
    - Common causes are diabetic ketoacidosis or type 1 (distal) or type 2 (proximal) renal tubular acidosis.
  - Metabolic alkalosis
    - Common causes are excessive vomiting (low urine chloride concentrations are commonly seen) or diuretic use.

8. Assess blood pressure if the source of hypokalemia is still unknown.
   - High rate of urinary potassium excretion and metabolic alkalosis
     - Normotensive
       - Measurement of the urine chloride concentration should be assessed to help determine cause.
         - Elevated urine chloride concentration is indicative of Gitelman's or Bartter's syndrome and diuretic use.
     - Hypertensive
       - Common causes are renovascular disease, primary mineralocorticoid excess, or diseases that mimic primary mineralocorticoid excess.
9. Determine if hypokalemia is acute (< 48 hours) or chronic (≥ 48 hours), if possible. If the duration or onset of hypokalemia is unknown, assume it is a chronic condition.

Goals of Therapy[12,31]

1. The goals of therapy are to return the serum potassium concentration to normal (≥ 3.5 mEq/L) and to prevent life-threatening conditions (paralysis, rhabdomyolysis, and cardiac arrhythmias).
2. Treatment of hypokalemia should center on determining the underlying cause or reducing/discontinuing the offending agent.

Management[12,20,21,31-33]

1. Hypokalemia is treated by the administration of either an oral or IV potassium supplement depending on the clinical scenario (Table 3-8 and Table 3-9).
2. In a patient with concomitant hypomagnesemia, magnesium should be replaced either orally or intravenously.
3. Oral potassium repletion is safer and preferred; however, if the patient is experiencing severe hypokalemia (symptomatic) or does not have a functioning GI tract, the IV route will need to be used.
   - Oral potassium formulations (capsule, tablet, or liquid) are available as chloride, bicarbonate, citrate, gluconate, and phosphate salts.
     - Regardless of the mode of administration, all formulations cause abdominal discomfort, nausea, and diarrhea.

Table 3-8. Commonly Used Oral Potassium Replacement Products.

Dosage Form	Brand Names	Strength	Clinical Considerations
		Enteral or oral administration	
Potassium bicarbonate			
Effervescent tablet for solution	Klor-Con/EF, K-Lyte	25 mEq	Dissolve in 90 mL of water; orange flavor
Potassium chloride			
Effervescent tablet for solution	K-Lor, Klor-Con	20 mEq/packet	Dissolve in 120 mL of water; fruit flavor
Powder for solution	Klor-Con/25	25 mEq/packet	Dilute in 120 mL of cold water or juice for administration; contains sorbitol, which may cause diarrhea
Solution		20 mEq/15 mL 40 mEq/15 mL	
Potassium phosphate			
Tablet for solution	K-Phos	500 mg (3.7 mEq potassium)	Dissolve in 90 mL of water
Powder for solution	Phos-NaK	250 mg (7.1 mEq potassium, 8 mmol phosphorus) per packet	Dilute in 75 mL of water; fruit flavor
Tablet	K-Phos No. 2	2.3 mEq potassium, 8 mmol phosphorus per tablet	
		Oral administration only	
Potassium chloride			
Capsule, extended-release, microencapsulated	Micro K	8 mEq/600 mg 10 mEq/750 mg	Swallow whole; capsules may be opened and contents sprinkled on applesauce and swallowed immediately without chewing
Tablet, extended-release	Micro K	8 mEq/600 mg 10 mEq/750 mg 20 mEq/1500 mg	Swallow whole; do not crush or chew; larger tablet size with higher doses; difficult to swallow; potential noncompliance issues
Tablet, extended-release, microencapsulated	Klor-Con M10 Klor-Con M15 Klor-Con M20	10 mEq/750 mg 15 mEq/1125 mg 20 mEq/1500 mg	Tablet may be broken in half; whole tablet may be dissolved in 120 mL water or ½ tablet in 60 mL of water
Tablet, extended-release, wax matrix	Klor-Con	8 mEq/600 mg 10 mEq/750 mg	Do not crush or chew; swallow whole

Table 3-9. Treatment of Hypokalemia.[12,31,a]		
Severity of Hypokalemia	**Oral Replacement Dosage[b]**	**IV Replacement Dosage[c]**
Mild (3–3.5 mEq/L)	20–80 mEq/d divided into 2 or 4 doses	IV treatment not recommended unless GI tract nonfunctional
Moderate (2.5–2.9 mEq/L)	40–120 mEq/d divided into 3 or 4 doses	20–40 mEq
Severe (< 2.5 mEq/L)	IV treatment recommended initially	40–80 mEq

GI, gastrointestinal; IV, intravenous.

[a]Dosing applies to patients with normal renal function or receiving continuous renal replacement therapy; patients with renal insufficiency should receive ≤ 50% of the initial empiric dose.

[b]Monitor for gastrointestinal tolerance; may require IV replacement if oral potassium not tolerated.

[c]Maximum infusion rate = 20 mEq/h.

- Tablets are often difficult to swallow, and the solution (even with a 1:5 dilution with water and enteral nutrition) has a reported osmolality > 4000 mOsm/kg, which contributes to diarrhea and abdominal discomfort

4. IV repletion corrects hypokalemia more rapidly, but adverse effects may include thrombophlebitis, arrhythmias, and hyperkalemia.
   - IV potassium formulations are available as chloride, acetate, or phosphate salts.
     - The most commonly used formulation is potassium chloride.
     - Potassium acetate should be used when correction of acidemia is desired and liver function is adequate to convert acetate to bicarbonate.
     - Potassium phosphate should be used when correcting coexisting hypokalemia and hypophosphatemia.
   - IV potassium infusions can be infused at a rate of 10 mEq/h to minimize adverse effects such as thrombophlebitis in a peripheral vein. If the patient has central venous access, IV potassium infusions may be infused at a maximum rate of 20 mEq/h; in these cases, continuous cardiac monitoring is required.

5. Management of hypokalemia is usually determined by the severity of symptoms, serum potassium deficit, acid-base status, and GI and kidney

function. The degree of potassium supplementation is divided into 3 categories: mild, moderate, and severe hypokalemia (Table 3-9).

- Mild (serum potassium 3–3.5 mEq/L) can usually be treated with a dietary or oral supplement but may require IV replacement if the patient has a nonfunctioning GI tract. The decision to use IV replacement depends on whether the patient can tolerate oral formulations, along with their adverse effects, and is compliant with medication.

- Moderate (serum potassium 2.5-2.9 mEq/L) can usually be treated with an oral supplement but may require IV replacement if the patient has a nonfunctioning GI tract. The decision to use IV replacement depends on whether the patient is symptomatic (ie, ECG changes), the severity of illness, and the cause of hypokalemia.

- Severe (serum potassium < 2.5 mEq/L) treatment with IV potassium is generally necessary especially if the patient is experiencing ECG changes.

- Potassium dosing is largely empiric because serum concentrations usually do not correlate with total body potassium stores. See Table 3-9.

Diagnostic Approach to Hypokalemia[12,34-36]

1. Assess serum potassium concentration.

   - In most cases, loss of potassium is apparent and secondary to vomiting, diarrhea, or diuretic therapy. For hospitalized patients, it can also be related to a reduction in dietary potassium intake either orally, enterally, or intravenously.

   - If no cause is apparent, assess urinary potassium excretion.

     - Measurement of potassium excretion in a 24-hour urine collection is ideal, but not practical.

     - In critically ill or patients with severe hypokalemia, random measurement of the urine potassium concentration (also include urine osmolality and serum osmolality for TTKG) or urine potassium:creatinine ratio in a spot urine sample can be used.

     - Common causes of urinary potassium excretion include diuretic therapy and primary aldosteronism or mineralocorticoid excess.

2. Assess the patient's serum magnesium concentration.

    - Hypomagnesemia is frequently observed in refractory hypokalemia.
    - Magnesium plays an important role in the regulation of intracellular potassium.
    - Treatment of hypomagnesemia should be in conjunction with potassium to avoid further delays in the management of refractory hypokalemia because magnesium reduces renal potassium excretion.
    - Common causes are diuretic use, alcoholism, malabsorption syndrome, and cisplatin and aminoglycoside (ie, gentamicin, tobramycin, amikacin) therapy.

3. Estimate the total body potassium deficit.

    - For every 0.3 mEq/L decrease in serum potassium concentration, the total body potassium deficit is approximately 100 mEq.

4. Assess the patient's acid-base status.

    - Asymptomatic patient with metabolic acidosis and a low rate of urinary potassium excretion.
        - Common causes are GI potassium loss or laxative use.
    - Metabolic acidosis with renal potassium wasting.
        - Common causes are diabetic ketoacidosis and type 1 (distal) or type 2 (proximal) renal tubular acidosis.

5. Assess the patient's blood pressure.

    - Normotensive patient with metabolic alkalosis and renal potassium wasting.
        - Common causes are diuretic use, vomiting, or Gitelman's or Bartter's syndrome.
    - Hypertensive patient with metabolic alkalosis and renal potassium wasting.
        - Common causes are mineralocorticoid excess or disease states that mimic mineralocorticoid excess, and renovascular disease.

6. Treatment should address the underlying cause and reduce/remove causative medication(s).

7. Potassium should be replaced either orally or intravenously based on the serum potassium level and severity of symptoms.

8. If the causative agent cannot be discontinued, daily oral potassium maintenance therapy should be prescribed (eg, potassium chloride 20 mEq orally daily).

Monitoring[12,20,21,31]

1. The degree of monitoring should reflect the severity of hypokalemia and ensure appropriate rate of potassium correction without posing a risk to the patient.

2. Asymptomatic patients treated conservatively may require assessment of potassium levels every 24–72 hours to ensure that the serum potassium is not being overcorrected too quickly.

3. Patients with mildly to moderately symptomatic hypokalemia should have a routine serum potassium level obtained every 24–48 hours; in addition, the serum potassium level should be measured within 2–8 hours after completion of therapy.

4. Patients with symptomatic severe hypokalemia who are being aggressively treated with IV potassium preparations should have serum potassium levels monitored at least every 12 hours and 1–2 hours after completion of IV therapy.

5. Patients at risk for hypokalemia should have regular follow-up (eg, every 3–6 months) with their primary care physician to monitor serum potassium levels, especially in the presence of medications or comorbidities that may precipitate hypokalemia.

Hyperkalemia

Prevalence and Mortality[30,37]

1. An estimated 1%–10% of all hospitalized patients will have hyperkalemia (serum potassium > 5 mEq/L), with 1% of these patients experiencing severe hyperkalemia (serum potassium ≥ 6 mEq/L).

2. Mortality ranges from 14% to 41% in hospitalized patients with hyperkalemia.

3. The prevalence of hyperkalemia in patients with end-stage renal disease (ESRD) is 5%–10% and contributes to 2%–5% of deaths in this patient population.

4. The prevalence of hyperkalemia (serum potassium ≥ 5.8 mEq/L) in the general medicine outpatient setting is approximately 1%.

Risk Factors[30,38,39]

1. Patients with underlying CKD or ESRD are more likely to experience hyperkalemia.

2. RAAS inhibitor therapies frequently cause hyperkalemia, especially in patients with heart failure and CKD.

3. Diabetes mellitus and cardiovascular disease are the most common comorbidities in patients with CKD.

Etiology[20,21,23]

1. Potassium supplementation, AKI, and CKD are the most common causes of hyperkalemia, but numerous other etiologies need to be considered in addition to these (Figure 3-8).

2. Hyperkalemia can also result secondary to medications (Figure 3-6).

3. Patients can have pseudohyperkalemia secondary to traumatic blood draws and hemolysis of blood samples causing release of potassium.

4. Patients with poorly controlled diabetes can experience hyperkalemia secondary to hyperosmolarity and hyperglycemia causing potassium to shift out of the cells.

5. Increased dietary intake is rarely the cause of hyperkalemia unless patients have CKD.

Clinical Presentation[12,21,23,40]

1. Clinical manifestations of hyperkalemia are cardiac and neurological in nature.

2. The majority of patients are asymptomatic until serum potassium concentrations exceed 5.5 mEq/L.

Figure 3-8. Nonmedication Causes of Hyperkalemia.[20,29]

Increased Potassium Load	Decreased Renal Potassium Excretion	Transcellular Shift
Exogenous • High potassium containing food, salt substitutes, stored blood, protein calorie supplements, and geophagia Endogenous • Hemolysis, exercise, gastrointestinal bleeding, catabolic states, rhabdomyolysis, and tumor lysis syndrome	Chronic kidney disease Acute kidney injury Impairment of distal renal tubular secretion Primary renal tubular secretory defect • Systemic lupus erythematosus, sickle cell disease, obstructive uropathy, post kidney transplantation, amyloidosis, tubulointerstitial nephritis, papillary necrosis Primary hypoaldosteronism Congenital adrenal hyperplasia Primary hyporeninism Hyporeninemic hypoaldosteronism Adrenal insufficiency Primary Infectious destruction of adrenal gland • *Mycobacterium avium intracellulare*, human immunodeficiency virus, cytomegalovirus, *Mycobacterium tuberculosis* Decrease in distal sodium delivery • Heart failure, cirrhosis, salt-wasting nephropathy	Hyperglycemia Acute hemolysis Vigorous exercise Fluoride poisoning Hyperkalemic periodic paralysis Acute metabolic acidosis

3. Signs and symptoms include muscle twitching, weakness, ECG changes (eg, tall-peaked T-waves, prolonged PR-interval, widened QRS complex, shortened QT-interval, A-V conduction blockade), and arrhythmias (eg, bradycardia, ventricular fibrillation, asystole).

4. No correlation exists between the degree of hyperkalemia and severity of symptoms; however, life-threatening arrhythmias are more likely in patients with a rapid rise of serum potassium.

Diagnosis/Diagnostic Tests[12,37,41]

1. Serum potassium should be closely monitored every 6–12 hours and an ECG obtained.

2. Assessment should include the patient's past medical and surgical history, and the medication and dietary supplement history should be evaluated for causes of hyperkalemia.

3. Initial laboratory tests should include a basic metabolic profile, serum magnesium, serum calcium, BUN, serum creatinine, serum phosphorus, complete blood count, and serum glucose.

   - Exclude pseudohyperkalemia to ensure that the potassium level is not artificially elevated secondary to a traumatic blood draw, leukocytosis, thrombocytosis, a hemolyzed blood sample, or potassium-containing infusions or parenteral nutrition (PN) being administered through the line from which the blood sample was obtained.

4. An evaluation should be done to determine if hyperkalemia is acute (< 48 hours) or chronic (≥ 48 hours), if possible. If the duration or onset of hyperkalemia is unknown, assume it is a chronic condition.

5. An assessment of 24-hour urine potassium excretion provides little utility in patients with stable chronic hyperkalemia; however, it may be beneficial in acute hyperkalemia.

   - Potassium excretion > 80–100 mEq/d is indicative of the use of a salt substitute.

6. In patients with persistent hyperkalemia that has an unknown etiology, the presence of hypoaldosteronism and other possible factors should be evaluated.

   - Obtain measurements of the plasma renin activity and plasma aldosterone level and evaluate the response of the TTKG to fludrocortisone.

Goals of Therapy[12]

1. The goals of therapy are to prevent and avoid the adverse cardiac effects of hyperkalemia, reverse any current symptoms, and return the serum potassium level to normal (3.5–5 mEq/L) while avoiding overcorrection.

2. The underlying cause should be determined and any exogenous sources of potassium should be discontinued.

Management[12,29,37]

1. Hyperkalemia is treated by administering medications that promote intracellular distribution of potassium or agents that enhance potassium excretion (Table 3-10).

Table 3-10. Agents Used for the Treatment of Hyperkalemia.[12]

Treatment	Dosing Regimen	Time to Onset	Duration of Effect	Mechanism of Action and Effects
Calcium gluconate[a,b]	1–2 g (4.65–9.3 mEq of calcium) IV over 5–10 min	1–2 min	10–30 min	Antagonizes cardiac conduction abnormalities
Sodium bicarbonate[a]	50–100 mEq IV over 2–5 min	30 min	2–6 h	Increases serum pH; redistributes potassium intracellularly
Regular insulin[a] (± dextrose)	5–10 units IV (± 50 mL of 50% dextrose infusion)	15–45 min	2–6 h	Redistributes potassium intracellularly
50% dextrose	50 mL (25 g) IV over 5 min	30 min	2–6 h	Increases insulin release, redistributes potassium intracellularly, prevents hypoglycemia when concurrent regular insulin administration
Furosemide	20–40 mg IV × 1	5–15 min	4–6 h	Increases renal potassium loss
Sodium polystyrene sulfonate[c]	15–60 g orally or rectally	1 h	4–6 h	Resin exchanges sodium for potassium; increases fecal potassium elimination
Albuterol	10–20 mg nebulized over 10 min	30 min	1–2 h	Stimulates sodium-potassium pump; redistributes potassium intracellularly
Hemodialysis	2–4 h	Immediate	Variable	Removes potassium from plasma

IV, intravenously

[a]First-line therapy regimen for a hyperkalemic emergency.

[b]Dose can be repeated in 5 minutes if electrocardiogram abnormalities persist. Calcium chloride can be given (1 g = 13.6 mEq of calcium) but can cause venous irritation if administered peripherally.

[c]Should not be used for hyperkalemic emergency because effects may not be seen for several hours. Removes 0.5–1 mEq of potassium per 1 g of sodium polystyrene sulfonate.

2. Patients should be treated emergently if they are experiencing ECG changes (peaked T-waves) and have an elevated serum potassium > 5.5 mEq/L.

   - Emergent treatment agents include IV calcium gluconate or calcium chloride, regular insulin with IV dextrose, and IV sodium bicarbonate, paired with continuous cardiac monitoring and admission to a telemetry-monitored bed.

3. Patients with severe hyperkalemia (serum potassium > 6.5 mEq/L) without ECG changes should still be treated aggressively with emergent agents.

   - Emergent treatment agents include IV calcium gluconate or calcium chloride, regular insulin with IV dextrose, and IV sodium bicarbonate, paired with continuous cardiac monitoring and hospital admission.

4. Treatment of hyperkalemia is divided into 3 categories: antagonism of the cardiac effects, rapid reduction in potassium concentration by redistribution intracellularly, and removal of potassium from the body.

   - Antagonism of the cardiac effects
     - IV calcium gluconate or calcium chloride
   - Redistribution of potassium intracellularly
     - Regular insulin with IV dextrose, IV sodium bicarbonate, and albuterol nebulization
   - Removal of potassium through the body
     - Furosemide, sodium polystyrene sulfonate oral or rectally, and hemodialysis

5. Any medications or underlying causes contributing to hyperkalemia should be discontinued or addressed.

Diagnostic Approach to Hyperkalemia[12,37,41]

1. Assess the need for emergency treatment.

   - Presence of ECG changes.
   - Severely elevated serum potassium level (> 6 mEq/L).
     - Assess the possible causes with careful evaluation of medications, dietary changes, dietary supplements, risk factors for AKI or CKD, acid-base status, urine output, blood pressure, and volume status.

- Exclude pseudohyperkalemia to ensure that the potassium level is not artificially elevated secondary to a traumatic blood draw, leukocytosis, thrombocytosis, a hemolyzed blood sample, or potassium-containing infusions or PN being administered through the line from which blood sample was obtained.

2. Determine if hyperkalemia is acute (< 48 hours) or chronic (≥ 48 hours), if possible. If the duration or onset of hyperkalemia is unknown, assume it is a chronic condition.

3. Note that measurement of 24-hour urine potassium excretion provides little utility in patients with stable chronic hyperkalemia; however, it may be beneficial in acute hyperkalemia.

4. In patients with persistent hyperkalemia that has an unknown etiology, evaluate the presence of hypoaldosteronism and other possible factors.

   - Obtain measurements of plasma renin activity and the plasma aldosterone level and evaluate the response of the TTKG to fludrocortisone.

5. Plan treatment to address the underlying cause and/or removal of causative medication(s).

6. Tailor the treatment regimen used for hyperkalemia based on the severity and acuity of the patient's hyperkalemia.

Monitoring[12,29]

1. The degree of monitoring (eg, every 1–6 hours) should reflect the severity of hyperkalemia and ensure the appropriate rate of potassium correction without posing a risk to the patient.

2. In symptomatic patients with hyperkalemia (> 5.5 mEq/L), the serum potassium level should be monitored every 1–6 hours during treatment, and the patient should be admitted to a telemetry unit.

3. After resolution of symptoms, the serum potassium level should be monitored every 4–12 hours until it is in the normal range (3.5–5 mEq/L).

4. In critically ill adult patients, potassium should be routinely monitored every 24–48 hours.

5. Patients at risk for hyperkalemia should have regular follow-up (eg, every 1–3 months) with their primary care physician to monitor serum potassium levels and renal function (eg, BUN, serum creatinine),

especially in the presence of medications or comorbidities that may precipitate hyperkalemia.

Patient/Family Counseling

1. Ensure that the patient and caregivers are educated and aware of the daily potassium allowance necessary to maintain nutrition based on the patient's comorbidities.

2. Screen all medications for their ability to potentially cause or exacerbate potassium disorders. These medications should be carefully reviewed by the primary physician for medical necessity, and the risk/benefit of continuing or discontinuing such medications should be discussed with the patient.

3. Report any excessive fluid losses, abnormal behavior, or signs or symptoms of potassium disorders to the patient's primary physician immediately.

4. Adjust dietary intake to include or exclude products high in potassium based on the patient's underlying potassium disorder. The patient and caregivers should be instructed how to properly read a nutrition label and interpret the potassium content. Always verify the patient's daily potassium allowance with the managing physician.

Foods High in Potassium[28]

1. Dried figs, dried fruits (eg, apricots, prunes, dates)

2. Molasses

3. Seaweed

4. Nuts

5. Bran cereals, wheat germ

6. Lima beans

7. Dark leafy greens, spinach, chard

8. Potatoes, parsnips, pumpkin, winter squash

9. Bananas, cantaloupe, kiwis, nectarines, oranges/orange juice

10. Avocados, artichokes, beets, tomatoes, carrots, cauliflower, broccoli

11. Vegetable juice, tomato/tomato juice

12. Ground beef, steak, pork, veal, lamb

Clinical Application

Patient Scenario 1

A 37-year-old woman with a history of hypertension and asthma presents to the ED with a 2-day history of increasing shortness of breath and wheezing. Patient states that she has had to use her rescue inhaler frequently over the last couple of days. The patient takes the following medications: atenolol 25 mg twice a day, hydrochlorothiazide 25 mg daily, and an albuterol inhaler as needed. She is 66 inches tall and weighs 65 kg.

In the ED, she is treated with nebulized albuterol every 15 minutes for 3 doses. The patient is admitted to a general medicine floor and is started on albuterol and ipratropium inhalation every 4 hours, levofloxacin 500 mg orally daily, and an oral prednisone taper. Her atenolol is stopped to ensure it is not contributing to her asthma exacerbation. On day 2 of hospitalization, the patient begins to experience weakness, fatigue, and severe muscle cramps. Vital signs, a physical examination, ECG, and laboratory values are obtained.

- Vital signs
    - Pulse, 56 beats/min
    - Respirations, 18 breaths/min
    - Blood pressure, 132/83 mm Hg
    - Temperature, 36.8 °C (98.2 °F)
- Physical examination
    - General: Alert, oriented
    - Eye: Pupils are equal, round, and reactive to light
    - Respiratory: Lungs are clear to auscultation
    - Cardiovascular: bradycardic, regular rhythm
    - Abdominal: Soft, nontender
    - Neurologic: Alert, oriented
- ECG
    - Bradycardia

- Laboratory results
  - Potassium, 2.9 mEq/L
  - Sodium, 132 mEq/L
  - CO_2, 24 mEq/L
  - Magnesium, 1.2 mEq/L
  - Glucose, 98 mg/dL
  - BUN, 18 mg/dL
  - Serum creatinine, 0.7 mg/dL

1. Assess the serum potassium level and determine if the patient is experiencing symptoms.
   - The patient's serum potassium level is considered moderately low (2.9 mEq/L), and she is experiencing weakness, muscle cramps, and fatigue, which are symptoms of hypokalemia.
2. Assess the patient's past medical and surgical history, medications, and laboratory parameters for causes of hypokalemia.
   - The patient has been receiving albuterol and hydrochlorothiazide, which are medications known to cause hypokalemia.
   - The patient's magnesium level is low and could also be contributing to the patient's hypokalemia.
3. Treatment options include the following:
   - Potassium supplementation
     - IV supplementation due to the presence of symptoms.
     - Potassium chloride 40 mEq IV piggyback administered centrally or peripherally at 10 mEq/h for 1 dose.
   - Magnesium supplementation
     - Patient should receive IV magnesium supplementation concurrently to ensure that the correction of hypokalemia is not delayed and to reduce renal potassium excretion.
     - Magnesium should be administered at 4 g IV piggyback once over 4 hours.

4. Monitoring

   - Serum potassium measurement should be obtained 1–2 hours after completion of the potassium IV therapy because she was symptomatic.

   - After resolution of symptoms and if the potassium serum level is within the normal range, potassium can be monitored every 12–24 hours during hospitalization.

5. The medication regimen should be tailored to decrease the risk of hypokalemia, and follow-up care should be arranged with the patient's primary care provider for routine monitoring.

Patient Scenario 2

A 52-year-old man presents to the ED with a chief complaint of weakness, nausea, and malaise for the past 2 days; however, the weakness became profoundly worse this morning upon waking. The patient was unable to stand up to get out of bed and had to have his wife help him to the bathroom. The patient's wife called 9-1-1, and the patient was brought to the hospital via ambulance. Patient had been otherwise healthy until 3 weeks ago when he suffered an acute myocardial infarction. During that admission, the patient was diagnosed with hypertension and hyperlipidemia. The following oral medications were prescribed: lisinopril 20 mg twice a day, metoprolol 50 mg twice a day, atorvastatin 40 mg at bedtime, aspirin 81 mg daily, and clopidogrel 75 mg daily.

By the time the patient arrived at the ED today, his weakness had progressed from the lower extremities to his upper extremities. He also was experiencing numbness and tingling bilaterally in his lower extremities and nausea. Patient denies any chest pain or shortness of breath.

- Vital signs

  - Pulse, 66 beats/min

  - Respirations, 21 breaths/min

  - Blood pressure, 152/83 mm Hg

  - Temperature, 36.3°C (97.4°F)

- Physical examination
    - General: Alert, oriented
    - Eye: Pupils are equal, round, and reactive to light
    - Respiratory: Lungs are clear to auscultation
    - Cardiovascular: Normal rate, regular rhythm
    - Abdominal: Mild diffuse tenderness
    - Neurologic: Alert, oriented
- ECG
    - Changes noted from prior ECG examination by the physician were peaked T-waves, PR interval increase (172 milliseconds), and QRS interval increase (120 milliseconds).
- Laboratory results
    - Potassium, 9.1 mEq/L
    - Sodium, 127 mEq/L
    - CO_2, 24 mEq/L
    - Glucose, 95 mg/dL
    - BUN, 31 mg/dL
    - Serum creatinine, 2.5 mg/dL

1. Assess the need for emergency treatment for hyperkalemia.
    - Patient's potassium level is considered severely elevated (> 6 mEq/L), and ECG changes are present (peaked T-waves, prolonged PR-interval, and increased QRS duration).
2. Exclude the possibility of pseudohyperkalemia.
    - Patient is experiencing signs and symptoms of hyperkalemia.
    - The venipuncture was not traumatic, and the blood sample was not reported as hemolyzed.

3. Assess any underlying causes or causative agents.

   - Patient was recently started on a RAAS inhibitor (lisinopril) and is experiencing AKI (serum creatinine 2.5 mg/dL).

4. Consider treatment options

   - Emergent cardiac stabilization

     - Administer calcium gluconate 1000 mg intravenously once, which may be repeated in 5 minutes if ECG changes persist.

   - Redistribution of potassium intracellularly

     - Administer dextrose 50% (25 g) intravenously with regular insulin 10 units intravenously once.

   - Removal of potassium through the body

     - Administer sodium polystyrene sulfonate 30 g rectally once.

5. Monitoring

   - Serum potassium should be monitored every 1–6 hours during treatment, and the patient should be admitted to a telemetry unit.

   - After resolution of symptoms, serum potassium level and renal function can be monitored every 4–12 hours.

   - Once the acute event has resolved, serum potassium level and renal function should be monitored every 24–48 hours during hospitalization.

6. The medication regimen should be tailored to decrease the risk of hyperkalemia, and follow-up care should be arranged with the patient's primary care provider for routine monitoring.

Magnesium

Overview

The predominant magnesium disorder encountered in clinical practice is hypomagnesemia, which is significant because it may contribute to higher mortality rates in hospitalized patients. Serum magnesium determinations are poor reflections of total body stores. The primary etiologies of hypomagnesemia are renal and GI losses, with renal losses being primarily drug induced. Clinical manifestations of hypomagnesemia are commonly the result of other concurrent electrolyte abnormalities, such as hypokalemia and hypocalcemia. Hypermagnesemia is less commonly seen and is often iatrogenic or related to excessive magnesium administration in the presence of underlying renal insufficiency and/or failure. Identifying the etiology and treatment strategies for specific magnesium disorders will aid the clinician in restoring magnesium homeostasis and preventing adverse consequences.

1. Homeostasis and physiological function[42-58]

- The normal serum magnesium range is 1.5–2 mEq/L (1.8–2.4 mg/dL).
- Magnesium is the second most common intracellular cation and the fourth most abundant cation in the body.
- Magnesium is a cofactor in oxidative-phosphorylation reactions in mitochondria.
- Magnesium catalyzes enzymatic processes and activates phosphatases concerning transfer, storage, and utilization of adenosine triphosphate (ATP).
- Magnesium is important for maintenance of the sodium-potassium-adenosine triphosphatase pump and cell membrane electrolyte composition (calcium)/action potential.
- Magnesium is important for glucose utilization and DNA, protein, and fat synthesis.
- The body's magnesium is distributed in the bone (53%), skeletal muscle (27%), soft tissues (19%), and ECF (1%).
- Total body distribution of magnesium consists of 25 mEq/kg (1750–2000 mEq) in the normal adult.
- Magnesium serves as a structural component of bone.
- Magnesium is essential in neuromuscular transmission, cardiovascular excitability, vasomotor tone, muscle contraction, and parathyroid hormone (PTH) secretion and synthesis.

2. Dietary intake[47,48,51,59]

- Adequate intake for infants and the recommended dietary allowance for adults, adolescents, and children (Table 3-11) vary by age and sex.

Table 3-11. Magnesium: Adequate Intake for Infants and Recommended Dietary Allowances for Children, Adolescents, and Adults.[59]

Age	Male	Female	Pregnancy	Lactation
		Adequate intake, mg		
Birth to 6 mo	30	30	–	–
7–12 mo	75	75	–	–
		Recommended dietary allowance, mg		
1–3 y	80	80	–	–
4–8 y	130	130	–	–
9–13 y	240	240	–	–
14–18 y	410	360	400	360
19–30 y	400	310	350	310
31–50 y	420	320	360	320
≥ 51 y	420	320	–	–

- The average American diet contains 16–30 mEq (200–350 mg) of magnesium per day.
- Oral magnesium absorption is approximately 30%–50% (8–15 mEq/d) and occurs primarily in the jejunum and ileum (alkaline environment).
- Absorptive capacity may be as low as 25% on a high magnesium diet and as high as 75% on a low magnesium diet (inversely related to intake).
    - Intestinal absorption of magnesium is impaired by high phosphate diets and high fiber foods containing phytate.
    - Dietary magnesium intake rarely leads to a clinically significant increase in bowel movements; only when supplemental oral or enteral magnesium products are used does the contribution to potential diarrhea become problematic.

3. Excretion[40,44,48,52,53]

- The kidneys excrete 35%–45% of daily oral magnesium intake (8–10 mEq/d or 100–120 mg/d) to maintain homeostasis (Table 3-12).

Table 3-12. Renal Handling of Magnesium.[56]

Site	Magnesium[a]
Glomerulus	70%–80% filtered
Proximal tubule	20%–30% reabsorbed
Ascending loop of Henle	50%–60% reabsorbed
Distal tubule	5% reabsorbed
Fractional excretion	3%–5%
Renal threshold	Serum magnesium range

[a]Small increases in serum magnesium result in increased excretion, because the reabsorptive capacity is normally at its maximum (95%).[47,48,60,61]

- Protein intake > 90 g/d may increase renal magnesium excretion.
- Circadian rhythm of magnesium renal excretion occurs maximally at night (urinary magnesium measurement should be done over 24 hours rather than with a spot collection).
- About 1%–2% of endogenous magnesium is normally eliminated in the feces.

Hypomagnesemia

Prevalence and Mortality[42–45,62–72]

1. Hypomagnesemia has been reported in 6.9%–47% of hospitalized patients (serum magnesium < 1–1.48 mEq/L) and 9%–68% of ICU patients (serum magnesium < 1–1.5 mEq/L).

2. Hypomagnesemic patients have higher mortality rates compared with normomagnesemic patients (17%–46% vs 6%–25%, respectively).

Etiologies and/or Risk Factors

1. GI and renal-associated losses of magnesium are the most common causes of hypomagnesemia (Figure 3-9).

2. Intracellular redistribution due to diabetic ketoacidosis, hyperthyroidism, and acute myocardial infarction is another cause of hypomagnesemia.

Clinical Presentation[52,82] (Figure 3-10)

1. Hypomagnesemia is primarily associated with other electrolyte abnormalities (hypokalemia, hypocalcemia) or concomitant medical problems.

Figure 3-9. Etiologies of Hypomagnesemia.[42,48-50,73-78]

Gastrointestinal

Reduced intake

- Protein-calorie malnutrition
- Prolonged intravenous fluid or nutrition support without added magnesium
- Alcoholism
- Anorexia

Reduced absorption

- Malabsorption syndromes
- Short bowel syndrome
- Intestinal bypass
- Acute pancreatitis
- Patiromer

Increased loss

- Diarrhea (ulcerative colitis, Crohn's disease, colonic neoplasms)
- Laxative abuse
- Bulimia or excessive emesis
- Gastric suctioning
- Intestinal and biliary fistulas

Renal

Drug-induced

- Alcohol (ethanol)
- Loop diuretics (furosemide, torsemide, bumetanide)
- Hydrochlorothiazide > 50 mg/d
- Amphotericin B
- Aminoglycosides
- Cisplatin
- Carboplatin
- Oxaliplatin
- Ifosfamide
- Cyclosporine
- Tacrolimus
- Foscarnet
- Cetuximab
- Proton pump inhibitors (eg, omeprazole)
- Pentamidine
- Ticarcillin
- Digoxin

Other

- Renal tubular acidosis
- Hypercalcemic states including malignancies
- Postobstructive diuresis
- Diuretic phase of acute tubular necrosis
- Hereditary renal magnesium wasting
- Hyperaldosteronism
- Renal transplantation
- Glucosuria-induced osmotic diuresis in diabetes mellitus

Other

Intracellular redistribution

- Diabetic ketoacidosis
- Hyperthyroidism
- Acute myocardial infarction

Miscellaneous

- Burns
- Pregnancy and lactation
- Exchange transfusion
- Cardiopulmonary bypass
- Theophylline overdose

Figure 3-10. Clinical Manifestations of Hypomagnesemia.[42,49,54,79-81]

Neuromuscular	Cardiac	Metabolic	Central Nervous System
• Muscle fasciculations • Tremors • Hyperreflexia • Paresthesias • Muscle weakness • Positive Chvostek's and Trousseau's signs • Myalgias • Choreoathetosis • Tetany • Myoclonic jerks	• Premature ventricular beats • Ventricular fibrillation • Ventricular tachycardia • Torsades de pointes • Predisposition to digoxin-mediated arrhythmias • Supraventricular arrhythmias • PR prolongation • QT prolongation	• Hypokalemia • Hypocalcemia	• Nystagmus • Seizures • Depression • Agitation • Psychosis • Disorientation • Confusion • Hallucinations • Irritability • Restlessness

2. Only 15% of ICU/hospitalized patients with serum magnesium < 1 mEq/L (1.2 mg/dL) had muscle fasciculations, tremor, and irritability.

   - All had concurrent hypocalcemia ≤ 6.7 mg/dL, but symptoms resolved after magnesium treatment in 3 of 4 patients.

   - None had positive Chvostek's or Trousseau's signs, ECG changes, or cardiac arrhythmias.

Diagnosis/Diagnostic Tests[49,52,55,69]

1. Total body magnesium is not correlated with any single laboratory test, making diagnosis difficult.

2. Past medical history and medication/dietary supplement history (past and current) should be assessed when evaluating hypomagnesemia.

3. Magnesium deficiency may be present with a normal serum magnesium level.

   - The cellular effects of decreased serum magnesium are difficult to predict based on level alone (acute vs chronic).

- Only 9% of pulmonary ICU patients had hypomagnesemia (≤ 1.4 mEq/L [1.7 mg/dL]) compared with 47% of other pulmonary ICU patients with decreased muscle magnesium and normomagnesemia.

4. Urinary magnesium < 1–2 mEq (12–24 mg) in 24 hours

   - This level reflects a magnesium-deficient state.
   - It may develop within 7 days after decreased magnesium intake.
   - With normal renal function, decreased urinary magnesium may occur before decreased serum magnesium.

Goals of Therapy[55,83,84]

1. Correct serum magnesium (> 1.5 mEq/L) and maintain serum magnesium within normal limits (1.5–2 mEq/L or 1.8–2.4 mg/dL).
2. Treat and prevent symptomatic hypomagnesemia (Torsades de pointes, refractory ventricular fibrillation/ventricular tachycardia, generalized tonic-clonic seizures).
3. *Identify and manage as appropriate all concurrent causes of* hypomagnesemia (medical history, medication/dietary supplement history) in addition to correcting hypomagnesemia.

Management[48,55,83-90]

IV Replacement

1. IV replacement is preferred to oral replacement in the setting of GI intolerance (ie, diarrhea, nausea/vomiting) and symptomatic hypomagnesemia.
2. Commercially available salts of IV magnesium exist in chloride and sulfate form (Table 3-13).
3. Initial treatment involves 16 mEq (2 g) of magnesium sulfate as a 20% solution (5% dextrose or 0.9% NaCl) given intravenously over 1 minute,

Table 3-13. Magnesium Parenteral Products.

Product	Available Solutions	Concentration, mEq/mL
Magnesium chloride	20%	2
Magnesium sulfate	50%	4.06

Table 3-14. Intravenous Guidelines for Treatment of Hypomagnesemia.[a]

Degree of Hypomagnesemia	Serum Magnesium Range	Treatment in First 24 h
Mild	1.3–1.5 mEq/L (1.5–1.8 mg/dL)	0.5 mEq/kg
Moderate	0.8–1.2 mEq/L (1–1.4 mg/dL)	1 mEq/kg
Severe	< 0.8 mEq/L (< 1 mg/dL)	2 mEq/kg

[a]Patients with urine output > 0.5 mL/kg/h, normal blood urea nitrogen/serum creatinine, based on ideal body weight, and magnesium sulfate infused intravenously over 24 hours. Clinical judgment should be used in renal insufficiency (25%–50% of above recommendations).

followed by an appropriate regimen based on the serum magnesium level (Table 3-14).

4. Additional 0.5 mEq/kg/d of IV magnesium sulfate for 3–5 days may be required since magnesium repletion of tissues is slow.
   - Monitor blood pressure, heart rate, respiratory rate, arterial O_2 saturation, deep tendon reflexes, urine output, and ECG.
     - No change in heart rate or mean arterial blood pressure occurred after 0.3 mEq/kg intravenously over 10 minutes, followed by 0.2 mEq/kg/h in 8 patients without cardiac disease, but a prolongation of the PR-interval was observed on ECG.
   - Expect elevated serum magnesium in the first 24 hours, based on literature.
     - After receiving 80 mEq magnesium chloride intravenously over 8 hours, followed by an additional 80 mEq over the next 16 hours, patients had serum magnesium increase from 1.7 to 3.2 mEq/L.
     - After a dose of 0.3 mEq/kg (based on ideal body weight) intravenously over 10 minutes, followed by 0.08 mEq/kg/h for 24 hours (mean dose 163 mEq), patients' serum magnesium increased from 1.7 to 3.5 mEq/L, with no serious adverse effects occurring.
   - Additional dosing is based on true magnesium deficit state vs acute hypomagnesemia (based on serum magnesium level).
   - Addition of magnesium sulfate 8–16 mEq/L to maintenance IV fluids may also be instituted to provide maintenance doses after 3–5 days of replacement.
5. About 50% of magnesium dose may be excreted despite the presence of a total body deficit, because as serum magnesium increases, the renal threshold for magnesium absorption is exceeded.

Table 3-15. Magnesium Oral/Enteral Products.[a]			
Magnesium Salt	**Brand Name/ Dosage**	**Elemental Magnesium per Dose, mEq**	**Elemental Magnesium per Dose, mg**
Chloride	Slow-Mag 535 mg	5 mEq/enteric coated tablet	64 mg/enteric coated tablet
Citrate	300 mL (generic)	167 mEq/300 mL	2000 mg/300 mL
Gluconate	Mag-G 500 mg	2.3 mEq/tablet	27 mg/tablet
Oxide	500 mg (generic)	25 mEq/tablet	300 mg/tablet
Protein complex	133 mg (generic)	12 mEq/tablet	133 mg/tablet
Sulfate	50% oral solution	4 mEq/mL	48 mg/mL
Hydroxide	Milk of Magnesia 311 mg (tablet) and 400 mg/5 mL (suspension)	11 mEq/tablet and 2.8 mEq/mL suspension	130 mg/tablet and 33 mg/mL suspension

[a]Chloride, gluconate, and protein complex salts may cause less diarrhea. Oxide salt is more insoluble and may induce diarrhea at higher doses. The citrate and sulfate salts are generally not used because of potential to induce diarrhea. Retention of enteric-coated magnesium tablets has occurred in patients with gastroparesis.[88]

Oral Replacement

1. The ideal dose and salt of oral or enteral magnesium (Table 3-15) is often a process of trial and error because most replacement products are limited by the frequency of bowel movements or the presence of either new or chronic diarrhea/ostomy output (Figure 3-11).

2. For patients who remain hypomagnesemic despite oral or enteral supplementation, amiloride (oral potassium-sparing diuretic) in doses of 5–20 mg/d may be effective in reducing renal magnesium losses.

Diagnostic Approach to Hypomagnesemia[78,87-89]

1. Identify predisposed patients/patients at risk.

    - Individuals with alcoholism, diabetes, malnutrition, or congestive heart failure

    - Patients receiving loop diuretics (furosemide, torsemide, bumetanide) or hydrochlorothiazide > 50 mg/d, amphotericin B, aminoglycosides, piperacillin, cisplatin, carboplatin, oxaliplatin, ifosfamide, cyclosporine, tacrolimus, patiromer, foscarnet, cetuximab, proton pump inhibitors (eg, omeprazole)

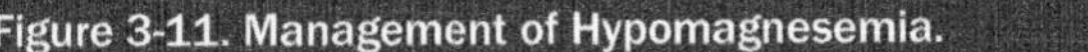

Figure 3-11. Management of Hypomagnesemia.

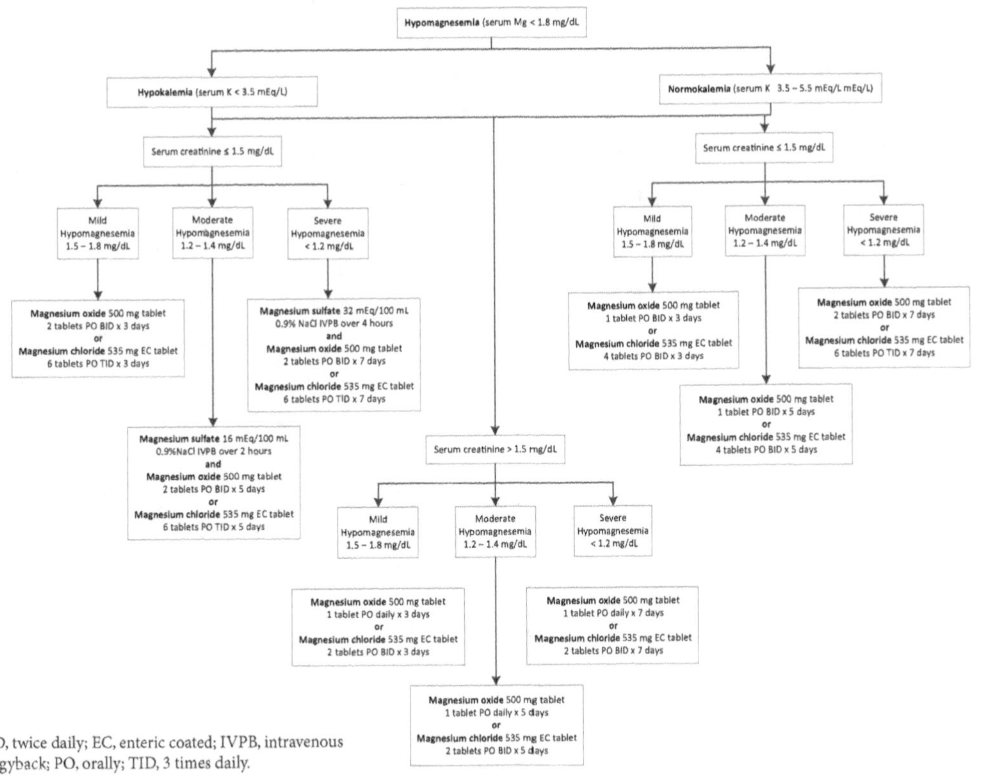

- **Hypomagnesemia** (serum Mg < 1.8 mg/dL
  - **Hypokalemia** (serum K < 3.5 mEq/L)
    - Serum creatinine ≤ 1.5 mg/dL
      - Mild Hypomagnesemia 1.5 – 1.8 mg/dL → **Magnesium oxide** 500 mg tablet 2 tablets PO BID x 3 days **or** **Magnesium chloride** 535 mg EC tablet 6 tablets PO TID x 3 days
      - Moderate Hypomagnesemia 1.2 – 1.4 mg/dL → **Magnesium sulfate** 16 mEq/100 mL 0.9%NaCl IVPB over 2 hours **and** **Magnesium oxide** 500 mg tablet 2 tablets PO BID x 5 days **or** **Magnesium chloride** 535 mg EC tablet 6 tablets PO TID x 5 days
      - Severe Hypomagnesemia < 1.2 mg/dL → **Magnesium sulfate** 32 mEq/100 mL 0.9% NaCl IVPB over 4 hours **and** **Magnesium oxide** 500 mg tablet 2 tablets PO BID x 7 days **or** **Magnesium chloride** 535 mg EC tablet 6 tablets PO TID x 7 days
  - **Normokalemia** (serum K 3.5 – 5.5 mEq/L mEq/L)
    - Serum creatinine ≤ 1.5 mg/dL
      - Mild Hypomagnesemia 1.5 – 1.8 mg/dL → **Magnesium oxide** 500 mg tablet 1 tablet PO BID x 3 days **or** **Magnesium chloride** 535 mg EC tablet 4 tablets PO BID x 3 days
      - Moderate Hypomagnesemia 1.2 – 1.4 mg/dL → **Magnesium oxide** 500 mg tablet 1 tablet PO BID x 5 days **or** **Magnesium chloride** 535 mg EC tablet 4 tablets PO BID x 5 days
      - Severe Hypomagnesemia < 1.2 mg/dL → **Magnesium oxide** 500 mg tablet 2 tablets PO BID x 7 days **or** **Magnesium chloride** 535 mg EC tablet 6 tablets PO TID x 7 days
  - Serum creatinine > 1.5 mg/dL
    - Mild Hypomagnesemia 1.5 – 1.8 mg/dL → **Magnesium oxide** 500 mg tablet 1 tablet PO daily x 3 days **or** **Magnesium chloride** 535 mg EC tablet 2 tablets PO BID x 3 days
    - Moderate Hypomagnesemia 1.2 – 1.4 mg/dL → **Magnesium oxide** 500 mg tablet 1 tablet PO daily x 5 days **or** **Magnesium chloride** 535 mg EC tablet 2 tablets PO BID x 5 days
    - Severe Hypomagnesemia < 1.2 mg/dL → **Magnesium oxide** 500 mg tablet 1 tablet PO daily x 7 days **or** **Magnesium chloride** 535 mg EC tablet 2 tablets PO BID x 7 days

BID, twice daily; EC, enteric coated; IVPB, intravenous piggyback; PO, orally; TID, 3 times daily.

- Patients with unexplained hypocalcemia or hypokalemia not responding to reasonable supplementation
- Up to 19% of patients receiving digoxin with hypomagnesemia may experience ventricular ectopy.

2. Follow serial serum magnesium concentrations routinely in hospitalized patients (Figure 3-12).

3. Avoid rapid IV infusions (< 8 hours) in patients with systolic blood pressure < 90 mm Hg, heart rate < 60 beats/min, and second or third degree atrioventricular block.

4. Make a general estimate of the change in serum magnesium after IV replacement in patients with normal renal function, approximately 0.1 mg/dL (or 0.1 mEq/L depending on how the laboratory reports it) for each 8 mEq administered (8 mEq of magnesium sulfate = 1 g of magnesium sulfate).

Monitoring

1. The degree of monitoring should reflect the severity of hypomagnesemia and the underlying cause of the disorder.

2. Acute, asymptomatic mild to moderate hypomagnesemia requires at least daily measurements of serum levels to ensure the serum magnesium is slowly improving. Several days of replacement may be necessary to achieve normal serum magnesium concentrations.

3. Symptomatic patients who are receiving aggressive magnesium replacement should have serum magnesium levels monitored every 1–6 hours based upon serum concentrations and symptoms. Once levels are normalized, assessments every 1–3 days while hospitalized are appropriate.

Hypermagnesemia

Prevalence and Mortality[63,64,91]

1. Hypermagnesemia (reported as > 1.9 mEq/L) has been reported in 4%–9.3% of hospitalized patients.

2. Patients with hypermagnesemia have higher mortality rates compared with normomagnesemic ICU patients (38% vs 8%, respectively).

Figure 3-12. Assessment of Hypomagnesemia.

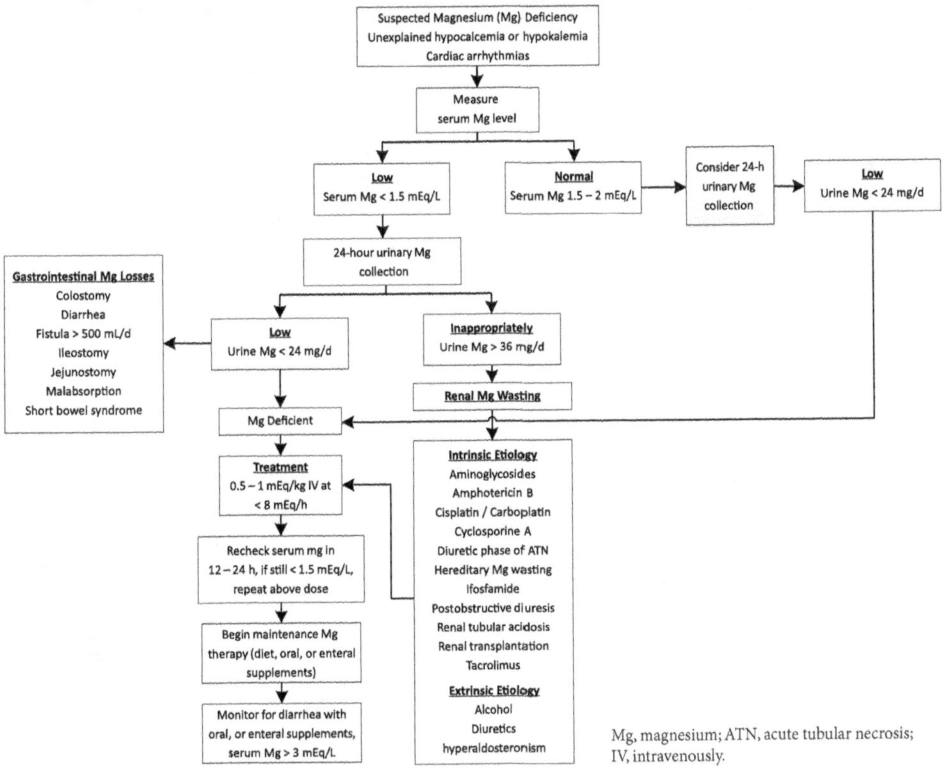

Mg, magnesium; ATN, acute tubular necrosis; IV, intravenously.

Figure 3-13. Etiologies of Hypermagnesemia.

Renal	Iatrogenic
• AKI • CKD or ESRD	• Infants delivered by mothers treated with high-dose magnesium for eclampsia • Excess administration in intravenous fluids or parenteral nutrition • Diabetic ketoacidosis • Primary hyperparathyroidism • Tumor lysis syndrome

AKI, acute kidney injury; CKD, chronic kidney disease; ESRD, end-stage renal disease.

Etiologies and/or Risk Factors[92-94]

1. Hypermagnesemia is attributed to renal and nonrenal/iatrogenic causes, with renal injury and excessive supplementation as the most common etiologies (Figure 3-13).

Clinical Presentation[92-96]

1. Clinical symptoms generally do not occur until serum levels exceed 4 mEq/L (4.8 mg/dL) (Table 3-16).

2. Magnesium levels have been observed as high as 45 mEq/L in neonates and 19.7 mEq/L in adults.

Table 3-16. Manifestations of Hypermagnesemia.

System Affected	Manifestation
Neuromuscular	Loss of deep tendon reflexes
Cardiopulmonary	Hypotension ECG changes (including cardiac arrest) Apnea
Central nervous system	Somnolence Paralysis Coma

ECG, electrocardiogram.

3. When serum magnesium levels exceed 15 mEq/L, coma and parasympathetic blockade are evident, requiring mechanical ventilation, and clinically mimic a central brainstem herniation syndrome.

Diagnosis/Diagnostic Tests[93,95]

1. Asymptomatic laboratory diagnosis is frequently observed when magnesium is administered therapeutically (laboratory tests done shortly after magnesium IV infusion).

    - Serum magnesium > 2.4 mEq/L (> 2.9 mg/dL)

2. Symptomatic patients are generally those with loss of deep tendon reflexes and subsequently observed elevated serum magnesium (mostly iatrogenic).

3. Hypermagnesemia follows inappropriate administration of IV magnesium (including its use in PN).

Goals of Therapy

1. Correct serum magnesium level (≤ 2.4 mEq/L) and maintain a serum magnesium within normal limits (1.5–2 mEq/L or 1.8–2.4 mg/dL).

2. Treat and prevent symptoms relating to the neuromuscular, cardiopulmonary, and central nervous systems.

3. Identify and manage as appropriate all concurrent causes of hypermagnesemia (medical history, medication/dietary supplement history).

Management/Diagnostic Approach

1. Identify predisposed patients/patients at risk.

    - Individuals with AKI or CKD or ESRD
    - Patients receiving magnesium-containing IV solutions or PN
    - Patients receiving oral or enteral magnesium products including over-the-counter products (eg, magnesium citrate or magnesium hydroxide)

2. Remove or discontinue any magnesium-containing IV solutions or medications.

    - For symptomatic patients, calcium chloride or gluconate 1–2 g intravenously over 5–10 minutes may acutely reverse the symptoms of magnesium excess.

- Hemodialysis can also rapidly lower serum magnesium levels for anuric patients.

- IV furosemide may also rapidly lower serum magnesium levels for nonoliguric patients.

3. Routinely follow serial serum magnesium concentrations.

Monitoring

1. Acute asymptomatic patients should have their serum magnesium concentrations assessed every 1–3 days.

2. Symptomatic patients who are being aggressively treated should have serum magnesium levels monitored every 1–6 hours based upon serum concentrations and symptoms. If hemodialysis is used, assess serum concentrations after dialysis. Once serum magnesium is normalized, assessments every 1–3 days while the patient is hospitalized is appropriate. Continuous ECG and blood pressure monitoring should be employed for rapid identification of untoward cardiac effects.

Patient/Family Counseling

1. Ensure that the patient and caregivers are educated and aware of the daily magnesium allowance necessary to maintain nutrition based on the patient's comorbidities.

2. Screen all medications for their ability to potentially cause or exacerbate magnesium disorders. These medications should be carefully reviewed by the primary physician for medical necessity, and the risk/benefit of continuing or discontinuing such medications should be discussed with the patient.

3. Report any excessive GI losses (eg, diarrhea, large ostomy output), abnormal behavior, or signs or symptoms of magnesium disorders to the patient's primary physician immediately.

4. Adjust dietary intake to include or exclude products high in magnesium based on the patient's underlying magnesium disorder. The patient and caregivers should be instructed how to properly read a nutrition label and interpret the magnesium content. Always verify the patient's daily magnesium allowance with the managing physician.

Foods High in Magnesium[96]

1. Almonds, cashews, peanuts
2. Boiled spinach
3. Breakfast cereal (including instant oatmeal)
4. Soymilk (plain or vanilla)
5. Black beans (cooked)
6. Edamame
7. Peanut butter (smooth)
8. Bread (whole wheat)
9. Avocados, potato (baked), brown rice (cooked)
10. Yogurt (plain and low fat)
11. Kidney beans (canned)
12. Banana
13. Atlantic salmon (cooked)
14. Milk (cow)

Medications That May Contribute to Magnesium Disorders[42,48–50,73–78]

Numerous medications can predispose patients to magnesium disorders, which necessitates a comprehensive medication review. The patient and caregivers should be counseled on those medications associated with the potential to precipitate magnesium disorders. Signs and symptoms of magnesium disorders should also be communicated. Discussions involving healthcare providers, the patient, and caregivers should be undertaken to ascertain the risk vs benefit of continuing specific therapies or adjusting the treatment regimen (eg, discontinue offending medication, adjust medication dosing, initiate supplementation) to limit possible untoward effects. Table 3-17 provides a list of medications with their overall mechanism leading to hypomagnesemia. Hypermagnesemia is primarily attributed to oversupplementation or excessive intake of magnesium with or without organ dysfunction.

Table 3-17. Drugs and Medications Commonly Associated With Hypomagnesemia.

Symptoms	Drugs and Medications
Decrease intestinal absorption	Alcohol (ethanol)
	Proton pump inhibitors (use > 3 mo)
	Patiromer
Increase gastrointestinal excretion	Alcohol (ethanol)
Increase renal excretion	Alcohol (ethanol)
	Loop diuretics
	Hydrochlorothiazide (> 50 mg/d)
	Amphotericin B
	Aminoglycosides
	Cisplatin, carboplatin, oxaliplatin
	Ifosfamide
	Cyclosporine, tacrolimus
	Foscarnet
	Cetuximab
	Pentamidine
	Ticarcillin, piperacillin
	Digoxin

Clinical Application

Patient Scenario 1

A 41-year-old man with a history of colitis presents to the ED 2 weeks after receiving a total colectomy with ileostomy. His chief complaint consists of weakness, muscle soreness, fatigue, confusion, and a 3-day history of high ostomy output ranging between 6–8 L/d. Patient states that he has been noncompliant with his prescribed diet and drinks several sugary drinks per day. In addition, he has been taking the following medications: acetaminophen/codeine 300/30 mg by mouth every 6 hours as needed for pain, potassium chloride liquid 20 mEq by mouth daily, and magnesium oxide tablets 500 mg by mouth twice daily. In the ED, he is treated with IV magnesium, IV potassium chloride, and IV 0.9% NaCl.

- Vital signs
  - Pulse, 110 beats/min
  - Respirations, 14 breaths/min

- Blood pressure, 98/70 mm Hg
- Temperature, 37 °C (98.6 °F)
- Weight, 75 kg (165 lb)
- Height, 157.5 cm (62 in)
- Body mass index, 30.2 kg/m^2
- Ideal body weight, 54.6 kg (120 lb)

- Physical examination
  - General: Ill appearing and confused
  - Eye: Pupils are equal, round, and reactive to light
  - Respiratory: Lungs are clear to auscultation
  - Cardiovascular: Tachycardic, regular rhythm
  - Abdominal: No tenderness, hyperactive bowel sounds, ostomy appliance in place with liquid contents
  - Neurologic: Cranial nerves II–XII intact
- ECG
  - Sinus tachycardia
- Laboratory results
  - Sodium, 139 mEq/L
  - Potassium, 3.1 mEq/L
  - Chloride, 101 mEq/L
  - CO_2, 26 mEq/L
  - Magnesium, 1.1 mEq/L
  - Calcium, 7.8 mg/dL
  - Glucose, 97 mg/dL
  - BUN, 16 mg/dL
  - Serum creatinine, 0.9 mg/dL

1. Assess the serum magnesium level and determine if the patient is experiencing symptoms.
   - Patient's magnesium is low, and the patient is experiencing confusion, high ostomy output, hypokalemia, and muscle weakness.
2. Assess the patient's past medical history, medications, and laboratory parameters for causes of hypomagnesemia.
   - The patient's magnesium level is low and is attributed to GI losses as evidenced by high ostomy output.
   - The patient has been taking oral magnesium oxide 500 mg by mouth twice daily; this product is known to increase stool output.
   - In addition, high osmolarity liquid medications (ie, potassium chloride liquid) are known to cause gastric discomfort and loose stools.
   - Concurrent hypokalemia is associated with hypomagnesemia.
3. Consider the following treatment options:
   - Oral magnesium
     - Patient should avoid oral magnesium products known to cause loose stools and diarrhea.
     - Oral replacement should be reserved for mild and asymptomatic cases of hypomagnesemia; IV replacement should be used in this patient.
     - Chloride, gluconate, and protein complex salt forms of oral magnesium cause less diarrhea than oxide.
   - IV magnesium
     - Patient should receive IV magnesium sulfate or chloride.
     - Weight-based dosing should be used in this symptomatic patient.
     - Ideal body weight should be used to dose magnesium; however, actual body weight should be used when actual body weight is less than ideal body weight.
     - IV fluids should be administered if signs and symptoms of volume depletion are present.
   - Concurrent correction of potassium and calcium should occur (see potassium and calcium sections).

4. Monitor.

   - Serum magnesium should be monitored every 6–8 hours during treatment, and the patient should be admitted to a telemetry unit for cardiac monitoring.

   - After resolution of symptoms, magnesium can be monitored every 12–24 hours.

5. Tailor the medication regimen to decrease the risk of hypermagnesemia and arrange follow-up care with the patient's primary care provider for routine monitoring.

6. Treat and manage the high ostomy output or diarrhea if it continues after stopping magnesium oxide and potassium chloride liquid.

Patient Scenario 2

A 68-year-old woman with a history of constipation and dyslipidemia presents to the ED with a 3-day history of acute constipation, abdominal pain, and somnolence. The patient's family member states that she has been drinking a bottle of magnesium citrate (296 mL) twice daily for the past 2 days without any resulting bowel movement. The patient takes the following medications: atorvastatin 20 mg by mouth daily and magnesium citrate 1 bottle (296 mL) by mouth as needed for constipation.

In the ED, she is treated with IV calcium and a bolus of 1 L 0.9% NaCl with IV furosemide 20 mg, and she is placed on cardiac telemetry. In addition, a computed tomography scan of the abdomen and pelvis is diagnostic of a large bowel obstruction.

- Vital signs

  - Pulse, 52 beats/min

  - Respirations, 12 breaths/min

  - Blood pressure, 78/51 mm Hg

  - Temperature, 37 °C (98.6 °F)

- Physical examination

  - General: Ill appearing

  - Eye: Pupils are equal, round, and reactive to light.

- Respiratory: Lungs are clear to auscultation.
- Cardiovascular: Bradycardia, regular rhythm
- Abdominal: Tenderness in all 4 quadrants, abdominal distention
- Neurologic: Somnolent, absent deep tendon reflexes

- ECG
  - Sinus bradycardia
- Laboratory results
  - Sodium, 143 mEq/L
  - Potassium, 4.8 mEq/L
  - Chloride, 104 mEq/L
  - CO_2, 30 mEq/L
  - Magnesium, 6.1 mEq/L
  - Glucose, 87 mg/dL
  - BUN, 90 mg/dL
  - Serum creatinine, 2.9 mg/dL

1. Assess the serum magnesium level and determine if the patient is experiencing symptoms.
   - Patient's magnesium is elevated, and the patient is experiencing somnolence, bradycardia, hypotension, and loss of deep tendon reflexes.
2. Assess the patient's past medical history, medications, and laboratory parameters for causes of hypermagnesemia.
   - The patient has been taking 1 bottle of magnesium citrate twice daily for the past 2 days.
   - The patient's magnesium level is high and is attributed to acute renal failure along with overconsumption of a magnesium-containing over-the-counter medication.

3. Consider the following treatment options:
   - IV calcium
     - Patient should receive 1–2 g of calcium gluconate or 1 g of calcium chloride intravenously as soon as possible in the presence of acute signs and symptoms of hypermagnesemia.
   - In the case of anuria and symptomatic hypermagnesemia, hemodialysis should be considered.
   - Administer IV fluids if signs and symptoms of volume depletion are present.
   - Consider an increased dose of a loop diuretic (ie, furosemide) to further increase the excretion of magnesium (in oliguric patients receiving IV fluids).
4. Monitor
   - Serum magnesium should be monitored every 4–6 hours during treatment, and the patient should be admitted to a telemetry unit for cardiac monitoring.
   - After resolution of symptoms, magnesium can be monitored every 12–24 hours.
5. Tailor the medication regimen to decrease the risk of hypermagnesemia and arrange follow-up care with the patient's primary care provider for routine monitoring.

Calcium

Overview

Calcium plays numerous important roles in the body, including bone metabolism, coagulation, and neuromuscular function. Asymptomatic hypocalcemia is a relatively benign electrolyte disorder in the acute setting; however, prolonged hypocalcemia may lead to derangements with bone-mineral metabolism and endocrine diseases. Symptomatic hypocalcemia requires aggressive calcium replacement. Hypercalcemia is primarily seen in patients with malignancies and hyperparathyroidism. Total serum calcium interpretation should always take serum albumin level and acid-base status into consideration. Correct identification of calcium disorders and knowledge of the pathophysiology behind these disorders and the available treatment strategies allow the clinician to provide safe, effective patient care.

1. Homeostasis and physiological function[12,97-103]

  - Normal total calcium range is 8.6–10.2 mg/dL (2.15–2.55 mmol/L); ionized calcium 4.4–5 mg/dL (1.1–1.25 mmol/L).

  - Calcium is the most prevalent cation in the body.

  - Calcium is essential for bone metabolism, nerve conduction, muscle contraction, intracellular signaling, functionality of cell membranes, coagulation cascade, and regulation of secretory functions.

  - Calcium's total body distribution is more than 99% in bone.

  - Serum distribution accounts for 1% of all calcium and is found partially in the ionized (free) state (40%–50%), bound to small anions (10%–15%), and bound to plasma proteins (40%–50%).

  - The majority of plasma protein binding occurs with albumin (80%).

  - Calcium homeostasis is regulated by vitamin D, phosphorus, and the hormones PTH and calcitonin (Figure 3-14).

    - In response to decreases in serum calcium concentrations, PTH is secreted to stimulate bone resorption, renal calcium resorption, and renal production of 1,25-dihydroxycholecalciferol (also called 1,25-dihydroxyvitamin D_3 or calcitriol).

    - 1,25-Dihydroxycholecalciferol stimulates bone resorption and enhances GI absorption of calcium and phosphorus.

    - In response to high serum calcium concentrations, calcitonin is secreted to counter PTH effects, inhibit bone resorption, and promote osteoblastic activity.

2. Dietary intake[99,105-108]

  - Oral/enteral nutrition (recommended dietary allowances)

    - Oral/enteral nutrition (recommended dietary allowances)—adequate intake for infants and recommended dietary allowance for adults, adolescents, and children (Table 3-18) vary by age and sex

  - Parenteral nutrition, 10–15 mEq/d (adults)

Figure 3-14. Calcium Homeostasis and Feedback Mechanisms.

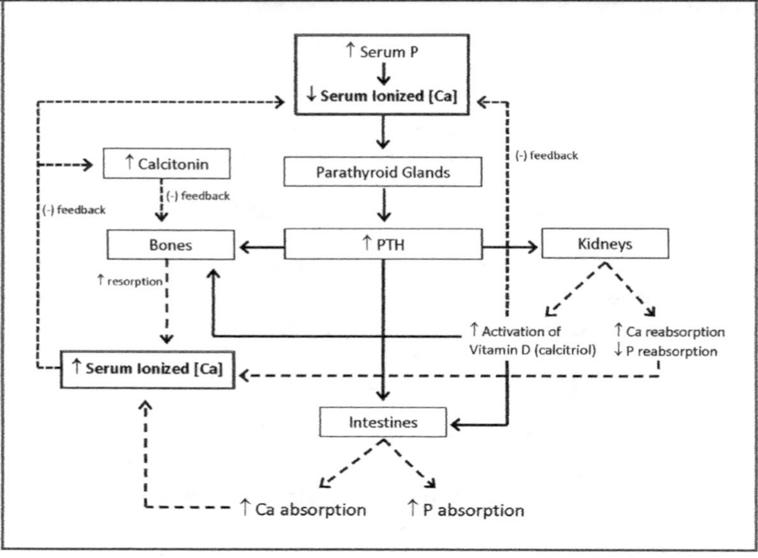

Ca, calcium; P, phosphorus; PTH, parathyroid hormone.

Reprinted with permission from Kraft MD. Phosphorus and calcium: a review for the adult nutrition support clinician. *Nutr Clin Pract*. 2015;30(1):21-33.

Table 3-18. Calcium: Adequate Intake for Infants and Recommended Dietary Allowances for Children, Adolescents, and Adults.[105]

Age	Male	Female	Pregnancy	Lactation
		Adequate intake, mg		
Birth to 6 months	260	200	–	–
7–12 mo	260	260	–	–
		Recommended dietary allowance, mg		
1–3 y	700	700	–	–
4–8 y	1000	1000	–	–
9–13 y	1300	1300	–	–
14–18 y	1300	1300	1300	1300
19–50 y	1000	1000	1000	1000
50–70 y	1000	1200	–	–
≥ 71 y	1200	1200	–	–

- Absorption
    - Small intestine absorbs 30%–35% of dietary intake.
    - Absorption is enhanced by vitamin D.

3. Excretion[99,107]
    - About 98% of calcium is reabsorbed by the kidneys.
    - The primary route of excretion is by the kidneys.
        - Reabsorption in proximal tubule, 60%–70%
        - Reabsorption in ascending loop of Henle, 20%–25%
        - Reabsorption in distal convoluted tubule, 5%–10%

Hypocalcemia

Prevalence[108-110]

1. The reported incidence of hypocalcemia based on the serum calcium level varies widely from 18% of hospitalized patients to 85% of patients in the ICU.
2. Vitamin D deficiency is the most common cause in the primary care setting.
3. Based on serum ionized calcium level, hypocalcemia varies between 15% and 88% of ICU patients.

Etiologies and/or Risk Factors[12] (Figure 3-15)

1. Hypocalcemia is most commonly due to hypoalbuminemia but may also be due to other electrolyte abnormalities, renal impairment, hypoparathyroidism, critical illness, pancreatitis, or medications.
2. Drug-induced causes of hypocalcemia are presented in Figure 3-16.

Clinical Presentation[12,100,101] (Table 3-19)

1. Clinical manifestations of hypocalcemia depend on both the degree of hypocalcemia and the rate of decline in serum calcium concentration. Acute is considered as ≤ 48 hours.
2. Mild to moderate acute hypocalcemia (total serum calcium 7.5–8.5 mg/dL [1.9–2.1 mmol/L] or ionized serum calcium 4–4.5 mg/dL [1–1.12 mmol/L]) may present with paresthesias, muscle cramps, mental status changes, Chvostek's sign, Trousseau's sign, and hypotension.

Figure 3-15. Etiologies of Hypocalcemia.[12,98-101,107,108,111,112]

Low PTH	High PTH	Other
Destruction or partial/total surgical removal of parathyroid glands	Vitamin D deficiency	Medications
Autoimmune	Vitamin D resistance	• Aminoglycosides
Altered parathyroid gland development	Chronic kidney disease	• Amphotericin B
Altered regulation of PTH	PTH resistance	• Bisphosphonates
Hungry-bone syndrome (post parathyroidectomy)	Extravascular calcium deposition	• Calcitonin
Infiltration of parathyroid gland	Hyperphosphatemia (over supplementation)	• Cholestyramine
Hypomagnesemia	Muscle breakdown	• Cisplatin
	Osteoblastic metastases	• Cinacalcet
	Acute pancreatitis	• Citrate (large volumes of banked blood products)
	Sepsis	• Corticosteroids
	Tumor lysis syndrome	• Cyclophosphamide
	Hypomagnesemia post surgery (citrate administration)	• Estrogens
		• Foscarnet
		• Intravenous amino acids (long-term exposure at high doses)
		• Loop diuretics
		• Mithromycin
		• Pentamidine
		• Phenytoin
		• Phenobarbital
		• Phosphate salts
		• Sodium EDTA
		Fluoride toxicity
		Respiratory alkalosis
		Hypoalbuminemia
		Small bowel surgery

EDTA, ethylenediaminetetraacetic acid; PTH, parathyroid hormone.

3. Severe acute hypocalcemia (total serum calcium < 7.5 mg/dL [< 1.9 mmol/L] or ionized serum calcium < 4 mg/dL [< 1 mmol/L]) will manifest as tetany, acute heart failure, and arrhythmias.

4. Chronic hypocalcemia may present with signs and symptoms affecting the central nervous system and integumentary system.

Figure 3-16. Mechanisms of Drugs Commonly Associated With Calcium Disorders.[101,103,107,113–116]

Hypocalcemia	Hypercalcemia
Decrease intestinal absorption • Corticosteroids • Proton pump inhibitors • Histamine-2 receptor antagonists • Low PTH • Cisplatin (high doses) • Loop diuretics • Aminoglycosides • Amphotericin B • Cyclophosphamide • Pentamidine • Cinacalcet Calcium chelators • Citrate (large volumes of banked blood products) • Sodium EDTA • Foscarnet Drug-induced vitamin D deficiency • Phenytoin • Phenobarbital • Cholestyramine (result of bile acid salt depletion) Increase renal losses • Loop diuretics • Corticosteroids • Calcitonin Decrease bone resorption • Bisphosphonates • Calcitonin • Estrogens • Mithromycin	Increase intake or intestinal absorption • Calcium supplements • Vitamin D (in excess) • Lithium Increase bone resorption • Vitamin A • Lithium Increase renal reabsorption • Thiazide diuretics • Lithium • Teriparatide PTH suppression reset • Lithium Enhanced PTH action • Theophylline (toxicity) Increase surge of PTH-related protein by tumor • Tamoxifen

EDTA, ethylenediaminetetraacetic acid; PTH, parathyroid hormone.

Table 3-19. Manifestations of Hypocalcemia.[12,98-100,108,111]

System Affected	Manifestations
Neuromuscular	Chvostek's sign Trousseau's sign Paresthesias Muscle cramps Muscle spasms Tetany Laryngeal spasms
Cardiac	QT prolongation Arrhythmias Bradycardia Hypotension
Central nervous system	Seizures Depression Anxiety Confusion Hallucinations
Integumentary system	Hair loss Grooved nails Brittle nails Eczema

Diagnosis/Diagnostic Tests[12,98,103]

1. Assessment of albumin status

2. Total serum calcium < 8.6 mg/dL (< 2.15 mmol/L)

   - For serum albumin < 4 g/dL, an adjusted total serum calcium calculation should be performed: Corrected total serum calcium (mg/dL) = measured total serum calcium (mg/dL) + [0.8 mg/dL × (4 g/dL − measured albumin (g/dL))]. If total serum calcium is measured in units of millimoles per liter, then a factor of 0.2 mmol/L should be used in place of 0.8 mg/dL.

3. Ionized serum calcium < 4.5 mg/dL (< 1.12 mmol/L)

   - Assessment of ionized serum calcium level should be used in the critical care setting because albumin-adjusted calcium estimations are not reliable. Underlying causes include the presence of severe hypoalbuminemia related to critical illness and/or alterations in serum pH.

   - Ionized serum calcium is inversely correlated with serum pH.

Goals of Therapy

1. The overall goals of therapy are to return serum calcium concentration to normal (total calcium 8.6–10.2 mg/dL or 2.15–2.55 mmol/L) and prevent life-threatening conditions (tetany, cardiac arrhythmias, acute heart failure).

2. Use of the correction equation should be assessed for appropriateness. Obtain ionized calcium in critically ill patients, especially if total serum calcium < 7 mg/dL (< 1.75 mmol/L).

3. Total serum calcium should be corrected to ≥ 8.6 mg/dL (≥ 2.15 mmol/L) or ionized serum calcium to > 4.5 mg/dL (> 1.12 mmol/L) and maintained within normal limits.

4. All concurrent causes of hypocalcemia (medical history, medication/dietary supplement history) should be identified and managed appropriately.

Management[12,98,101,103,107–109,111,117]

1. Oral supplementation appropriate for asymptomatic or mild to moderate hypocalcemia (total serum calcium 7.5–8.5 mg/dL [1.9–2.1 mmol/L]).

2. IV calcium

   - Intermittent IV boluses should be considered in patients with symptomatic or severe hypocalcemia, total serum calcium < 7.5 mg/dL (< 1.9 mmol/L) or ionized serum calcium < 4 mg/dL (< 1 mmol/L), and normal renal function (Table 3-20).

   - Symptomatic hypocalcemia is a medical emergency and should be managed with 1 g of calcium chloride or 2–3 g of calcium gluconate given intravenously over 5–10 minutes.

   - Asymptomatic hypocalcemia should be managed with 2–4 g of calcium gluconate given over 2–4 hours, respectively (1 g/h).

Table 3-20. Calcium Parenteral Products.[12,101,108]

Product[a]	Available Solutions	Elemental Calcium Content per 1000 mg of Solution	Route of Administration
Calcium gluconate	10%	92 mg (4.65 mEq)	Peripheral/central
Calcium chloride	10%	272 mg (13.6 mEq)	Central

[a]To reduce the risk of forming an insoluble solution, calcium products should not be added to intravenous solutions containing bicarbonate or phosphate. Calcium gluconate is less likely to cause injury if extravasated. In nonemergent situations, calcium chloride should be administered through a central venous catheter; maximum infusion rate should not exceed 1.4 mEq of calcium per minute in symptomatic patients.

Figure 3-17. Treatment of Refractory/Severe Hypocalcemia.[99,108,111]

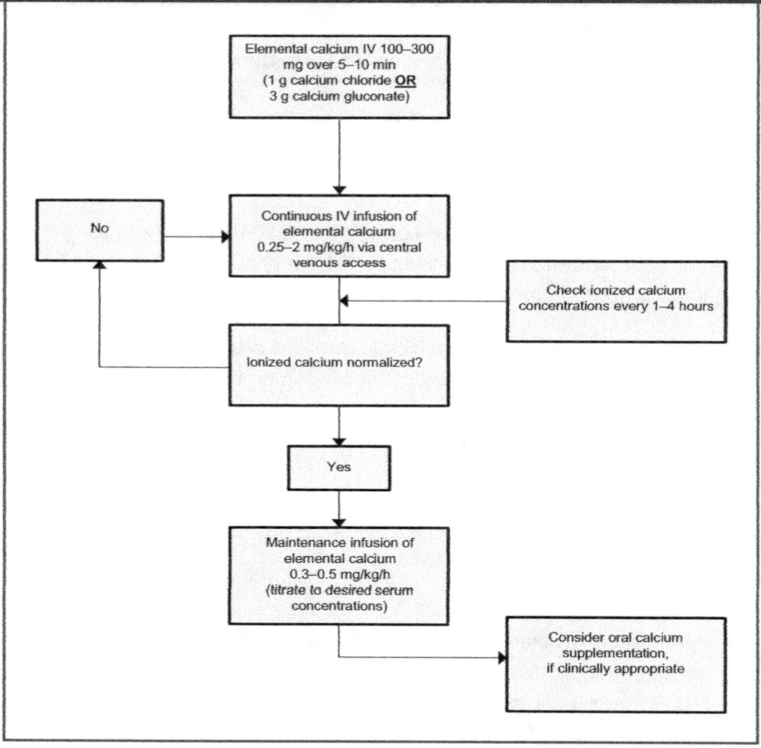

Elemental calcium IV 100–300 mg over 5–10 min (1 g calcium chloride **OR** 3 g calcium gluconate)

Continuous IV infusion of elemental calcium 0.25–2 mg/kg/h via central venous access

Check ionized calcium concentrations every 1–4 hours

Ionized calcium normalized?

No

Yes

Maintenance infusion of elemental calcium 0.3–0.5 mg/kg/h (titrate to desired serum concentrations)

Consider oral calcium supplementation, if clinically appropriate

3. Refractory hypocalcemia should be treated with a continuous infusion of elemental calcium (Figure 3-17).

   - Ionized serum calcium monitoring should occur every 1–4 hours during continuous infusions.

4. Chronic mild to moderate or asymptomatic hypocalcemia should be treated with oral agents.

   - Initial doses are 1–4 g of elemental calcium per day in divided doses (Table 3-21).

   - Vitamin D preparations, such as ergocalciferol (vitamin D_2) or cholecalciferol (vitamin D_3), should be considered in patients with vitamin D deficiency or hypoparathyroidism.

Table 3-21. Calcium Oral/Enteral Products.[12]

Calcium Salt	Elemental Calcium Content per 1000 mg	Elemental Calcium
Citrate	10.5 mEq (210 mg)	21%
Carbonate	20 mEq (400 mg)	40%
Acetate	12.7 mEq (253 mg)	25%
Gluconate	4.65 mEq (92 mg)	9%

Diagnostic Approach to Hypocalcemia[98-103,107-109,111,118,119]

1. Underlying conditions and offending medications should be identified and addressed.

2. Ionized serum calcium level should be followed in critically ill patients and corrected total serum calcium determined in patients with hypoalbuminemia (< 4 g/L).

3. Ionized serum calcium level is altered in critically ill patients with acid-base imbalances.

4. When IV therapy proves effective, oral calcium agents should be considered (if route of administration permits) and started while transitioning off the IV therapy.

5. If hypomagnesemia is present, magnesium should be corrected before calcium replacement is begun.

6. Oral calcium products may interact with concurrently administered oral/enteral medications (Table 3-22).

7. Oral calcium citrate is preferred in patients with achlorhydria.

8. Measurements of serum phosphorus, vitamin D metabolites (25-hydroxyvitamin D), alkaline phosphatase, intact PTH, and magnesium should be performed.

9. Adverse effects of oral calcium and vitamin D supplementation should be monitored.

    - Hypercalcemia and hypercalciuria are prevalent in hypoparathyroid patients.

    - Hypercalciuria can lead to nephrolithiasis, nephrocalcinosis, and CKD.

    - Thiazide diuretics can decrease urinary calcium concentration and lead to hypercalcemia.

Table 3-22. Calcium Affecting the Action of Medication.[119]

Oral/Enteral Medication[a]	Effect on Medication Activity
Tetracyclines	Decrease
Fluoroquinolones	Decrease
β-Blockers	Decrease
Diuretics	Increase
Estrogens	Increase
Bile acid sequestrants	Decrease
Bisphosphonates	Decrease
Thyroxine (levothyroxine)	Decrease
Antiepileptics	Decrease
Digoxin (digitalis)	Increase

[a]This list is not comprehensive; consult a pharmacist for a full list of calcium–medication interactions.

10. Laboratory monitoring of total serum calcium levels should be performed when hypocalcemia is suspected, with subsequent ionized serum calcium (when available) being the preferred laboratory monitoring parameter for treatment management (eg, daily to 3 times weekly).

11. Patients receiving digoxin may not respond despite therapeutic digoxin levels in the setting of hypocalcemia because digoxin is known to increase calcium uptake by cardiac muscle cells.

Monitoring

1. The degree of monitoring should reflect the severity of hypocalcemia and the underlying cause of the disorder.

2. Asymptomatic patients treated conservatively with oral replacement may require assessments every 24–48 hours (inpatient) or every 2–3 months (outpatient).

3. Acute, symptomatic patients who are being aggressively treated should have levels monitored every 4–6 hours until normal serum concentrations are obtained and symptoms are resolved. After such time, every 24–48 hours while hospitalized is appropriate.

Hypercalcemia

Prevalence[99,101,120]

1. Hypercalcemia occurs in approximately 15% of acutely ill patients with a 17%–58% occurrence in cancer patients.

Etiologies and/or Risk Factors[101] (Figure 3-18)

1. Hyperparathyroidism is responsible for 40% of hypercalcemia cases.

2. Malignancy accounts for 30%–40%.

3. Other causes include immobilization, granulomatous disease, and medications.

4. Drug-induced causes of hypercalcemia can be found in Figure 3-16.

Figure 3-18. Etiologies of Hypercalcemia.[12,99,101,103,107,121,122]

Hyperparathyroidism	Malignancy	Other
Primary	Solid organ tumors	Medications
Secondary (long term)	Multiple myeloma	• Excess calcium intake
Tertiary	Lymphoma	• Lithium
	Leukemia	• Thiazide diuretics
		• Vitamin D
		• Vitamin A
		• Teriparatide
		• Theophylline
		• Tamoxifen
		• Al^{3+}/Mg^{2+}-containing antacids
		Granulomatous disease
		Hyperthyroidism
		Adrenal insufficiency
		Paget's disease
		Prolonged immobilization
		Milk alkali syndrome
		Chronic kidney disease

Clinical Presentation[12,101,107] (Table 3-23)

1. Hypercalcemia may be characterized as mild to moderate with a total serum calcium of 10.3–12.9 mg/dL (2.57–3.22 mmol/L) or severe at ≥ 13 mg/dL (≥ 3.25 mmol/L).

2. Patients with mild to moderate hypercalcemia are often asymptomatic.

3. Hypercalcemic crisis is defined by a total serum calcium > 15 mg/dL (> 3.75 mmol/L), AKI, and mental status changes.

Table 3-23. Manifestations of Hypercalcemia.[98,99,107,121,123,124]

System Affected	Manifestations
Cardiac	Bradycardia
	Arrhythmias with ECG changes
	Hypertension
	Digitalis toxicity
Central nervous system	Fatigue
	Altered mental status
	Coma
	Ataxia
	Weakness
	Hypertonia
	Psychosis
	Depression
Renal	Nephrolithiasis
	Nephrocalcinosis
	Acute renal injury
	Polyuria
	Polydipsia
Gastrointestinal	Nausea
	Vomiting
	Anorexia
	Pancreatitis
	Constipation
	Peptic ulcer disease

ECG, electrocardiogram.

Diagnosis/Diagnostic Tests[12,98,103]

1. Assessment of serum albumin level

2. Total serum calcium > 10.2 mg/dL (> 2.55 mmol/L)

3. Ionized serum calcium > 5.2 mg/dL (> 1.3 mmol/L)

   - Assessment of ionized serum calcium should be used in the critical care setting.

   - Ionized serum calcium is inversely correlated with serum pH.

Goals of Therapy

1. The overall goals of therapy are to return serum calcium concentration to normal (total calcium 8.6–10.2 mg/dL or 2.15–2.55 mmol/L) and prevent life-threatening conditions (cardiac arrhythmias, coma, AKI).

2. Appropriateness for correction equation should be assessed and/or the ionized serum calcium obtained.

3. Total serum calcium should be corrected if ≤ 10.2 mg/dL (≤ 2.55 mmol/L) and total serum calcium maintained within normal limits.

4. All concurrent causes of hypercalcemia (medical history, medication/dietary supplement history) should be identified and managed as appropriate.

Management[12,101,120–127]

1. IV fluids, 0.9% NaCl infused at 200–300 mL/h over 24–48 hours, followed by loop diuretics (furosemide, bumetanide) after hypovolemia correction

   - 0.9% NaCl restores intravascular fluids losses from hypercalcemia and initially decreases total serum calcium since sodium promotes calciuresis at the distal nephron.

   - Loop diuretics block calcium reabsorption in the ascending loop of Henle.

2. Bisphosphonates (pamidronate, zolendronic acid, ibandronate)

   - These compounds inhibit farnesyl pyrophosphate synthase enzyme of mevalonate pathway in osteoclasts to reduce total serum calcium.

   - They require up to 2 days before a reduction in total serum calcium is observed; therefore, they should be combined with other therapies listed above.

   - In addition, they require caution in the presence of renal impairment.

3. Calcitonin

- Reserve use of calcitonin for symptomatic patients with severe hypercalcemia.

- Compared with other available agents for the treatment of hypercalcemia, calcitonin has a rapid onset of action (within 12–24 hours) following subcutaneous or intramuscular injection by reducing osteoclastic bone resorption and promoting calciuresis.

- Calcitonin is associated with frequent occurrence of tachyphylaxis within 48 hours, limiting its long-term effectiveness.

- It is beneficial with Paget's disease.

- The intranasal dosage form lacks efficacy in hypercalcemia.

4. Other therapies

- Denosumab

    - This drug should be reserved for patients with hypercalcemia of malignancy with bisphosphonate failure or refractory hypercalcemia.

    - Denosumab inhibits the maturation, survival, and function of osteoclasts.

- Calcimimetics

    - Cinacalcet is available for treatment of hypercalcemia associated with parathyroid carcinoma and hypercalcemia associated with primary hyperparathyroidism, both indications are designed as a FDA orphan drug for these conditions.

- Corticosteroids

    - These drugs are only useful if the tumor responsible for hypercalcemia is inherently corticosteroid responsive.

- Hemodialysis with low calcium dialysate solution

    - This type of hemodialysis is reserved for patients with renal impairment or as salvage therapy when other therapies have failed or are contraindicated.

Diagnostic Approach to Hypercalcemia[98,99,101,102,118,123-126]

1. Identify and address underlying conditions and offending medications.
2. Follow ionized serum calcium in critically ill patients and follow corrected total serum calcium in patients with hypoalbuminemia (< 4 g/dL).
3. Note that ionized serum calcium level is altered in critically ill patients with acid-base imbalances.
4. Consider PTH measurement to rule out PTH-mediated causes of hypercalcemia.
5. Know that IV 0.9% NaCl followed by loop diuretics is considered the first-line therapy.
    - Caution is needed in heart failure and/or renal failure.
    - Loop diuretics cause hypomagnesemia and hypokalemia, which need close monitoring with total serum calcium.
6. Consider IV bisphosphonate therapy in hypercalcemia related to malignancies and consider denosumab for IV bisphosphonate failure.
7. Be aware that calcitonin therapy is associated with tachyphylaxis.
8. Consider oral bisphosphonate therapy for long-term management of hypercalcemia.
9. Use caution in the context of metastatic calcification when correcting hypophosphatemia with IV phosphate during hypercalcemia.
10. Consider hemodialysis in patients who are nonresponsive to traditional therapies, have renal failure, or have contraindications to other therapies.

Monitoring

1. Chronic, asymptomatic patients on cinacalcet therapy should have serum calcium concentrations performed weekly.
2. Acute, asymptomatic patients should have assessments completed every 24–48 hours.

3. Acute, severe, or symptomatic patients should have levels monitored every 4–24 hours until normal serum concentrations are obtained and symptoms are resolved. After such time, every 24–48 hours while hospitalized is appropriate.

Patient/Family Counseling

1. Ensure that the patient and caregivers are educated and aware of the daily calcium intake necessary to maintain nutrition based on the patient's comorbidities.

2. Screen all medications for their ability to potentially cause or exacerbate calcium disorders. The risks and benefits of continuing or discontinuing medications should be discussed with the patient and caregivers. All medications found to be medically unnecessary or to have a higher risk over benefit ratio should be discontinued.

3. Report any abnormal behavior or signs/symptoms of calcium disorders to the patient's clinician immediately.

4. Adjust dietary intake to include or exclude products high in calcium based on the patient's underlying calcium disorder. The patient and caregivers should be instructed on how to properly read a nutrition label and interpret the calcium content. Always verify the patient's daily calcium requirement with the managing clinician.

Foods High in Calcium[96]

1. Milk and milk products (eg, yogurt, cheese, buttermilk, cottage cheese, sour cream)

2. Green leafy vegetables (eg, broccoli, collards, kale, mustard greens, turnip greens, bok choy, Chinese cabbage)

3. Salmon and sardines (canned with soft bones)

4. Soymilk (fortified)

5. Seeds (eg, sunflower, tahini)

6. Nuts (eg, almonds, Brazil nuts)

7. Blackstrap molasses

8. Calcium-fortified foods (eg, orange juice, cereals, breads, tofu)

Medications That May Contribute to Calcium Disorders

Numerous medications can predispose patients to calcium disorders, which necessitates a comprehensive medication review. The patient and caregivers should be counseled on those medications associated with the potential to precipitate calcium disorders. Discussions involving healthcare providers, the patient, and caregivers should be undertaken to ascertain the risk vs benefit of continuing specific therapies or adjusting the treatment regimen (eg, discontinuing the offending medication, adjusting medication dosing, initiating supplementation) to limit possible untoward effects. Figure 3-16 provides a list of medications with their overall mechanism leading to calcium disorders.

Clinical Application

Patient Scenario 1

A 39-year-old man (85 kg) presents to his primary care physician for an annual physical. Upon review of symptoms, he states that he is more fatigued than usual and his mood has not been the best. He attributes this to working long hours at the office and not getting outside for his daily 3-mile run. His vital signs are normal (heart rate 70 beats per minute, blood pressure 130/84 mm Hg, respiratory rate 14 breaths per minute, afebrile). Past medical history is significant for hypothyroidism and seasonal allergies. Daily home medications include levothyroxine 50 mcg orally and loratadine 10 mg orally as needed for allergy symptoms. Significant laboratory results are as follows:

- Calcium, 7.6 mg/dL
- Phosphorus, 3.9 mg/dL
- Magnesium, 1.9 mEq/dL
- Albumin, 3.9 g/dL
- Serum 25-hydroxyvitamin D, 13 ng/mL (deficient < 20 ng/mL, insufficient 20–30 ng/mL)

1. Assess the serum calcium level—mild to moderate hypocalcemia.
    - Serum calcium of 7.6 mg/dL
2. Assess signs and symptoms related to calcium disorder.
    - Fatigue and depressed mood

3. Identify and address underlying conditions and offending medications

    - Vitamin D deficiency is the cause of hypocalcemia. Likely causes of this deficiency are decreased vitamin D intake and limited sun exposure due to working long hours in an office. No medication causes identified.

4. Treatment of hypocalcemia due to vitamin D deficiency includes the following:

    - Oral vitamin D replacement: Vitamin D (in the form of either D_2 or D_3) 50,000 IU orally once weekly for 8 weeks to achieve a 25-hydroxyvitamin D level > 30 ng/mL. At that time, maintenance treatment of 1500–2000 IU/d should be provided.[129]

    - Sensible sun exposure, especially during the hours of 10:00 am and 3:00 pm, is also effective in the treatment of vitamin D deficiency.

    - Oral calcium therapy: 1–4 g of elemental calcium per day in divided doses. Any calcium supplement is appropriate for use.

    - Dietary education should be provided to the patient and caregiver(s) to help increase intake of foods rich in vitamin D and calcium.

5. Monitoring

    - Serum calcium and 25-hydroxyvitamin D measurements after 2–6 months of treatment for deficiency.

Patient Scenario 2

A 52-year-old woman (70 kg) presents to the ED with altered mental status, vomiting, and abdominal and back pain. Her husband reports that the patient has complained of a headache and nausea over the past week, which have limited her oral intake of both fluids and food. Her vital signs are as follows: heart rate, 98 beats per minute; blood pressure, 90/56 mm Hg; respiratory rate, 16 breaths per minute; and temperature, 37.7 °C (99.8 °F). Past medical history is significant for breast cancer (8 years post surgery and chemoradiation) and hypertension. Home oral medications include lisinopril 10 mg daily and hydrochlorothiazide 12.5 mg daily. Bone lesions noted on abdominal x-ray suggestive of metastatic disease.

- Sodium, 143 mEq/L
- Potassium, 3.6 mEq/L
- BUN, 25 mg/dL

- Serum creatinine, 1.1 mg/dL
- Glucose, 88 mg/dL
- Calcium, 13.1 mg/dL
- Phosphorus, 2.6 mg/dL
- Albumin, 3.8 g/dL

1. Assess the serum calcium level—Severe hypercalcemia.
   - Serum calcium of 13.1 mg/dL
2. Assess signs and symptoms related to calcium disorder.
   - Altered mental status, nausea and vomiting, headache, pain, and decreased appetite
3. Identify and address underlying conditions and offending medications.
   - Due to history of breast cancer and abdominal x-ray findings, a full workup should be completed to assess for disease recurrence/ metastatic disease.
   - Use of hydrochlorothiazide predisposes this patient to hypercalcemia. Discontinue therapy and adjust medication regimen for hypertension management if needed since she may be hypovolemic from hypercalcemia. Her lisinopril should also be held with her current blood pressure since it may reduce her renal blood flow as well.
4. Treatment of hypercalcemia of malignancy includes the following:
   - IV fluid administration: 0.9% NaCl at 200–300 mL/h over 24–48 hours.
   - Loop diuretics may be added: furosemide 40 mg intravenously every 6–12 hours or as needed.
   - Calcitonin 4 IU/kg subcutaneously every 12 hours for 1–3 days until bisphosphonate can lower total serum calcium.
   - Bisphosphonate therapy: zolendronic acid 4 mg intravenously over 15 minutes for 1 dose.

5. Monitor the following:

- Vital signs, inputs and outputs, renal function (BUN, serum creatinine), signs and symptoms of fluid overload, and serum electrolytes.
- Measure total serum calcium frequently during fluid administration to assess response to therapy and daily during hospital stay. After hospital discharge, measure total serum calcium every 1–2 weeks.

Phosphorus

Overview

Phosphorus is an essential element of all body tissues and is necessary for a variety of body functions. Disturbances in homeostasis may signify and cause a multitude of clinical disorders.

Generally most disturbances are mild and asymptomatic; however, when they are severe, understanding the physiologic significance and influential factors of phosphorus disorders will impact treatment and management. Phosphorus disorders are encountered frequently and occur in almost every area of clinical practice.

1. Homeostasis and physiological function[130-134]

- Normal serum phosphorus range is generally 2.5–4.5 mg/dL or 0.8–1.5 mmol/L.
- Most laboratories measure elemental phosphorus, but most phosphorus in the body exists in the form of phosphate (PO_4); the terms phosphorus and phosphate are often used interchangeably.
- Phosphorus is a primary anion of the human body and makes up approximately 1% of the total body weight. Approximately 85% of the body's phosphorus is located in the bones and teeth, 14% in the cells, and < 1% is within the ECF.
- Phosphorus is a vital component of all body tissues and has a wide variety of key functions, including formation of energy-storing substances such as ATP; formation of red blood cell 2,3-diphosphoglycerate, which facilitates oxygen delivery to the tissues; metabolism of carbohydrates, protein, and fat; and maintenance of normal pH, neurologic function, and muscular function.

- Serum phosphorus level is determined by a combination of factors, including dietary intake, intestinal absorption, bone resorption and deposition, distribution between ICF and ECF compartments, and renal excretion.

- Phosphorus balance is closely tied to calcium homeostasis.

2. Dietary intake[130,133–136]

- Thirty-one milligrams of elemental phosphorus is equal to 1 mmol of phosphate.

- The average adult intake for a Western diet is 1000–1600 mg/d.

- About two-thirds of phosphate is actively absorbed from the proximal small intestine, predominately in the jejunum.

- Absorption is increased by the presence of vitamin D and moderate amounts of calcium.

- Phosphorus absorption is diminished in the presence of a large amount of calcium or aluminum in the intestine (eg, antacids) due to *formation of insoluble phosphate compounds.*

3. Excretion[132,133,135]

- About 90% of serum phosphorus is filterable at the renal glomerulus, with active reabsorption predominately by the proximal tubules in the kidneys.

- Renal transport is saturable, pH dependent, and requires sodium ions.

- PTH inhibits the reabsorption of phosphorus throughout the nephron. Interactions between PTH and serum phosphorus are mutually regulatory since increasing the serum phosphorus levels stimulate PTH secretion, thereby promoting renal phosphorus excretion.

- Fibroblast growth hormone 23 is secreted by the osteocytes and osteoblasts in response to a phosphorus load, and it induces greater urinary fractional excretion of phosphorus.

- Excreted phosphorus is primarily found in the urine, with the remainder eliminated via stool.

Hypophosphatemia

Prevalence and Mortality[134,137,138]

1. An estimated 2.2%–3.1% of hospitalized patients will have moderate hypophosphatemia (serum phosphorus 1–2 mg/dL), and 0.2%–0.4% will have severe hypophosphatemia (serum phosphorus < 1 mg/dL).
   - Approximately 45% of all hospital cases are reported to occur in critically ill patients.
   - Hypophosphatemia occurs more frequently in diabetic ketoacidosis, sepsis, trauma, burns, and renal replacement therapy and in the postoperative period.
2. Mortality depends on the acuity and severity of depletion.
   - Mild and transient hypophosphatemia is generally asymptomatic and is not accompanied by long-term complications.
   - Acute severe hypophosphatemia can manifest as widespread organ dysfunction and has been reported to predict up to an 8-fold increased mortality rate in patients with sepsis.
   - Multiple studies have shown an association between hypophosphatemia and increased mortality, but it remains unclear whether hypophosphatemia leads to mortality or is merely a marker for severity of illness.

Risk Factors[138]

1. Hypophosphatemia secondary to intracellular shifts is more likely to occur in respiratory alkalosis, after a carbohydrate load, with PN containing inadequate phosphate, in nutrition recovery, and during androgen therapy.
2. Hypophosphatemia secondary to urinary losses include hypomagnesemia; hypokalemia; hyperparathyroidism; use of diuretics such as acetazolamide, thiazides, or loop diuretics; diuretic phase of acute tubular necrosis; and Fanconi's syndrome.
3. Hypophosphatemia is more likely with a reduction of intestinal absorption secondary to malabsorption disorders, vomiting, diarrhea, prolonged gastric suctioning, and the use of aluminum antacids and phosphate binders.

4. Other possible risk factors include alcoholism and acute alcohol withdrawal, diabetic ketoacidosis, vitamin D deficiency, mannitol use, liver transplantation, and severe burns.

Etiology[134,137]

1. Hypophosphatemia can be caused by 3 different mechanisms: decreased intestinal intake or absorption, increased renal losses, or internal redistribution (Table 3-24).

Table 3-24. Common Causes of Hypophosphatemia.[134,137]

Mechanism	Cause
Decreased intestinal intake or absorption	Malnutrition Phosphate-binding agents Vitamin D deficiency Secretory diarrhea Steatorrhea Vomiting Malabsorption Pancreatic exocrine insufficiency Nasogastric suctioning
Increase renal losses	Metabolic acidosis Diuretics Volume expansion Corticosteroids Kidney disorders (tubular) Hereditary syndromes Malignancy-induced through PTH-related protein Hyperparathyroidism
Internal redistribution (shifts into the cells)	Acute without depletion • Respiratory alkalosis • Dextrose and insulin release/administration • Catecholamines Acute with depletion • Recovery from malnutrition (refeeding syndrome) • Recovery from diabetic ketoacidosis • Rapid cell uptake/proliferation (hungry bone syndrome, acute leukemia)

PTH, parathyroid hormone.

Clinical Presentation[12,134,137-144]

1. Most symptoms result from decreases in cellular functions that require energy, ATP, and 2,3-diphosphoglycerate.

2. Generally, an acute change in serum phosphorus to < 1 mg/dL is more commonly associated with symptoms compared to chronic changes. Common clinical manifestations are

   - Respiratory: respiratory muscle dysfunction, decreased O_2 delivery
   - Cardiac: decreased contractility; arrhythmias, chest pain, cardiomyopathy
   - Hematologic: hemolysis, leukocyte and platelet dysfunction, thrombocytopenia
   - Endocrine: insulin resistance
   - Neuromuscular: myopathy, peripheral nerve paresthesias, rhabdomyolysis, seizures, altered mental status, coma

3. Chronic depletion occurs over several weeks to years. It can be asymptomatic, but individuals may exhibit memory loss, osteomalacia, bone loss/fractures, and arthralgia.

Diagnosis/Diagnostic Tests[12,134,137-139]

1. Hypophosphatemia is defined as a serum phosphorus < 2.5 mg/dL.

   - Mild hypophosphatemia: 2–2.4 mg/dL
   - Moderate hypophosphatemia: 1–1.9 mg/dL
   - Severe hypophosphatemia: < 1 mg/dL

2. PTH level may be normal or elevated in hyperparathyroidism or vitamin D deficiency.

   - PTH secretion results in increased movement of phosphorus out of the bone as well as increased urinary excretion of phosphorus.

3. Serum 25-hydroxyvitamin D levels may be low or inappropriately normal.

   - Adequate vitamin D status enhances absorption of phosphorus in the small intestine.

4. Serum magnesium may be decreased because of increased urinary excretion of magnesium during hypophosphatemia.

5. Alkaline phosphatase may be elevated with the increased osteoblast activity.

6. X-ray studies may reveal the skeletal changes typical of osteomalacia or bone fractures seen in chronic hypophosphatemia.

Goals of Therapy

1. Therapeutic goals include returning the serum phosphorus concentration to normal (2.5–4.5 mg/dL) and resolving symptoms of hypophosphatemia.

2. Treatment should be directed at the underlying cause.

Management[12,141–149]

1. Phosphorus replacement for treatment of acute depletion can be given either enterally or intravenously (Table 3-25).

2. Oral repletion is safer, but the absorption of oral supplements can be unpredictable, and higher doses lead to intolerance with GI symptoms such as abdominal cramping and diarrhea.

Table 3-25. Select Oral/Enteral and Intravenous Phosphorus Replacements.[137,148,149]

Preparation (Dosage)	Phosphate Content	Sodium Content	Potassium Content
Oral preparations[a]			
Skim milk, 1 cup (240 mL)	250 mg (8 mmol)	126 mg (5.5 mmol)	406 mg (10 mEq)
Phos-NaK (powder for solution, 1 packet)	250 mg (8 mmol)	160 mg (6.9 mmol)	280 mg (7.1 mEq)
K-Phos Neutral (tablet, 250 mg) Phospha 250 Neutral (tablet, 250 mg)	250 mg (8 mmol)	298 mg (13 mmol)	45 mg (1.1 mEq)
K-Phos No. 2 (tablet, 250 mg)	250 mg (8 mmol)	134 mg (5.8 mmol)	88 mg (2.3 mEq)
Intravenous preparations[b]			
Sodium phosphate (1 mL)	11 mg (3 mmol)	4 mEq	0
Potassium phosphate (1 mL)	11 mg (3 mmol)	0	4.4 mEq

[a]Phosphorus, 31 mg = 1 mmol; sodium, 23 mg = 1 mmol (1 mEq); potassium, 39 mg = 1 mmol (1 mEq).

[b]Sodium phosphate, 1 mmol = 1.33 mEq sodium; potassium phosphate, 1 mmol = 1.47 mEq potassium.

3. IV repletion corrects hypophosphatemia more rapidly, but adverse effects may include thrombophlebitis, hypocalcemia, arrhythmias, ectopic calcification, and AKI.

   - IV phosphate formulations are available as potassium or sodium salts.

     - Potassium phosphate can be used in patients with concurrent hypokalemia; otherwise, sodium phosphate is the preferred salt because it contains approximately one-third the amount of aluminum as potassium phosphate (especially important in neonates).

     - Patients experiencing volume overload or hypernatremia or those requiring sodium restriction should be evaluated for possible complications before the use of the sodium phosphate salt.

   - Total IV phosphate dose should be infused over 4–6 hours and not more than 7 mmol phosphate per hour to minimize adverse effects such as calcium/phosphate precipitation. Limiting the administration to 7 mmol phosphate per hour would be approximately 10 mEq potassium per hour if potassium phosphate is used and would be appropriate for patients not on telemetry. Thrombophlebitis may develop if potassium phosphate is infused in a peripheral vein.

4. Severity of hypophosphatemia is important in determining the urgency and mode of treatment. Generally, treatment is based on the degree of depletion, presence of symptoms, and ability to tolerate enteral supplementation. Hypophosphatemia treatment is divided into 3 categories: mild, moderate, and severe.

   - Mild hypophosphatemia (serum phosphorus 2–2.4 mg/dL) can usually be treated by increasing dietary intake or using an oral phosphate supplement.

   - Moderate hypophosphatemia (serum phosphorus 1–1.9 mg/dL) can usually be treated with a dietary/oral phosphate supplement, but may require IV replacement. The decision to replace by IV depends on if hypophosphatemia is symptomatic, the severity of illness, and the underlying cause of depletion.

   - Severe hypophosphatemia (serum phosphorus < 1 mg/dL) generally necessitates treatment with IV phosphate.

   - IV therapy is also indicated in a patient who cannot tolerate or is unable to ingest oral medications or in a patient in whom enteral access is lacking.

   - Phosphate dosing has a wide therapeutic index because serum concentrations usually do not correlate with total body stores and dosing is primarily based upon degree of severity. Suggested dosing is provided in Table 3-26.

Table 3-26. Treatment of Hypophosphatemia.[12,138-148,a]

Degree of Hypophosphatemia	Oral/Enteral Phosphate Replacement Dosage[b]	IV Phosphate Replacement Dosage[c]
2-2.4 mg/dL (mild, asymptomatic)	1000-2000 mg/d divided into 4 or 5 doses	0.08-0.16 mmol/kg
1-1.9 mg/dL (moderate, asymptomatic)	1000-2000 mg/d divided into 4 or 5 doses	0.16-0.32 mmol/kg
1-1.5 mg/dL (moderate, symptomatic) or < 1 mg/dL (severe, symptomatic)	IV treatment recommended	0.32-1 mmol/kg

IV, intravenous.

[a]In patients with normal renal function or receiving continuous renal replacement therapy; patients with renal insufficiency should receive ≤ 50% of the initial empiric dose.

[b]Monitor for gastrointestinal intolerance, may require IV replacement if oral phosphate not tolerated.

[c]Maximum infusion rate = 7 mmol phosphate per hour.

Diagnostic Approach to Hypophosphatemia[12,139,140,149]

1. The cause of the hypophosphatemia should be identified and corrected.

- The cause of depletion is often evident from the patient history and assessment (Table 3-24).
- Physical examination identifies consequences and suggests potential risks and possible causes.
  - Symptoms may be nonspecific, but generalized muscle weakness and fatigue are common in chronic depletion.
  - Careful assessment of skeletal structure for signs of weakness, pathological fractures or pseudofractures, and skeletal deformities is needed. Bone pain may also be present.
  - Assess for severe muscle pain because it may indicate rhabdomyolysis.
  - Note any rachitic features (eg, distention of bone-cartilage junctions in ribs) in adults because these features suggest chronic hypophosphatemia since childhood.
  - Assess nutrition status with a weight history detailing the degree and duration of weight loss and a nutrition intake history evaluating inadequate or imbalanced nutrient intake. This assessment will help identify malnutrition and risk of refeeding syndrome with nutrition recovery.

- Review medication history. Drugs such as insulin; laxatives; diuretics, including acetazolamide, thiazides, or loop diuretics; antacids; magnesium supplements; and phosphate binders are commonly associated with hypophosphatemia.

- Laboratory assessment should include the evaluation of other electrolytes and renal function.
  - Serum electrolytes including magnesium and calcium, glucose, BUN, serum creatinine should be assessed because many causes of hypophosphatemia such as refeeding with malnutrition, renal tubular disease, diabetic ketoacidosis, and hungry bone syndrome after parathyroidectomy often result in other electrolyte deficiencies.
  - Serum creatine kinase levels should also be assessed if muscle pain is present.
  - When musculoskeletal symptoms, hypomagnesemia, and/or hypoalbuminemia are present, or if the cause is still unknown, ionized calcium, PTH, and 25-hydroxyvitamin D levels should be assessed.
- If further assessment is warranted, then measurement of urinary phosphorus excretion should assist with determining if the cause is due to renal phosphorus wasting.
  - The ratio of the maximum rate of tubular phosphate reabsorption to the GFR (TmP/GFR) requires the measurement of phosphorus and creatinine in a fasting serum sample and second voided urine sample in the morning. TmP/GFR approximates the fraction of filtered phosphorus that appears in the urine.

$$\text{TmP/GFR (mg/dL)} = \left\{1 - \left[\left(\frac{\text{urine phosphorus}}{\text{serum phosphorus}}\right) \times \left(\frac{\text{serum creatinine}}{\text{urine creatinine}}\right)\right]\right\} \times \text{serum phosphorus}$$

Note: Urine and serum values are in mg/dL units

  - TmP/GFR reference range is 2.5–4.2 mg/dL.
  - A TmP/GFR < 2.5 mg/dL indicates renal phosphorus wasting and may warrant evaluation of serum fibroblast growth factor 23.
    - Serum fibroblast growth factor 23 is produced by mesenchymal tumors associated with osteomalacia and the gene responsible for hereditary hypophosphatemic rickets.

2. Treatment should also include addressing the underlying cause. Removal of causative medication(s) and the development of a nutrition plan to treat deficiencies need to be included in treatment strategies.

3. Route of replacement, either oral/enterally or intravenously, depends on the severity and presence of symptoms.

4. If patients are at risk for refeeding syndrome (see Chapter 5), hypophosphatemia should be corrected PRIOR to initiation of any form of nutrition support.

Monitoring[12,139,140,148,149]

1. The degree of monitoring should reflect the severity of hypophosphatemia and the underlying cause of the disorder.

2. Asymptomatic patients treated conservatively with oral replacement may require assessment of daily levels to ensure that the serum phosphorus level is improving.

3. Symptomatic or mechanically ventilated patients who are being aggressively treated with IV phosphate should have serum phosphorus levels monitored 2–4 hours after infusion to ensure response and assist with need for additional supplementation.

4. Patients at risk for acute hypophosphatemia, such as those who are critically ill or malnourished individuals at risk for refeeding syndrome, should have serum phosphorus levels monitored every 12–24 hours.

5. Patients with chronic depletion should have serum ionized calcium, magnesium, phosphorus, potassium, and creatinine monitored monthly until stable, then every 3 months with alkaline phosphatase and PTH measurements every 6–12 months.

Hyperphosphatemia

Prevalence and Mortality[136,150,153]

1. Hyperphosphatemia is rare in the general population, but it is a common disorder in patients with CKD.

2. Elevation can occur at any age, but it is more common with advanced age. The incidence is directly related to the presence and severity of renal compromise.

3. It is associated with increased cardiovascular disease morbidity and mortality in both the general and CKD populations.

4. Increases in serum phosphorus levels have also been associated with left ventricular hypertrophy, development of secondary hyperparathyroidism, and CKD progression and are linked to arterial calcifications.

Risk Factors[154]

1. Risk is greatest when renal impairment is present and the body has lost the ability to regulate phosphate balance via renal excretion.

Etiology[136,150–155]

1. Hyperphosphatemia occurs primarily from 3 different mechanisms: an increased phosphorus load, a primary increase in renal phosphate reabsorption, and a decrease in renal phosphorus excretion.
   - An increased load of either exogenous or endogenous phosphorus will overwhelm renal phosphorus excretion. Common causes are the following:
     - Excessive exogenous intake can occur with administration of any phosphate supplements, use of enemas and laxatives containing phosphate, or vitamin D excess with increased GI phosphorus absorption. IV lipid emulsions contain 15 mmol phosphate/L and may contribute in patients with AKI or CKD.
     - Increased endogenous phosphorus release from the ICF occurs in conditions such as neoplastic disease (eg, leukemia and lymphoma), tumor lysis syndrome, chemotherapy, increased tissue catabolism, massive hemolysis, and rhabdomyolysis. Traumatic crush injuries also cause a large endogenous load of phosphorus that overwhelms the renal threshold.
     - Other causes that shift serum phosphorus from the ICF to the ECF include lactic acidosis, diabetic ketoacidosis, and respiratory acidosis.
   - Elevation secondary to increased tubular reabsorption of phosphorus results from deficiencies in PTH or fibroblast growth hormone 23 or resistance to their actions.
     - Conditions that cause increased tubular reabsorption include hypoparathyroidism, vitamin D toxicity, familial tumoral calcinosis, use of bisphosphonates, and acromegaly.
   - Decreased urinary phosphorus excretion is most commonly found in AKI and CKD.
     - When GFR falls to $< 20–25$ mL/min, urinary phosphorus excretion is usually not enough to offset phosphorus dietary intake.

2. Pseudohyperphosphatemia (false or factitious hyperphosphatemia) is a laboratory error caused by interference with analytical methods. Such errors may occur in the context of hyperglobulinemia due to multiple myeloma, Waldenstrom's macroglobulinemia, or monoclonal gammopathy; hyperlipidemia; hemolysis; liposomal amphotericin B therapy; or blood sample contamination with heparin or tissue plasminogen activator.

   - In these scenarios, the serum phosphorus level can be determined by using a different analyzer.

Clinical Presentation

1. Clinical manifestations of hyperphosphatemia are few and nonspecific. They include anorexia, nausea, vomiting, muscle weakness, hyperreflexia, tetany, and tachycardia.

2. Most symptoms that do occur are nearly the same as for hypocalcemia because of the inverse relationship that exists between calcium and phosphorus (see hypocalcemia sections).

3. *Soft tissue and vascular calcifications can occur when the serum calcium-*phosphorus product exceeds 55 mg^2/dL^2. These calcifications may involve the joints, skin, and soft tissues as well as the cornea, lung, and kidney.

   Calcium-phosphorus product (mg^2/dL^2) = Total serum calcium × Serum phosphorus

   Note: Serum values are in mg/dL units and total serum calcium should *not* be corrected for hypoalbuminemia.

   - Ideally, serum phosphorus levels should be ≤ 4.5 mg/dL in patients with stage 3–5 CKD.

Diagnosis/Diagnostic Tests[136,154]

1. Hyperphosphatemia is defined as a serum phosphorus > 4.5 mg/dL. Improper handling can lead to hemolysis of a sample and pseudohyperphosphatemia.

2. Assessment of total serum calcium level is useful in evaluating potential consequences of treatment and diagnosing the primary problem. Serum ionized calcium should be evaluated with concurrent hypoalbuminemia.

3. PTH and 25-hydroxyvitamin D levels assist with determining the cause of hyperphosphatemia.

4. BUN and serum creatinine levels will help determine renal function and if the kidneys are appropriately eliminating phosphorus.

5. X-ray studies may reveal skeletal changes resulting from osteodystrophy (defective bone development) in chronic hyperphosphatemia.

6. ECG changes such as prolonged QT-interval, which is characteristic of hypocalcemia, establish the severity of symptoms and guide treatment strategies.

7. Hyperphosphatemia should be classified as acute (usually associated with symptomatic hypocalcemia secondary to a large phosphorus load) or chronic (commonly associated with renal function decline).

Goals of Therapy[154]

1. Therapeutic goals include returning serum phosphorus concentration to normal (2.5–4.5 mg/dL), and resolving symptoms of hyperphosphatemia, which may include those related to hypocalcemia.

2. Treatment should be directed at the underlying cause.

Management[136,152–156]

1. Acute hyperphosphatemia in an individual with normal renal function is most often related to an acute phosphorus load. This sharp rise in serum level is also more pronounced in a patient with CKD or dehydration because they are more susceptible to complications. When severe and symptomatic, acute hyperphosphatemia can be life threatening.

   - Treatment is aimed at increasing renal phosphorus excretion by extracellular volume expansion with 0.9% NaCl IV infusion.

   - All external phosphorus sources should be discontinued if possible (eg, IV lipid emulsion or propofol).

   - Use of a loop diuretic may be concomitantly administered to aid in renal elimination in patients without hypotension or volume depletion.

   - An elevated serum phosphorus level resolves rapidly (6–12 hours) because phosphorus is readily cleared with normal kidney function.

   - Closely monitor total serum calcium levels for potential hypocalcemia. Serum ionized calcium should be evaluated with concurrent hypoalbuminemia and hypocalcemia symptoms.

   - Hemodialysis may be indicated in patients with symptomatic hypocalcemia or severe hyperphosphatemia (> 12 mg/dL).

2. Phosphorus retention associated with AKI commonly seen with tumor lysis syndrome is usually treated with dietary intake restriction or oral phosphate binders. Additional treatment measures include hydration with 0.9% NaCl infusion, dialysis, or hemofiltration.

3. Treatment of chronic hyperphosphatemia consists of dietary restriction and use of oral phosphate-binding medications to increase elimination of phosphorus from the GI tract (Table 3-27).

4. In dialysis patients, hyperphosphatemia may also be managed by adjusting the dialysis dose and/or schedule.

Diagnostic Approach to Hyperphosphatemia[152-159]

1. Once hyperphosphatemia is suspected, a thorough patient history, comprehensive metabolic laboratory panel, and physical assessment should be obtained.

2. Patient history should include a review of factors that influence homeostasis including:

    - Increased intake
        - Excessive administration of supplements containing phosphorus
        - Increased intake of vitamin D supplements
    - Decreased renal function
        - AKI or CKD
        - Hypoparathyroidism
        - Volume depletion/dehydration
    - Extracellular shifts or release from intracellular space
        - Respiratory acidosis
        - Metabolic acidosis
        - Neoplastic disease (leukemia, lymphoma)
        - Tumor lysis syndrome
        - Recent chemotherapy
        - Increased tissue catabolism
        - Rhabdomyolysis or crush injury

Table 3-27. Common Phosphate-Binding Agents.[12,136,154,155,157]

Binder Available Form	Mineral Content	Initial Daily Dose[a]	Recommended Maximum Dose[a,b]	Potential Advantages	Potential Disadvantages
Aluminum hydroxide: tablets, 300 mg, 600 mg; suspension, 320 mg/5 mL	100 to > 200 mg Al per dose	300–600 mg, 3–4 times daily	30 mL every 4 h	Effective for short-term use, inexpensive	Risk of bone, hematological, and neurological toxicity; not recommended for long-term use
Calcium acetate: tablet, 667 mg; caplet, 667 mg	250 mg elemental Ca/g	1334 mg, 3 times daily	2668 mg, 3 times daily (avoid hypercalcemia)	Effective, inexpensive	May contribute to hypercalcemia; oversuppression of PTH, promote vascular calcification, or both
Calcium carbonate: tablet, capsule, liquid, and powder; various strengths	400 mg of elemental Ca/g	1000–2000 mg, 3 times daily	2000 mg, 3 times daily (avoid hypercalcemia)	Effective, inexpensive, readily available	May contribute to hypercalcemia; oversuppression of PTH, promote vascular calcification, or both
Magnesium hydroxide: tablets, 311 mg; liquid, 400 and 800 mg/5 mL	420 mg of elemental Mg/g	300–600 mg, 3 times daily	1200 mg, 4 times daily (avoid hypermagnesemia)	Effective, inexpensive, readily available	Risk of hypermagnesemia; long-term effect not known; diarrhea common
Sevelamer: tablets, 400 mg, 800 mg; powder packet, 400 mg	None	800–1600 mg, 3 times daily	3200 mg, 3 times daily (max total daily dose studied 13–14 g)	Effective, no Ca or metal content; not absorbed; reduces LDL-cholesterol;	Expensive; GI side effects
Lanthanum carbonate: chewable tablet, 500, 750, 1000 mg	500, 750, and 1000 mg of elemental La per tablet	500 mg, 3 times daily	1500 mg, 3 times daily	Effective, does not contain Ca or Mg	Expensive; potential for accumulation in bone and other tissues
Sucroferric oxyhydroxide: chewable tablets, 500 mg	500 mg of Fe per tablet	500 mg, 3 times daily	1000 mg, 3 times daily	Effective, does not contain Ca or Mg, very little, if any Fe absorption	Expensive; GI side effects; long-term effect not known

GI, gastrointestinal; LDL, low-density lipoprotein cholesterol; PTH, parathyroid hormone.

[a]Timing of doses should be with meals. The dosage should be adjusted to achieve the goal serum phosphorus level.

[b]May require higher doses in rare situations or in some patient with severe hyperphosphatemia and chronic kidney disease.

3. Laboratory assessment involves the following:
   - Assessment of the serum phosphorus level
     - A value > 4.5 mg/dL is diagnostic.
   - Careful examination of renal function
     - AKI or worsening CKD will diminish phosphorus excretion.
   - Assessment of the total serum calcium level
     - Because of the interrelationship between serum phosphorus and calcium, hypocalcemia (total serum calcium < 8.6 mg/dL or ionized calcium < 4.5 mg/dL) may be present and needs to be addressed and monitored as hyperphosphatemia is treated.
   - Further laboratory assessment to diagnose the etiology of hyperphosphatemia
     - Assessment of the serum PTH and vitamin D levels
       - PTH levels will assist with evaluation of parathyroid involvement.
       - 25-Hydroxyvitamin D levels assist with diagnosis of vitamin D intoxication or milk alkali syndrome.
     - Measurement of urinary phosphate levels in patients with normal renal function
       - Urinary phosphorus levels > 1500 mg/dL imply excess phosphorus load.
       - Urinary phosphorus levels < 1500 mg/dL suggest increased renal reabsorption.
4. If elevation is acute, especially with symptomatic hypocalcemia, prompt treatment including discontinuation of all external phosphorus sources should be carried out because this condition can be life threatening.
5. If chronic hyperphosphatemia is suspected, treatment depends on underlying cause (see Table 3-28).
   - Elevation in hypoparathyroidism results from increased renal phosphorus reabsorption, leading to elevated serum phosphorus levels. Treatment with oral calcium and vitamin D (calcitriol [1,25-dihydroxyvitamin D]) lowers serum phosphorus value but not always back to the normal range.

Table 3-28. Laboratory Findings for Common Causes of Chronic Hyperphosphatemia.[152]

Cause	Serum Phosphate	Serum Calcium	PTH	Renal Function (BUN, SCr Levels)	Vitamin D
Hypoparathyroidism	↑	↓	↓	↔	↔
Chronic kidney disease	↑	↓	↔, ↑	↑	↔, ↓
Vitamin D intoxication	↑	↑	↔	↔	↑
Milk alkali syndrome	↑	↑	↓	↔	↓
Familial tumoral calcinosis	↑	↔	↔	↔	↑

↑, increase; ↓, decrease; ↔, within normal limits; BUN, blood urea nitrogen; PTH, parathyroid hormone; SCr, serum creatinine.

- Hyperphosphatemia will occur in CKD and worsen with advancing stage.
  - The current recommendations are to initiate treatment when serum phosphorus levels are above the normal range.
  - The Kidney Disease: Outcomes Quality Initiative (KDOQI) 2017 clinical guidelines for bone metabolism and disease in CKD recommended targeting a normal serum phosphorus level.
  - Treatment strategies for hyperphosphatemia in renal failure patients include the following:

    1. Dietary restriction
        - Restrict dietary intake to 800–1000 mg/d.
        - Intensified dietary instruction from a registered dietitian with counseling on avoidance of food additives that contribute an extra phosphorus load is more successful in reaching phosphorus laboratory goals.
        - See the foods high in phosphorus section for a list of foods that should be avoided or limited.
    2. Phosphate binders
        - Binders are used in combination with dietary restriction.
        - They are generally classified as calcium-containing (calcium carbonate, calcium citrate or calcium acetate) or non–calcium-containing (sevelamer, lanthanum carbonate or sucroferric oxyhydroxide, and aluminum hydroxide).

- Calcium-based binders should be avoided in patients with hypercalcemia and vascular calcifications.
- Aluminum-based binders are no longer recommended for chronic treatment due to the systemic aluminum toxicity.

- Magnesium salts are not widely used due to lack of long-term studies, common GI side effects, and potential for hypermagnesemia.
    - See Table 3-27 for more information on phosphate binders as a treatment option.

3. Dialysis
    - Phosphorus removal varies among the different modalities of dialysis and duration of treatment.
    - Conventional, intermittent hemodialysis is largely inadequate for elimination of the total amount of phosphorus absorbed in 1 week from a standard protein intake.
    - *In CKD patients on dialysis, effective removal of phosphorus during dialysis treatment should be ensured.*
    - When usual dialysis prescription is not sufficient, an increase in frequency and/or duration of dialysis should be considered.

Monitoring[12,158,159]

1. In patients with acute elevations secondary to excessive phosphorus load or AKI, monitoring serum levels every 12–24 hours is sufficient. In patients who are severely ill, more frequent monitoring may be necessary.

2. Recommended monitoring parameters for CKD patients are listed in Table 3-29.

Patient/Family Counseling

1. Ensure that the patient and caregivers are educated and aware of the daily phosphorus intake necessary to maintain nutrition based on the patient's comorbidities.

2. All medications should be screened for their ability to potentially cause or exacerbate phosphorus disorders. The risks and benefits of continuing or discontinuing medications should be discussed with

Table 3-29. Monitoring Parameters.[159]

Disease State	Calcium and Phosphorus	Parathyroid Hormone	Alkaline Phosphatase
CKD stage 3	6–12 mo	Baseline and CKD progression	N/A
CKD stage 4	3–6 mo	6–12 mo	Annually or more frequently if PTH is elevated
CKD stage 5	1–3 mo	3–6 mo	Annually or more frequently if PTH is elevated
AKI	12–24 h	N/A	N/A

AKI, acute kidney injury; CKD, chronic kidney disease; PTH, parathyroid hormone.

the patient. All medications found to be medically unnecessary or having a higher risk than benefit should be discontinued.

3. Any excessive fluid losses, abnormal behavior, or signs or symptoms of phosphorus disorders should be reported to the patient's clinician immediately.

4. Dietary intake should be adjusted to include or exclude products high in phosphorus based on the patient's underlying phosphorus disorder. The patient and caregivers should be instructed on how to properly read a nutrition label and interpret the phosphorus content. Always verify the patient's daily phosphorus allowance with the managing clinician.

Foods High in Phosphorus[135]

1. Meats, especially organ meats

2. Fish

3. Poultry

4. Milk and milk products (eg, cheese, cottage cheese, ice cream)

5. Whole grains

6. Seeds (eg, pumpkin, sesame, sunflower)

7. Nuts (eg, Brazil nuts, peanuts)

8. Beans and peas (eg, tofu, baked beans)

9. Eggs and egg products

Figure 3-19. Medications Commonly Associated With Phosphorus Disorders.[134,137]

Hypophosphatemia	Hyperphosphatemia
Decrease intake or intestinal absorption	Increase administration or absorption
• Phosphate binders (see Table 3-25)	• Phosphorus supplements
Increase renal losses	• Phosphorus-containing laxatives and enemas
• Diuretics	• Vitamin D (in excess)
• Corticosteroids	Increase renal reabsorption
Transcellular (intracellular) shift	• Vitamin D (in excess)
• Glucose/dextrose	• Bisphosphonates (eg, pamidronate, zolendronate)
• Insulin	Cellular lysis
• Catecholamines	• Chemotherapy for leukemia or lymphoma

The source of dietary phosphorus is important because plant-derived foods are less bioavailable than animal-derived food or heavily processed foods.

Medications That May Contribute to Phosphorus Disorders

Please see Figure 3-19 for a list of medications of commonly associated with phosphorus disorders.

Clinical Application

Patient Scenario 1

A 79-year-old woman (54 kg) presents to the ED with a 2-day history of vomiting and dehydration. She is 8 weeks post colostomy and sigmoid resection secondary to a diverticulitis-related rupture. Her vital signs are normal (heart rate, 65 beats per minute; blood pressure, 126/82 mm Hg; respiratory rate, 15 breaths per minute; afebrile) on presentation, and she denies any fevers or chills. The patient has not taken any medications in the past 48 hours. She reports that she has not been able to eat solid foods for more than 2 weeks and has lost 20 pounds since surgery. Past medical history is significant for rheumatoid arthritis. She is admitted to the hospital and on day 2, PN is initiated. The next day, she is transferred to the unit after developing respiratory distress and requiring mechanical ventilation. Her laboratory results are as follows:

- Serum sodium, 140 mEq/L
- Serum potassium, 2.9 mEq/L
- Serum creatinine, 0.8 mg/dL
- BUN, 15 mg/dL
- Glucose, 125 mg/dL
- Serum phosphorus, 0.3 mg/dL

1. Assess the serum phosphorus level.
    - Serum phosphorus of 0.3 mg/dL: severe deficiency
2. Assess the patient for symptoms of hypophosphatemia.
    - Patient develops respiratory distress after 12 hours of PN therapy, requiring mechanical ventilation.
3. Treatment options include the following:
    - Based on the severity and presence of symptoms, IV phosphorus replacement at a dose of 0.32–1 mmol/kg should be infused. For this patient, IV dose would be approximately 18–54 mmol phosphate.
    - Hypokalemia is also present with serum potassium of 2.9 mEq/L. Use of potassium phosphate will allow for correction of both potassium and phosphorus in a single IV bag. For this patient, dose of potassium provided would be 27–79 mEq.
4. Monitoring includes the following:
    - Checking serum phosphorus 2 hours post infusion of replacement dose.
    - Repeat replacement if hypophosphatemia is still present. Dose should be based on the current laboratory value, not the original laboratory value.
    - Continue to check 2 hours post infusion and repeat replacement based on the current laboratory value until serum phosphorus is corrected.
    - If potassium phosphate is used for supplementation, the serum potassium should also be monitored.

Patient Scenario 2

A 63-year-old woman (60 kg) with stage 4 CKD presents with fasting laboratory measures of serum phosphorus, 6.5 mg/dL; total serum calcium, 8.8 mg/dL; serum creatinine, 1.9 mg/dL; serum PTH, 28 pg/mL; and serum 25-hydroxyvitamin D, 40 ng/mL. The patient's biannual food record shows sufficient protein intake of 1.1 g/kg/d and adequate energy intake of 31 kcal/kg/d. Her GFR is calculated to be approximately 27 mL/min. During her dietary interview, the patient reports eating processed food frequently and drinking soft drinks every day.

1. Serum phosphorus assessment
   - Serum phosphorus level in this patient is consistent with hyperphosphatemia.
2. Renal or external phosphorus load causes in differential diagnosis
   - External excess due to her history of consuming processed foods and soft drinks.
   - GFR of 27 mL/min consistent with diminished renal phosphorus excretion.
3. Treatment
   - Counsel patient on low phosphorus foods and encourage patient to minimize and eventually eliminate processed foods and soft drinks from diet. This patient may also benefit from targeted training on preparing suitable meals to assist with dietary adherence.
   - Total serum calcium level is within normal limits. A good phosphorus-binding treatment option is a calcium-containing binder such as calcium acetate 1334 mg (2 tablets) with meals 3 times daily or calcium carbonate 1–2 g with meals 3 times daily.
4. Monitoring
   - Follow-up on serum phosphorus and total serum calcium should be rechecked in 3 months.
   - If the PTH level is within normal limits, follow-up should be done in 12 months.

References

1. Whitmore SJ. Nutrition-focused evaluation and management of dysnatremias. *Nutr Clin Pract.* 2008;23(2):108–121.

2. Bruno JJ, Canada TW. Electrolyte disorders in the critically ill population. In: Erstad, B, ed. *Critical Care Pharmacotherapy.* 1st ed. Lenexa, KS: American College of Clinical Pharmacy; 2016:58–97.

3. Upadhyay A, Jaber BL, Madias NE. Incidence and prevalence of hyponatremia. *Am J Med.* 2006;119(7 suppl 1):S30–S35.

4. Anderson RJ, Chung HM, Kluge R, Schrier RW. Hyponatremia: a prospective analysis of its epidemiology and the pathogenetic role of vasopressin. *Ann Int Med.* 1985;102(2):164–168.

5. Hawkins RC. Age and gender as risk factors for hyponatremia and hypernatremia. *Clin Chim Acta.* 2003;337(1–2):169–172.

6. Hoorn EJ, Lindemans J, Zietse R. Development of severe hyponatraemia in hospitalized patients: treatment-related risk factors and inadequate management. *Nephrol Dial Transplant.* 2006;21(1):70–76.

7. Spasovski G, Vanholder R, Allolio B, et al; Hyponatraemia Guideline Development Group. Clinical practice guidelines on the diagnosis and treatment of hyponatremia [published correction appears in *Nephrol Dial Transplant.* 2014 Jun;40(6):924]. *Nephrol Dial Transplant.* 2014;29(suppl 2):i1–i39.

8. Androgue HJ, Madias NE. Hyponatremia. *N Engl J Med.* 2000;342(21):1581–1589.

9. Lin M, Liu SJ, Lim IT. Disorders of water imbalance. *Emerg Med Clin North Am.* 2005;23(3): 749–770.

10. Heitz U, Horne MM. *Fluid, Electrolyte, and Acid-Base Balance.* 5th ed. St. Louis, MO: Elsevier Mosby; 2005.

11. Sterns RH. The treatment of hyponatremia: first, do no harm. Am J Med 1990;88(6):557–560.

12. Kraft MD, Btaiche IF, Sacks GS, Kudsk KA. Treatment of electrolyte disorders in adult patients in the intensive care unit. *Am J Health Syst Pharm.* 2005;62(16):1663–1682.

13. Dillon RC, Merchan C, Altshuler D, Papadopoulos J. Incidence of adverse events during peripheral administration of sodium chloride 3%. *J Intensive Care Med* 2018;33(1):48–53.

14. Liamis G, Milionis H, Elisaf M. A review of drug-induced hyponatremia. *Am J Kidney Dis* 2008;52(1):144–153.

15. Yeates KE, Singer M, Morton AR. Salt and water: a simple approach to hyponatremia. *CMAJ* 2004;170(3);365–369.

16. Androgue HJ, Madias NE. Hypernatremia. *N Engl J Med.* 2000;342(20):1493–1499.

17. Alshayeb HM, Showkat A, Babar F, Mangold T, Wall BM. Severe hypernatremia correction rate and mortality in hospitalized patients. *Am J Med Sci.* 2011;341(5):356–360.

18. Arora SK. Hypernatremic disorders in the intensive care unit. *J Intensive Care Med.* 2013;28(1):37–45.

19. Rose BD, Post TW. *Clinical Physiology of Acid-Base and Electrolyte Disorders.* 5th ed. New York, NY: McGraw-Hill; 2001.

20. Schaefer TJ, Wolford RW. Disorders of potassium. *Emerg Med Clin North Am.* 2005;23(3): 723–747.

21. Mandel A. Hypokalemia and hyperkalemia. *Med Clin North Am.* 1997;81(3):611–639.

22. Theisen-Toupal J. Hypokalemia and hyperkalemia. *Hosp Med Clin.* 2015;4(1):34–50.

23. Gennari FJ. Disorders of potassium homeostasis hypokalemia and hyperkalemia. *Crit Care Clin.* 2002;18(2):273–288.

24. Jensen HK, Brabrand M, Vinholt PJ, Hallas J, Lassen AT. Hypokalemia in acute medical patients: risk factors and prognosis. *Am J Med.* 2015;128(1):60–67.e1.

25. Paice BJ, Paterson KR, Onyanga-Omara F, Donnelly T, Gray JM, Lawson DH. Record linkage of hypokalaemia in hospitalized patients. *Post Grad Med J.* 1986;62(725):187–191.

26. Cohn JN, Kowey PR, Whelton PK, Prisant LM. New guidelines for potassium replacement in clinical practice. *Arch Intern Med.* 2000;160(16):2429–2436.

27. Doig GS, Simpson F, Heighes PT, et al. Restricted versus continued standard caloric intake during the management of refeeding syndrome in critically ill adults: a randomised, parallel-group, multicentre, single-blind controlled trial. *Lancet Resp.* 2015;3(12):943–952.

28. Gennari FJ. Hypokalemia. *N Engl J Med.* 1998;339(7):451–458.

29. Evans KJ, Greenburg A. Hyperkalemia: a review. *J Intensive Care Med.* 2005;20(5):272–290.

30. Kovesdy CP. Management of hyperkalemia: an update for the internist. *Am J Med.* 2015;128(12):1281–1287.

31. Hoskote SS, Joshi SR, Ghosh AK. Disorders of potassium homeostasis: pathophysiology and management. *J Assoc Physicians India.* 2008;56:685–693.

32. Melikian AP, Cheng LK, Wright GJ, Cohen A, Bruce RE. Bioavailability of potassium from three dosage forms: suspension, capsule, and solution. *J Clin Pharmacol.* 1988;28(11):1046–1050.

33. Klang M, McLymont V, Ng N. Osmolality, pH, and compatibility of selected oral liquid medications with an enteral nutrition product. *JPEN J Parenter Enteral Nutr.* 2013;37(5):689–694.

34. Squires RD, Huth EJ. Experimental potassium depletion in normal human subjects. I. Relation of ionic intakes to the renal conservation of potassium. *J Clin Invest.* 1959;38(7):1134–1148.

35. Lin SH, Lin YF, Chen DT, Chu P, Hsu CW, Halperin ML. Laboratory tests to determine the cause of hypokalemia and paralysis. *Arch Intern Med.* 2004;164(14):1561–1566.

36. Schaefer M, Link J, Hannemann L, Rudolph KH. Excessive hypokalemia and hyperkalemia following head injury. *Intensive Care Med.* 1995;21(3):235–237.

37. Hollander-Rodriguez JC, Calvert JF. Hyperkalemia. *Am Fam Physician.* 2006;73(2):283–290.

38. Desai A. Hyperkalemia associated with inhibitors of the renin-angiotensin-aldosterone system: balancing risk and benefit. *Circulation.* 2008;118(16):1609–1611.

39. Khosla N, Kalaitzidis R, Bakris GL. Predictors of hyperkalemia risk following hypertension control with aldosterone blockade. *Am J Nephrol.* 2009;30(5):418–424.

40. Williams ME. Hyperkalemia. *Crit Care Clin.* 1991;7(1):155–174.

41. Wiederkehr MR, Moe OW. Factitious hyperkalemia. *Am J Kidney Dis.* 2000;36(5):1049–1053.

42. Whang R. Magnesium deficiency: pathogenesis, prevalence, and clinical implications. *Am J Med.* 1987;82(suppl 3A):24–29.

43. Whang R, Oei TO, Aikawa JK, et al. Predictors of clinical hypomagnesemia: hypokalemia, hypophosphatemia, hyponatremia, and hypocalcemia. *Arch Intern Med.* 1984;144(9):1794–1796.

44. Whang R, Ryder KW. Frequency of hypomagnesemia and hypermagnesemia: requested vs. routine. *JAMA.* 1990;263(22):3063–3064.

45. Desai TK, Carlson RW, Geheb MA. Prevalence and clinical implications of hypocalcemia in acutely ill patients in a medical intensive care setting. *Am J Med.* 1988;84(2):209–214.

46. Boyd JC, Bruns DE, Wills MR. Frequency of hypomagnesemia in hypokalemic states. *Clin Chem.* 1983;29(1):178–179.

47. Rude RK. Physiology of magnesium metabolism and the important role of magnesium in potassium deficiency. *Am J Cardiol.* 1989;63(14):31G–34G.

48. Cronin RE, Knochel JP. Magnesium deficiency. *Adv Intern Med.* 1983;28:509–533.

49. Berkelhammer C, Bear RA. A clinical approach to common electrolyte problems: 4. hypomagnesemia. *Can Med Assoc J.* 1985;132(4):360–368.

50. Gums JG. Clinical significance of magnesium: a review. *Drug Intell Clin Pharm.* 1987;21(3): 240–246.

51. Elin RJ. Assessment of magnesium status. *Clin Chem.* 1987;33(11):1965–1970.

52. Zaloga GP. Interpretation of the serum magnesium level. *Chest.* 1989;95(2):257–258.

53. Whang R, Flink EB, Dyckner T, Wester PO, Aikawa JK, Ryan MJ. Magnesium depletion as a cause of refractory potassium repletion. *Arch Intern Med.* 1985;145(9):1686–1689.

54. Seelig M. Cardiovascular consequences of magnesium deficiency and loss: pathogenesis, prevalence and manifestations—magnesium and chloride loss in refractory potassium repletion. *Am J Cardiol.* 1989;63(14):4G–21G.

55. Flink EB. Nutritional aspects of magnesium metabolism. *West J Med.* 1980;133(4):304–312.

56. Ryan MP. Diuretics and potassium/magnesium depletion: directions for treatment. *Am J Med.* 1987;82(suppl 3A):38–47.

57. Anast CS, Mohs JM, Kaplan SL, Burns TW. Evidence for parathyroid failure in magnesium deficiency. *Science.* 1972;177(4049):606–608.

58. Anast CS, Winnacker JL, Forte LR, Burns TW. Impaired release of parathyroid hormone in magnesium deficiency. *J Clin Endocrinol Metab.* 1976;42(4):707–717.

59. Rude RK. Magnesium. In: Coates PM, Betz JM, Blackman MR, Cragg GM, Levine M, Moss J, White JD, eds. *Encyclopedia of Dietary Supplements.* 2nd ed. New York, NY: Informa Healthcare; 2010:527–537.

60. Nicoll GW, Struthers AD, Fraser CG. Biological variation of urinary magnesium. *Clin Chem.* 1991;37(10 pt 1):1794–1795.

61. Rude RK, Bethune JE, Singer FR. Renal tubular maximum for magnesium in normal, hyperparathyroid, and hypoparathyroid man. *J Clin Endocrinol Metab.* 1980;51(6): 1425–1431.

62. Rude RK, Ryzen E. TmMg and renal Mg threshold in normal man and in certain pathophysiologic conditions. *Magnesium.* 1986;5(5–6):273–281.

63. Wong ET, Rude RK, Singer FR, Shaw ST. A high prevalence of hypomagnesemia and hypermagnesemia in hospitalized patients. *Am J Clin Pathol.* 1983;79(3):348–352.

64. Whang R, Aikawa JK, Oei TO, Hamiter T. The need for routine serum magnesium determination. *Clin Res.* 1977;25:154A.

65. Rubeiz GJ, Thill-Baharozian M, Hardie D, Carlson RW. Association of hypomagnesemia and mortality in acutely ill medical patients. *Crit Care Med.* 1993;21(2):203–209.

66. England MR, Gordon G, Salem M, Chernow B. Magnesium administration and dysrhythmias after cardiac surgery: a placebo-controlled, double-blind, randomized trial. *JAMA.* 1992;268(17):2395–2402.

67. Salem M, Kasinski N, Andrei AM, et al. Hypomagnesemia is a frequent finding in the emergency department in patients with chest pain. *Arch Intern Med.* 1991;151(11):2185–2190.

68. Chernow B, Bamberger S, Stoiko M, et al. Hypomagnesemia in patients in postoperative intensive care. *Chest.* 1989;95(2):391–397.

69. Fiaccadori E, Del Canale S, Coffrini E, et al. Muscle and serum magnesium in pulmonary intensive care unit patients. *Crit Care Med.* 1988;16(8):751–760.

70. Reinhart RA, Desbiens NA. Hypomagnesemia in patients entering the ICU. *Crit Care Med.* 1985;13(6):506–507.

71. Ryzen E, Wagers PW, Singer FR, Rude RK. Magnesium deficiency in a medical ICU population. *Crit Care Med.* 1985;13(1):19–21.

72. Zaloga GP, Wilkens R, Tourville J, Wood D, Klyme DM. A simple method for determining physiologically active calcium and magnesium concentrations in critically ill patients. *Crit Care Med.* 1987;15(9):813–816.

73. Chernow B, Smith J, Rainey TG, Finton C. Hypomagnesemia: implications for the critical care specialist. *Crit Care Med.* 1982;10(3):193–196.

74. Reinhart RA. Magnesium metabolism: a review with special reference to the relationship between intracellular and serum levels. *Arch Intern Med.* 1988;148(11):2415–2420.

75. Kroenke K, Wood DR, Hanley JF. The value of serum magnesium determination in hypertensive patients receiving diuretics. *Arch Intern Med.* 1987;147(9):1553–1556.

76. Schrag D, Chung KY, Flombaum C, Saltz L. Cetuximab therapy and symptomatic hypomagnesemia. *J Natl Cancer Inst.* 2005;97(16):1221–1224.

77. Furlanetto TW, Faulhaber GA. Hypomagnesemia and proton pump inhibitors: below the tip of the iceberg. *Arch Intern Med.* 2011;171(15):1391–1392.

78. Sterns RH, Grief M, Bernstein PL. Treatment of hyperkalemia: something old, something new. *Kidney Int.* 2016;89(3):546–554.

79. Knochel JP. Neuromuscular manifestations of electrolyte disorders. *Am J Med.* 1982;72(3):521–535.

80. Hall RC, Joffe JR. Hypomagnesemia: physical and psychiatric symptoms. *JAMA.* 1973;224(13):1749–1751.

81. Iseri LT, Freed J, Bures AR. Magnesium deficiency and cardiac disorders. *Am J Med.* 1975;58(6):837–846.

82. Kingston ME, Al-Siba'i MB, Skooge WC. Clinical manifestations of hypomagnesemia. *Crit Care Med. 1986;14(11):950–954.*

83. Flink EB. Therapy of magnesium deficiency. *Ann NY Acad Sci.* 1969;162(2):901–905.

84. Brown RO, Hak LJ. Hypomagnesemia in critically ill patients. *ACCP Report.* 1993; March: 6.

85. Kulick DL, Hong R, Ryzen E, et al. Electrophysiologic effects of intravenous magnesium in patients with normal conduction systems and no clinical evidence of significant cardiac disease. *Am Heart J.* 1988;115(2):367–373.

86. Feldstedt M, Boesgaard S, Bouchelouche P, et al. Magnesium substitution in acute ischaemic heart syndromes. *Eur Heart J.* 1991;12(11):1215–1218.

87. Sueta CA, Clarke SW, Dunlap SH, et al. Effect of acute magnesium administration on the frequency of ventricular arrhythmia in patients with heart failure. *Circulation.* 1994;89(2):660–666.

88. Chapron DJ, Korman LB, Barry WL. Gastric retention of enteric-coated magnesium chloride tablets. *Ann Pharmacother.* 1994;28(7–8):874–877.

89. Woods KL, Fletcher S, Roffe C, Haider Y. Intravenous magnesium sulphate in suspected acute myocardial infarction: results of the second Leicester Intravenous Magnesium Intervention Trial (LIMIT-2). *Lancet.* 1992;339(8809):1553–1558.

90. Bundy JT, Connito D, Mahoney MD, Pontier PJ. Treatment of idiopathic renal magnesium wasting with amiloride. *Am J Nephrol.* 1995;15(1):75–77.

91. Broner CW, Stidham GL, Westenkirchner DF, Tolley EA. Hypermagnesemia and hypocalcemia as predictors of high mortality in critically ill pediatric patients. *Crit Care Med.* 1990;18(9):921–928.

92. Ali A, Walentik C, Mantych GJ, et al. Iatrogenic acute hypermagnesemia after total parenteral nutrition infusion mimicking septic shock syndrome: two case reports. *Pediatrics.* 2003;112(1 pt 1):e70–e72.

93. Massry SG, Seelig MS. Hypomagnesemia and hypermagnesemia. *Clin Nephrol.* 1977;7(4): 147–153.

94. Rizzo MA, Fisher M, Lock JP. Hypermagnesemic pseudocoma. *Arch Intern Med.* 1993;153(9): 1130–1132.

95. Rude RK, Singer FR. Magnesium deficiency and excess. *Ann Rev Med.* 1981;32:245–259.

96. US Department of Agriculture, Agricultural Research Service. FoodData Central. https://fdc.nal.usda.gov. Accessed November 30, 2019.

97. Felsenfeld A, Rodriguez M, Levine B. New insights in regulation of calcium homeostasis. *Curr Opin Nephrol Hypertens.* 2013;22(4):371–376.

98. Bushinsky AD, Monk RD. Electrolyte quintet: calcium. *Lancet.* 1998;352(9124):305–311.

99. Olinger ML. Disorders of calcium and magnesium metabolism. *Emerg Med Clin N Am.* 1989;7(4):795–822.

100. Guise TA, Mundy GR. Clinical review 69: evaluation of hypocalcemia in children and adults. *J Clin Endocrinol Metab.* 1995;80(5):1473–1478.

101. French S, Subauste J, Geraci S. Calcium abnormalities in hospitalized patients. *South Med J.* 2012;105(4):231–237.

102. Dickerson RN, Alexander KH, Minard G, Croce MA, Brown RO. Accuracy of methods to estimate ionized and "corrected" serum calcium concentrations in critically ill multiple trauma patients receiving specialized nutrition support. *JPEN J Parenter Enteral Nutr.* 2004;28(3):133–141.

103. Ariyan CE, Sosa JA. Assessment and management of patients with abnormal calcium. *Crit Care Med.* 2004;32(4 suppl):S146–S154.

104. Kraft MD. Phosphorus and calcium: a review for the adult nutrition support clinician. *Nutr Clin Pract.* 2015;30(1):21–33.

105. Committee to Review Dietary Reference Intakes for Vitamin D and Calcium, Food and Nutrition Board, Institute of Medicine. *Dietary Reference Intakes for Calcium and Vitamin D.* Washington, DC: National Academy Press, 2010.

106. Ayers P, Adams S, Boullata J, et al; ASPEN. A.S.P.E.N. parenteral nutrition safety consensus recommendations. *JPEN J Parenter Enteral Nutr.* 2014;38(3):296–333.

107. Agus ZS, Wasserstein A, Goldfarb S. Disorders of calcium and magnesium homeostasis. *Am J Med.* 1982;72(3):473–488.

108. Zaloga GP. Hypocalcemia in critically ill patients. *Crit Care Med.* 1992;20(2):251–262.

109. Cooper MS, Gittoes NJL. Diagnosis and management of hypocalcaemia. *BMJ.* 2008;336(7656):1298–1302.

110. Zivin JR, Gooley T, Zager RA, Ryan MH. Hypocalcemia: a pervasive metabolic abnormality in the critically ill. *Am J Kidney Dis.* 2001;37(4):689–698.

111. Reber PM, Heath H III. Hypocalcemic emergencies. *Med Clin North Am.* 1995;79(1):93–106.

112. Juan D. Hypocalcemia: differential diagnosis and mechanisms. *Arch Intern Med.* 1979;139(10):1166–1171.

113. Liamis G, Milionis HJ, Elisaf M. A review of drug-induced hypocalcemia. *J Bone Miner Metab.* 2009;27(6):635–642.

114. Carroll MF, Schade DS. A practical approach to hypercalcemia. *Am Fam Physician.* 2003;67(9):1959–1966.

115. McPherson ML, Prince SR, Atamer ER, Maxwell DB, Ross-Clunis H, Estep HL. Theophylline-induced hypercalcemia. *Ann Intern Med.* 1986;105(1):52–54.

116. Arumugam GP, Sundravel S, Shanthi P, Sachdanandam P. Tamoxifen flare hypercalcemia: an additional support for gallium nitrate usage. *J Bone Miner Metab.* 2006;24(3):243–247.

117. Dickerson RN, Morgan LM, Croce MA, Minard G, Brown RO. Treatment of moderate to severe acute hypocalcemia in critically ill trauma patients. *JPEN J Parenter Enteral Nutr.* 2007:31(3):228–233.

118. Slomp J, van der Voort PH, Gerritsen RT, Berk JAM, Bakker AJ. Albumin-adjusted calcium is not suitable for diagnosis of hyper- and hypocalcemia in the critically ill. *Crit Care Med.* 2003;31(5):1389–1393.

119. Shapses SA, Schlussel YR, Cifuentes M. Drug-nutrient interactions that impact on mineral status. In: Boullata JI, Armenti VT, eds. *Handbook of Drug-Nutrient Interactions.* 2nd ed. New York, NY: Humana Press; 2010:537–571.

120. Zojer N, Keck AV, Pecherstorfer M. Comparative tolerability of drug therapies for hypercalcaemia of malignancy. *Drug Saf.* 1999;21(5):389–406.

121. Ralston SH, Coleman R, Fraser WD, et al. Medical management of hypercalcemia. *Calcif Tiss Int.* 2004;74(1):1–11.

122. Potts JT. Hyperparathyroidism and other hypercalcemic disorders. *Adv Intern Med.* 1996;41:165–212.

123. Lumachi F, Brunello A, Roma A, Basso U. Medical treatment of malignancy-associated hypercalcemia. *Curr Med Chem.* 2005;15(4):415–421.

124. Chisholm MA, Mulloy AL, Taylor AT. Acute management of cancer-related hypercalcemia. *Ann Pharmacother.* 1996;30(5):507–513.

125. Ahmad S, Kuraganti G, Steenkamp D. Hypercalcemic crisis: a clinical review. *Am J Med.* 2015;128(3):239–245.

126. Thosani S, Hu MI. Denosumab: a new agents in the management of hypercalcemia of malignancy. *Future Oncol.* 2015;11(21):2865–2871.

127. Food and Drug Administration. Cumulative list of orphan products designated and approved. https://www.accessdata.fda.gov/scripts/opdlisting/oopd/listResult.cfm. Accessed November 30, 2019.

128. Costa L, Lipton A, Coleman RE. Role of bisphosphonates for the management of skeletal complications and bone pain from skeletal metastases. *Support Cancer Ther.* 2006;3(3):143–153.

129. Holick MF, Binkley NC, Bischoff-Ferrari HA, et al; Endocrine Society. Evaluation, treatment, and prevention of vitamin D deficiency: an Endocrine Society clinical practice guideline [published correction appears in *J Clin Endocrinol Metab.* 2011 Dec;96(12):3908]. *J Clin Endocrinol Metab.* 2011;96(7):1911–1930.

130. Stoff JS. Phosphate homeostasis and hypophosphatemia. *Am J Med.* 1982;72(3):489–495.

131. Marks J, Debnam ES, Unwin RJ. The role of the gastrointestinal tract in phosphate homeostasis in health and chronic kidney disease. *Curr Opin Nephrol Hypertens.* 2013;22(4):481–487.

132. Penido MG, Alon US. Phosphate homeostasis and its role in bone health. *Pediatr Nephrol.* 2012;27(11):2039–2048.

133. Lederer E. Regulation of serum phosphate. *J Physiol.* 2014;592(18):3985–3995.

134. Gaasbeek A, Meinders AE. Hypophosphatemia: an update on its etiology and treatment. *Am J Med.* 2005;118(10):1094–1101.

135. Gallagher ML. The nutrients and their metabolism. In: Mahan LK, Escott-Stump S, Raymond JL, eds. *Krause's Food and the Nutrition Care Process.* 13th ed. St Louis, MO: Saunders Elsevier; 2012:105–110.

136. Tonelli M, Pannu N, Manns B. Oral phosphate binders in patients with kidney failure. *N Engl J Med.* 2010;362(14):1312–1324.

137. Geerse DA, Bindels AJ, Kuiper MA, Roos AN, Spronk PE, Schultz MJ. Treatment of hypophosphatemia in the intensive care unit: a review. *Crit Care.* 2010;14(4):R147.

138. Felsenfeld AJ, Levine BS. Approach to treatment of hypophosphatemia. *Am J Kidney Dis.* 2012;60(4):655–661.

139. Imel EA, Econs MJ. Approach to the hypophosphatemic patient. *J Clin Endocrinol Metab.* 2012;97(3):696–706.

140. Glendenning P, Bell DA, Clifton-Bligh RJ. Investigating hypophosphataemia. *BMJ.* 2014;348:g3172.

141. Andress DL, Vannatta JB, Whang R. Treatment of refractory hypophosphatemia. *South Med J.* 1982;75(6):766–767.

142. Vannatta JB, Andress DL, Whange R, Papper S. High-dose intravenous phosphorus therapy for severe complicated hypophosphatemia. *South Med J.* 1983;76(11):1424–1426.

143. Kingston M, Al-Siba'i MB. Treatment of severe hypophosphatemia. *Crit Care Med.* 1985;13(1):16–18.

144. Rosen GH, Boullata JI, O'Rangers EA, Enow NB, Shin B. Intravenous phosphate repletion regimen for critically ill patients with moderate hypophosphatemia. *Crit Care Med.* 1995;23(7):1204–1210.

145. Clark CL, Sack GS, Dickerson RN, Kudsk KA, Brown RO. Treatment of hypophosphatemia in patients receiving specialized nutrition support using a graduated dosing scheme: results from a prospective clinical trial. *Crit Care Med.* 1995;23(9):1504–1511.

146. Taylor BE, Huey WY, Buchman TG, Boyle WA, Coopersmith CM. Treatment of hypophosphatemia using a protocol based of patient weight and serum phosphorus level in a surgical intensive care unit. *J Am Coll Surg.* 2004;198(2):198–204.

147. Brown K, Dickerson RN, Morgan LM, Alexander KH, Minard G, Brown RO. A new graduated dosing regimen for phosphorus replacement in patient receiving nutrition support. *JPEN J Parenter Enteral Nutr.* 2006;30(3):209–214.

148. Kraft MD, Btaiche IF, Sack GS. Review of refeeding syndrome. *Nutr Clin Pract.* 2005;20(6): 625–633.

149. Shiber JR, Mattu A. Serum phosphate abnormalities in the emergency department. *J Emerg Med.* 2002;23(4):395–400.

150. Gonzalez-Parra E, Tuñón J, Egido J, Ortiz A. Phosphate: a stealthier killer than previously thought? *Cardiovasc Pathol.* 2012;21(5):372–381.

151. Nguyen TV, Wang A. Hyperphosphatemia: consequences and management strategies. *J Nurse Pract.* 2012;8(1):56–60.

152. Malberti F. Hyperphosphataemia: treatment options. *Drugs.* 2013;73(7):673–688.

153. Goldsmith D, Covic A. Oral phosphate binders in CKD—is calcium the (only) answer? *Clin Nephrol.* 2014;81(6):389–395.

154. Podd D. Hyperphosphatemia: understanding the role of phosphate metabolism. *JAAPA.* 2010;23(7):32–37.

155. Bhan I. Phosphate management in chronic kidney disease. *Curr Opin Nephrol Hypertens.* 2014;23(2):174–179.

156. Fouque D, Horne R, Cozzolino M, Kalantar-Zadeh K. Balancing nutrition and serum phosphorus in maintenance dialysis. *Am J Kidney Dis.* 2014;64(1):143–150.

157. Nastou D, Fernández-Fernández B, Elewa U, et al. Next generation phosphate binders focus on iron based binders. *Drugs.* 2014;74(8):863–877.

158. Kidney Disease: Improving Global Outcomes (KDIGO) CKD Workgroup. KDIGO 2012 clinical practice guideline for the evaluation and management of chronic kidney disease. *Kidney Int Suppl.* 2013;3(1):1–150.

159. Kidney Disease: Improving Global Outcomes (KDIGO) CKD Workgroup. KDOQI 2017 clinical practice guideline update for the diagnosis, evaluation, prevention and treatment of chronic kidney disease-mineral and bone disorder (CKD-MBD). *Kidney Int Suppl.* 2017;7(1):1–59.

CHAPTER 4

Acid-Base Homeostasis and Disorders

Identification and management of acid-base disorders together play a large role in providing safe and effective patient care. Understanding acid-base homeostasis is a vital step within this process. This chapter begins by providing an overview of acid-base physiology and then presents a stepwise process for evaluating arterial or venous blood gases and identifying specific acid-base disorders. This chapter covers diagnostic strategies first, followed by emphasis and review of the individual acid-base disorders.

Overview

Acid-Base Physiology[1]

For normal cell function, acid-base balance via metabolic and respiratory processes must be consistently maintained. The lungs, kidneys, and endogenous chemical buffer systems regulate acid-base homeostasis. The inability of these systems to balance acids and bases underlies the development of acid-base disorders. Acids are substances that can donate hydrogen ions (H^+), and bases are substances that can accept or combine with H^+.

1. pH: the concentration of H^+ in solution
    - pH is measured on a logarithmic scale ranging from 1 to 14.
    - A pH of 7 is considered neutral, while values < 7 are acidotic and values > 7 are alkalotic.
    - The normal physiologic pH range is 7.35–7.45. The body attempts to maintain pH tightly at 7.40.
2. Alterations in pH
    - Acidemia: pH < 7.35
    - Acidosis is a process associated with an increase in H^+ concentration (resulting in decreased pH).
    - Alkalemia: pH > 7.45
    - Alkalosis is a process associated with a decrease in H^+ concentration (resulting in increased pH).

Regulation of H^+ Concentration[1,2]

Most physiologic H^+ originates as a by-product or end-product of cellular metabolism. The concentration of H^+ must be tightly regulated to maintain a pH compatible with life (6.8–7.8). The process of H^+ regulation involves 3 sequential steps: (1) chemical buffering by extracellular and intracellular mechanisms, (2) control of the partial pressure of carbon dioxide (PCO_2) in the blood by alterations in the rate of ventilation, and (3) control of the serum bicarbonate (HCO_3^-) concentration by changes in renal H^+ excretion. Figure 4-1 illustrates the carbonic acid/HCO_3^- buffer system.

1. Chemical buffers are weak acid and base pairs that prevent large changes in the H^+ concentration. They provide immediate acid-base protection and compensation to prevent large changes in pH.
    - The carbonic acid/HCO_3^- buffer system is the principal extracellular buffer system.

Figure 4-1. Carbonic Acid/Bicarbonate Buffer System.

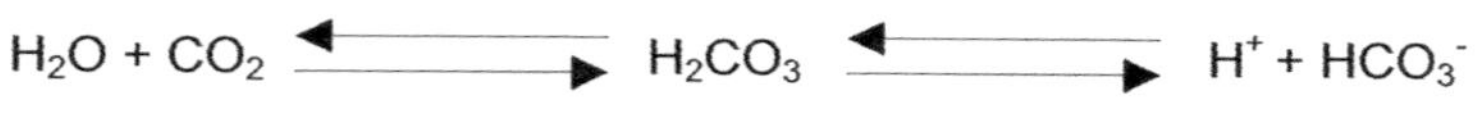

$$H_2O + CO_2 \rightleftarrows H_2CO_3 \rightleftarrows H^+ + HCO_3^-$$

- Phosphate promotes the excretion of H^+ in the renal tubules.
- Ammonium (NH_4^+) promotes greater renal excretion of H^+ from the renal tubules.
- Hemoglobin is an intracellular erythrocyte buffer and the most important protein buffer.

2. Lungs regulate PCO_2 by altering the rate and depth of ventilation to allow for excretion (ie, exhalation) of CO_2 generated by diet and cellular metabolism. This process compensates for acid-base disturbances within minutes.
3. Kidneys regulate acid-base status via alterations in renal H^+ excretion and HCO_3^- reabsorption. This process compensates for acid-base disturbances within 2–3 days.

Normal Blood Gas Values[1,2]

Laboratory assessment of acid-base status can be measured using blood gas analysis. Blood gas can be sampled either from venous or arterial blood, with reference ranges depending on the source. Arterial blood gas (ABG) analysis reflects the ability of the lungs to oxygenate blood, whereas venous blood gas analysis reflects tissue oxygenation. Table 4-1 provides normal adult values for both types of analysis.

1. pH measures H^+ concentration and reflects the acid-base status of the blood.
2. PCO_2 in the blood is the respiratory component of acid-base regulation.

Table 4-1. Adult Normal Blood Gas Values.

Measurement	Arterial	Venous
pH	7.40 (7.35–7.45)	7.36 (7.33–7.43)
PCO_2, mm Hg	35–45	41–51
PO_2, mm Hg	80–100	35–40
HCO_3^-, mEq/L	22–26	24–28
Base excess	−2 to +2	0 to +4
SO_2, %	95–100	70–75

PCO_2, partial pressure of carbon dioxide; PO_2, partial pressure of oxygen; SO_2, oxygen saturation.

3. The partial pressure of oxygen (PO_2) in the blood has no primary role in acid-base regulation; it reflects the ability of hemoglobin to carry oxygen.

4. Serum HCO_3^- is the major metabolic component of acid-base regulation.

    - To determine acid-base status, use either the calculated HCO_3^- from blood gas analysis or directly measured serum HCO_3^-.

    - The calculated HCO_3^- is typically 1–2 mEq/L lower than the measured serum value. Values outside this range may indicate an inaccurate measurement due to problems with blood collection, sample storage, or calibration of the blood gas analyzer. For these reasons, the measured serum HCO_3^- is preferred.

5. Base excess versus deficit represents the metabolic component status (ie, amount of excess or insufficient buffer) present in whole blood.

    - A large base excess is indicative of alkalosis.

    - A negative base excess (commonly referred to as a base deficit) indicates the absence of sufficient buffer in the blood, resulting in acidosis.

6. Oxygen saturation is the percentage of hemoglobin saturated with oxygen.

Role of Acid-Base Status on Oxygenation[2]

Oxygen's ability to bind to hemoglobin depends on many factors. Acid-base status and temperature are 2 factors that can affect oxygen saturation (Figure 4-2). Acidemia decreases oxygen's affinity for hemoglobin and may thus slightly increase the PO_2. Alkalemia increases oxygen's affinity for hemoglobin and thus results in a decrease in the PO_2. Essentially, acidemia makes the hemoglobin molecule more apt to release oxygen, whereas alkalemia makes the hemoglobin molecule less apt to release oxygen.

Figure 4-2. Hemoglobin-Oxygen Dissociation Curve Under Normal Conditions.

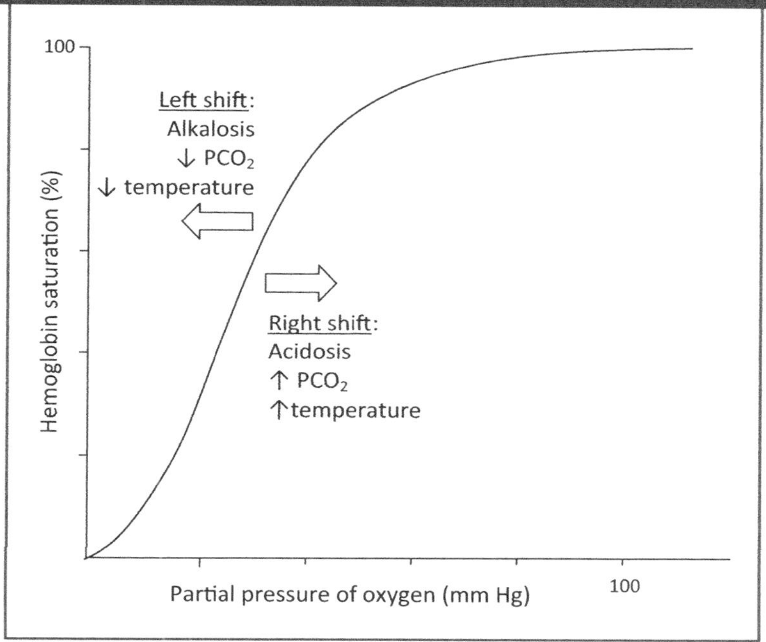

PCO_2, partial pressure of carbon dioxide.

Acid-Base Disorders

Prevalence[3–6]

1. Nine of every 10 patients in the intensive care unit experience acid-base disorders.

2. Approximately 8% of critically ill patients experience severe acid-base disorders (pH < 7.2).

3. Acid-base disorders have been associated with poorer clinical outcomes in multiple intensive care unit populations.

Stepwise Approach for the Assessment of Acid-Base Disorders[1]

A systematic approach to assessing ABGs is important in determining the acid-base status of a patient. The method presented here provides a structured approach for clinicians to assess a patient's acid-base status and subsequently make treatment recommendations. The following recommendations are not applicable when interpreting venous blood gases.

Step 1: Assess pH to determine the presence of acidemia or alkalemia.

The body attempts to tightly maintain pH at 7.40; however, the normal physiological pH range is 7.35–7.45.

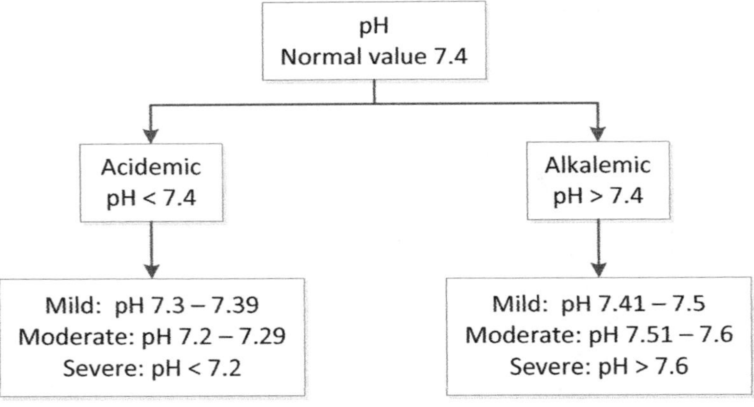

Step 2: Assess PCO_2.

PCO_2 is the respiratory component in acid-base regulation. The PCO_2 value is the *acid component* in the carbonic acid/HCO_3^- buffer system (normal range 35–45 mm Hg). Any rise in PCO_2 above 40 mm Hg indicates respiratory acidosis, and any fall in PCO_2 below 40 mm Hg normal indicates respiratory alkalosis.

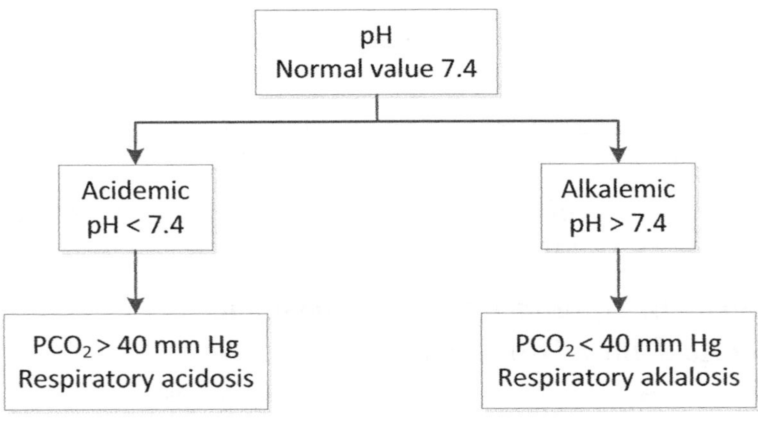

Step 3: Assess serum HCO_3^-.

HCO_3^- is the metabolic component in acid-base regulation. The HCO_3^- value is the *base component* in the carbonic acid/HCO_3^- buffer system (normal range 22–30 mEq/L). Any rise in HCO_3^- above 24 indicates metabolic alkalosis, and any fall in HCO_3^- below 24 indicates metabolic acidosis.

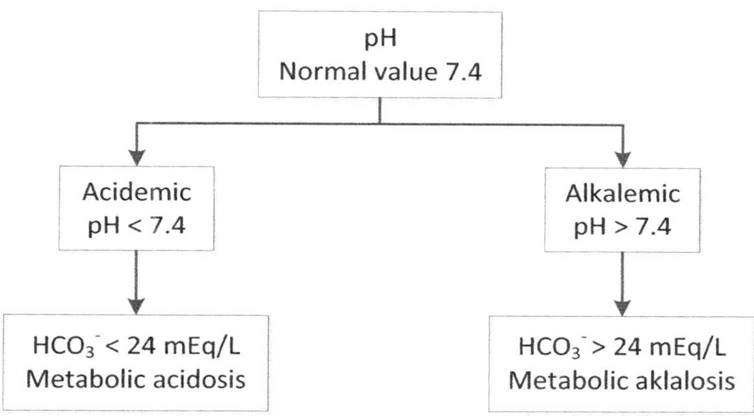

Step 4: If acidemic, calculate the anion gap (AG)[1,7-9]

The AG is an estimate of the difference between the measured and unmeasured major extracellular cations and anions (sodium [Na^+], HCO_3^-, and chloride [Cl^-]):

$$AG\ (mEq/L) = Na^+ - (Cl^- + HCO_3^-)$$

The normal range for a calculated AG is between 3 and 11 mEq/L; however, the normal range varies depending upon the specific analyzer utilized. The calculated AG represents a variety of unmeasured anions in the serum (eg, albumin, organic anions, phosphate, lactate, ketones).

1. Elevated unmeasured anion concentrations are frequently the cause of an AG metabolic acidosis.

2. For elevated AG, focus the assessment on identifying the most likely underlying cause of the altered unmeasured anion concentrations (see Metabolic Acidosis).

3. Hypoalbuminemia can cause a falsely decreased AG. The following formula can be used to correct the AG in hypoalbuminemia:

   Corrected AG = observed AG + 2.5 × [4.5 − measured albumin (g/dL)]

4. Delta ratio

- Determining the delta ratio may help during the assessment of elevated AG disorders to determine if another acid-base disorder exists.

- The delta ratio should not be the only analysis used to detect mixed acid-base disorders.

- Delta ratio = anion gap excess/HCO_3^- deficit = (measured AG − 12)/(24 − measured HCO_3^-), where 12 represents a normal AG value and 24 represents a normal serum bicarbonate value.

    - General rule is that for every millimole of acid present causing a 1-mEq increase of AG, the serum bicarbonate should drop by 1 mEq, leading to a delta ratio of 1.

    - Delta ratio = 0.8–1.2 indicates uncomplicated/pure AG metabolic acidosis.

    - Delta ratio < 0.8 indicates mixed AG gap and non-AG metabolic acidosis.

    - Delta ratio > 1.2 indicates AG metabolic acidosis and metabolic alkalosis.

Step 5: Determine if an acid-base disorder is acute (< 48 hours) or chronic (> 48 hours).

Step 6: Determine the occurrence of compensation for the primary disorder.

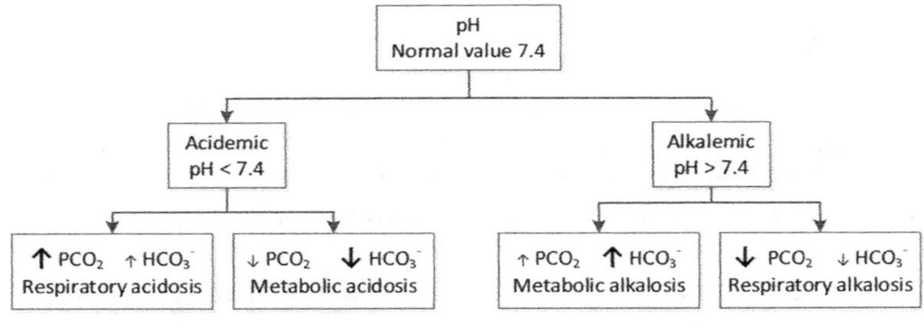

When a metabolic disorder occurs, the lungs will typically adjust the respiratory rate to either retain CO_2 (in metabolic alkalosis) or exhale CO_2 (in metabolic acidosis). If pulmonary function is not intact, this compensation may be less than expected. Alternatively, when a respiratory disorder occurs, the kidneys will adjust serum HCO_3^- by either increasing excretion (in respiratory alkalosis) or decreasing excretion (in respiratory

Table 4-2. Renal and Respiratory Compensation to Primary Acid-Base Disorders.[1]

Disorder	Primary Disturbance	Compensatory Response
Metabolic acidosis	↓ HCO_3^-	1.2 mm Hg decrease in PCO_2 for every 1 mEq/L fall in HCO_3^-
Metabolic alkalosis	↑ HCO_3^-	0.7 mm Hg increase in PCO_2 for every 1 mEq/L rise in HCO_3^-
Respiratory acidosis	↑ PCO_2	
Acute		1 mEq/L increase in HCO_3^- for every 10 mm Hg rise in PCO_2
Chronic		3 mEq/L increase in HCO_3^- for every 10 mm Hg rise in PCO_2
Respiratory alkalosis	↓ PCO_2	
Acute		2 mEq/L decrease in HCO_3^- for every 10 mm Hg fall in PCO_2
Chronic		4 mEq/L decrease in HCO_3^- for every 10 mm Hg fall in PCO_2

PCO_2, partial pressure of carbon dioxide.

acidosis). Unlike respiratory compensation, which begins almost immediately, metabolic compensation may take up to 3 days to occur. Disorders in renal function may affect compensation. A mixed disorder is the presence of 2 or more simple acid-base disorders at the same time. These disorders can be identified when values for either the expected PCO_2 (or HCO_3^-) or expected change in pH using the appropriate equations in Table 4-2 and Table 4-3 do not match upon calculation.

Step 7: Make a conclusion.

Figure 4-3 depicts the systematic approach described above, including all steps to accurately assess ABG and determine the acid-base status of a patient.

Table 4-3. Equations to Assess Adequate Compensation.

Disorder	Compensatory Response
Metabolic acidosis	Expected $PCO_2 = 40 - [1.2 \times (24 - \text{measured } HCO_3^-)]$
Metabolic alkalosis	Expected $PCO_2 = 40 + [0.7 \times (\text{measured } HCO_3^- - 24)]$
Respiratory acidosis	
Acute	Expected decrease in pH $= 0.08 \times [(\text{measured } Pco_2 - 40)/10]$
Chronic	Expected decrease in pH $= 0.03 \times [(\text{measured } Pco_2 - 40)/10]$
Respiratory alkalosis	
Acute	Expected increase in pH $= 0.08 \times [(40 - \text{measured } Pco_2)/10]$
Chronic	Expected increase in pH $= 0.03 \times [(40 - \text{measured } Pco_2)/10]$

PCO_2, partial pressure of carbon dioxide.

Figure 4-3. Stepwise Approach for the Diagnosis of Acid-Base Disorders.

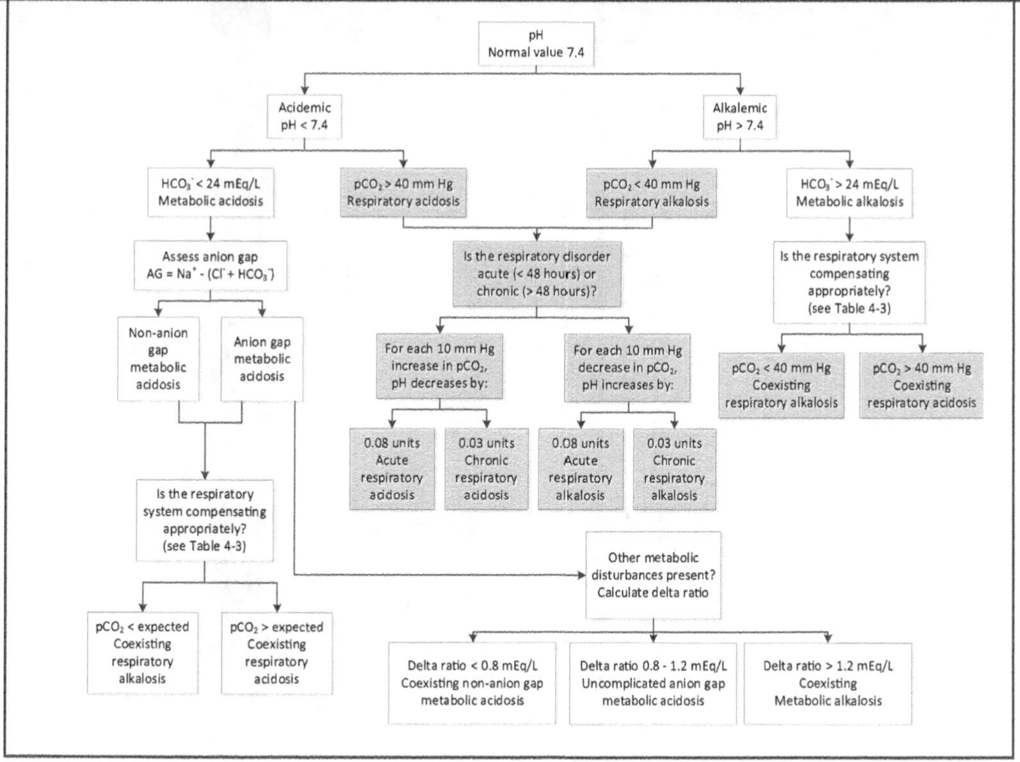

pH
Normal value 7.4

Acidemic
pH < 7.4

Alkalemic
pH > 7.4

HCO_3^- < 24 mEq/L
Metabolic acidosis

pCO_2 > 40 mm Hg
Respiratory acidosis

pCO_2 < 40 mm Hg
Respiratory alkalosis

HCO_3^- > 24 mEq/L
Metabolic alkalosis

Assess anion gap
AG = $Na^+ - (Cl^- + HCO_3^-)$

Is the respiratory disorder acute (< 48 hours) or chronic (> 48 hours)?

Is the respiratory system compensating appropriately? (see Table 4-3)

Non-anion gap metabolic acidosis

Anion gap metabolic acidosis

For each 10 mm Hg increase in pCO_2, pH decreases by:

For each 10 mm Hg decrease in pCO_2, pH increases by:

pCO_2 < 40 mm Hg
Coexisting respiratory alkalosis

pCO_2 > 40 mm Hg
Coexisting respiratory acidosis

0.08 units
Acute respiratory acidosis

0.03 units
Chronic respiratory acidosis

0.08 units
Acute respiratory alkalosis

0.03 units
Chronic respiratory alkalosis

Is the respiratory system compensating appropriately? (see Table 4-3)

Other metabolic disturbances present?
Calculate delta ratio

pCO_2 < expected
Coexisting respiratory alkalosis

pCO_2 > expected
Coexisting respiratory acidosis

Delta ratio < 0.8 mEq/L
Coexisting non-anion gap metabolic acidosis

Delta ratio 0.8 - 1.2 mEq/L
Uncomplicated anion gap metabolic acidosis

Delta ratio > 1.2 mEq/L
Coexisting Metabolic alkalosis

Respiratory Acid-Base Disorders

Primary respiratory acid-base disorders result from a condition, disease, or situation that leads to alterations in respiratory rate. Prompt, accurate identification and treatment are necessary to prevent significant morbidity and mortality. Unlike metabolic acid-base disorders, respiratory disorders are classified as either acute or chronic. Patients with acute respiratory acid-base disorders generally present with symptoms that are more prominent and require immediate, aggressive therapy.

Respiratory Acidosis[1,7]

1. Decrease in pH (< 7.4) as a result of a primary elevation of Pco_2 (> 40 mm Hg).

2. Acute respiratory acidosis develops over a period of <48 hours.

3. Chronic respiratory acidosis develops over a period of >48 hours.

4. Compensation occurs via the kidneys.

    - Renal compensation for acute respiratory acidosis begins within 6–12 hours; however, full compensation typically takes up to 3–5 days.

    - Compensation may not be complete if concomitant renal dysfunction is present.

Etiology and Risk Factors[7,10]

Respiratory acidosis results from disorders producing alterations in ventilatory control or gas exchange, increased production or decreased exhalation of CO_2, and respiratory muscle weakness. This ultimately leads to CO_2 retention and accumulation. Table 4-4 lists causes of respiratory acidosis.

1. Alterations in ventilatory control include diseases affecting central control of breathing and the use of sedating medications or neuromuscular blocking agents, leading to insufficient respiratory rate or drive.

2. Neuromuscular diseases, restrictive pulmonary disorders, and hypophosphatemia can result in muscle fatigue and resultant decrease in respiratory rate.

Table 4-4. Causes of Respiratory Acidosis.

Cause	Examples
Medications	Opioids (eg, fentanyl, hydromorphone, morphine, oxycodone, codeine)
	Anesthetics (eg, bupivacaine, mepivacaine)
	Sedatives (eg, alprazolam, diazepam, lorazepam, propofol)
	Neuromuscular blockers (eg, succinylcholine, vecuronium, cisatracurium, rocuronium, pancuronium)
Neuromuscular diseases/ abnormalities	Guillain-Barré syndrome
	Myasthenia gravis
	Multiple sclerosis
	Amyotrophic lateral sclerosis
	Central respiratory depression (eg, head injury, spinal cord injury, stroke)
	Hypophosphatemia
Metabolic	Overfeeding
Pulmonary/thoracic diseases/ conditions	Massive pulmonary embolus
	Acute respiratory distress syndrome
	Interstitial lung disease
	Flail chest
	Pleural disease
	Pneumothorax
	Pulmonary edema
	Severe pneumonia
	Smoke inhalation
	Chronic obstructive pulmonary disease
	Emphysema
	Bronchitis
	Asthma
	Sleep apnea
	Obesity hypoventilation syndrome
Airway obstruction	Foreign body
	Severe asthma attack/bronchospasm
	Aspiration
	Malignancy

3. Severe pulmonary disease can lead to both impaired gas exchange and ineffective breathing, leading to CO_2 retention.

4. Overfeeding total calories may result in increased hypercapnia due to an excess generation of CO_2 relative to O_2 consumption during carbohydrate metabolism.

5. Acute hypercapnia may occur due to upper airway obstruction or bronchospasm.

6. Renal insufficiency can result in impaired compensation.

Clinical Presentation[7]

1. Symptoms include anxiety, confusion, lethargy, delirium, increased heart rate, increased respiratory rate, diaphoresis, and cyanosis.

2. Patients with acute respiratory acidosis are often symptomatic, presenting with a greater alteration in pH compared with chronic respiratory acidosis.

3. Patients with chronic respiratory acidosis often do not present with symptoms. Minimal to no intervention may be required with chronic respiratory acidosis because it results from a chronic condition (eg, chronic obstructive pulmonary disease [COPD]) with acidosis indicative of patient adaptation to the disorder.

Diagnosis/Diagnostic Tests[11]

1. Complete a thorough patient history and physical, including a medication history upon presentation.

2. A toxicology panel may prove useful to guide treatment recommendations for patients with suspected drug use.

3. Obtain an ABG to determine the primary disorder and the presence of concomitant acid-base disorders.

4. Obtain serum chemistry panel to ascertain renal status and specific electrolyte abnormalities that may be the cause (eg, hypophosphatemia) or the result (eg, hyperkalemia) of respiratory acidosis.

5. Radiographic imaging (eg, chest radiography, computed tomography, magnetic resonance imaging) can be helpful in identifying abnormalities affecting respiration and/or ventilation (eg, infectious processes, malignancy, pulmonary embolism).

6. Obtain microbiology analysis (eg, sputum culture) in patients with suspected infectious processes to provide directed antimicrobial therapy.

7. Where available, determine the respiratory quotient (RQ) to assess for potential overfeeding (total calories). Increased CO_2 generation secondary to overfeeding may cause and/or worsen respiratory acidosis.

   - Obtain RQ through the use of a metabolic cart (indirect calorimetry) or specially designed ventilators.

   - $RQ = Vco_2/Vo_2$ (where Vco_2 is the volume of CO_2 produced, and Vo_2 is the volume of O_2 consumed).

   - An RQ > 1 indicates excess caloric intake (ie, overfeeding), which promotes fat synthesis.

8. Pulmonary function testing can help to identify and stage pulmonary disease.

Goals of Therapy

The goals of therapy in respiratory acidosis are to normalize pH, treat and/or optimize therapy of underlying conditions, and alleviate signs and/or symptoms related to respiratory acidosis.

Management[7,8,10,12–15]

The management strategies used for respiratory acidosis depend upon the severity of symptoms and the condition of the patient. Treat severe symptoms aggressively to safely restore acid-base homeostasis and prevent morbidity and mortality. Management of respiratory acidosis should focus on treating or removing the underlying cause and providing appropriate supportive care measures, which may include one or more of the following:

- Discontinue offending medication(s). Administer naloxone or flumazenil during cases of medication overdose to reverse the negative respiratory and cardiovascular effects of opioids or benzodiazepines, respectively.

- Provide adequate ventilation to aid in exhalation of excessive CO_2 and ensure adequate oxygen saturation. Intubation may be required to maintain airway patency or provide airway protection in cases of altered mental status, severe respiratory insufficiency, or respiratory failure.

Oxygen supplementation should be provided to patients when necessary either through noninvasive means (eg, nasal cannula, non-rebreather mask) for those with spontaneous breathing or via mechanical ventilation after intubation. Oxygen supplementation in patients with chronic respiratory acidosis resulting from COPD must be undertaken judiciously because respiratory acidosis can worsen with over-supplementation. Oxygen therapy should be titrated in these cases to a target oxygen saturation of 88%–92%. Bronchoscopy may also be necessary to clear airway secretions or obstructions to improve ventilation. Chest physiotherapy can be a useful noninvasive method to aid in movement and indirect clearance of respiratory secretions.

- Use inhaled bronchodilators (eg, albuterol, levalbuterol) in asthma and COPD to aid in dilation of airways for improved oxygenation and ventilation.

- Initiate empiric antibiotics upon presentation for those with suspected infections. Obtain cultures and sensitivities to aid with subsequent de-escalation of antimicrobial agents to only those necessary for successful eradication of the infection.

- *Use corticosteroid therapy (ie, prednisone and methylprednisolone)* during COPD and asthma exacerbations to decrease inflammation and improve patient symptoms.

- Centrally acting respiratory stimulants (eg, caffeine, theophylline) can be used short term in hypercapnia for stimulation of respiratory drive and elimination of excess CO_2.

- In cases of overfeeding, reduction of total caloric intake or provision is necessary. Where available, utilize indirect calorimetry to measure resting energy expenditure to guide the nutrition care plan.

Salvage therapy with sodium bicarbonate ($NaHCO_3$) infusion should be reserved for patients with profound respiratory acidosis (pH < 7.2) not responding to supportive therapies.

- $NaHCO_3$ infusions have no proven benefit for severe respiratory acidosis, but such therapy is used in clinical practice as a temporary measure while the etiology of respiratory acidosis is being evaluated.

- $NaHCO_3$ should be provided as 150 mEq in 1000 mL of sterile water for injection or dextrose 5% in water administered intravenously at a rate of 42–125 mL/h.

- Follow serial ABGs to detect inadvertent over-alkalinization.

Monitoring

Base the frequency and extent of monitoring on clinical status and underlying causes of respiratory acidosis. Monitoring may include but is not limited to the following:

1. ABG and serum chemistries
2. Vital signs (blood pressure, heart rate, respiratory rate, continuous pulse oximetry)
3. Neurological assessments
4. Microbiology cultures
5. Radiologic imaging based on clinical condition or suspicion of disease
6. Electrocardiography (ECG) monitoring

Respiratory Alkalosis[1,7,12,16]

1. An increase in pH (> 7.4) occurs as a result of a primary decrease in PCO_2 (< 40 mm Hg).
2. Acute respiratory alkalosis develops over a period of < 48 hours.
3. Chronic respiratory alkalosis develops over a period of > 48 hours.
4. Compensation occurs via the kidneys.
   - Renal compensation for acute respiratory alkalosis begins within 6–12 hours and may take up to 3–5 days to be complete.
   - Compensation may not be complete if concomitant renal dysfunction is present.

Etiology and Risk Factors[7,8,10,16]

Respiratory alkalosis results from conditions, diseases, or medications leading to an increase in the respiratory rate and resultant CO_2 exhalation. CO_2 levels consequently decrease, increasing pH. Table 4-5. provides causes of respiratory alkalosis grouped by the underlying mechanism.

1. Central nervous system conditions, pain, or anxiety leading to hyperventilation.
2. Acute asthma exacerbation or acute pulmonary disorders due to respiratory stimulation, hypoxia, or hypoxemia.

Table 4-5. Causes of Respiratory Alkalosis.

Cause	Examples
Medications (stimulate central nervous system respiration)	Xanthine derivatives (theophylline, aminophylline, caffeine) Nicotine Catecholamines (eg, epinephrine, norepinephrine, dopamine) Salicylate overdose
Central nervous system stimulation of respiration	Brain tumors Encephalitis, meningitis Head trauma Vascular accidents Anxiety Pain Fever Pregnancy
Hypoxia	High altitudes Hyperventilation Hypoxemia Pneumonia Pulmonary edema Severe anemia
Peripheral stimulation of respiration	Pulmonary embolus Asthma
Other	Thyrotoxicosis Cirrhosis

3. Living at a high altitude where oxygen concentrations are lower.
4. Pregnancy due to elevation in progesterone leading to increased ventilation and decreased PCO_2.
5. Salicylate use, the most common medication-related cause of respiratory alkalosis, due to direct stimulation of medullary chemoreceptors.
6. Other medications, such as theophylline and aminophylline that stimulate the respiratory drive and increase the ventilatory response to CO_2.
7. Renal insufficiency resulting in impaired compensation.
8. Hepatic encephalopathy (see Chapter 5).

Clinical Presentation[7]

1. Symptoms include nausea, vomiting, increased respiratory rate, dizziness, paresthesia, anxiety, chest pain/tightness, palpitations, and tetany.

2. Severe cases of acute respiratory alkalosis (developing within 48 hours) may present with confusion, syncope, or seizures due to cerebral vasoconstriction and decreased cerebral blood flow.

Diagnosis/Diagnostic Tests

1. Complete a thorough patient history and physical, including a medication history upon presentation.

2. Salicylate and theophylline serum levels can identify salicylate overdose or methylxanthine toxicity, respectively.

3. Obtain an ABG to determine the primary disorder and the presence of concomitant acid-base disorders.

4. Obtain serum chemistry to ascertain renal status and specific electrolyte abnormalities that may cause respiratory alkalosis (eg, hypokalemia, hypophosphatemia, hypocalcemia).

5. Obtain complete blood count to identify potential infection or presence of anemia.

6. As with respiratory acidosis, radiographic imaging (eg, chest radiography, computed tomography, magnetic resonance imaging) can be helpful in identifying infectious processes, malignancy, and pulmonary disorders (eg, pulmonary embolism).

7. Obtain microbiology analysis (eg, sputum culture) to identify infectious pathogens and guide antimicrobial therapy.

8. Obtain thyroid function tests (eg, thyrotropin, thyroxine) to rule out hyperthyroidism.

9. Obtain liver function tests or serum ammonia to determine if hepatic failure is an underlying cause.

Goals of Therapy

The goals of therapy in respiratory alkalosis are to normalize pH, treat and/or optimize therapy of underlying condition, and relieve and/or prevent associated symptoms.

Management[7,8,16]

The management strategies used for respiratory alkalosis depend upon the severity of symptoms and condition of the patient. Respiratory alkalosis is rarely life threatening; however, its presence may be the first sign of underlying cardiac or pulmonary illness prior to decompensation. Management of respiratory alkalosis should focus on treating or removing the underlying cause and providing appropriate supportive care measures. This process may include one or more of the following:

- Discontinuation of offending medication(s).

- For patients with anxiety or hyperventilation syndrome, reassurance with or without the use of a rebreathing device (eg, paper bag) is the first line recommendation. Sedatives and antidepressants may be required for severe anxiety attacks or those not responding to conservative treatment. β-Adrenergic blockers may be helpful to reduce or eliminate hyperventilation due to a hyperadrenergic state. Complete further investigation into psychological stress once anxiety or hyperventilation syndrome is under control.

- *Use analgesic agents in patients with inadequate sedation, pain, or both.*

- When hyperventilation occurs during mechanical ventilation, measures to slow the mechanical delivery of breaths and decrease the tidal volume can assist in reducing CO_2 excretion.

- Initiate empiric antibiotics upon presentation for patients with suspected infections. Obtain cultures and sensitivities with de-escalation of antimicrobial agents to only those necessary for successful eradication of infection.

Monitoring

Base the frequency and extent of monitoring on clinical status and underlying cause(s) of respiratory alkalosis. Monitoring may include but is not limited to the following:

1. ABG and serum chemistries (hypophosphatemia may be present because increased uptake of phosphate into the cells occurs with alkalosis)

2. Vital signs (blood pressure, heart rate, respiratory rate, continuous pulse oximetry)

3. Neurological assessments

4. Microbiology cultures

5. Radiologic imaging based on clinical condition or suspicion of disease

6. ECG monitoring

Metabolic Acid-Base Disorders

Primary metabolic acid-base disorders result from a condition, disease, or situation that leads to alterations in serum HCO_3^-. Prompt, accurate identification and treatment are necessary to prevent significant morbidity and mortality. Two subtypes of metabolic acid-base disorders exist. For metabolic acidosis, calculation of the AG helps to identify underlying causes and to guide therapy. For metabolic alkalosis, treatment should center on the classification of saline responsive or saline resistant.

Metabolic Acidosis[1,7]

1. Decreased pH (< 7.4) as a result of a primary decrease in serum HCO_3^- (< 24 mEq/L).

2. Respiratory compensation occurs rapidly by the lungs through increasing the respiratory rate (ie, hyperventilation). When concomitant pulmonary dysfunction is present, compensation may not be complete.

3. The first step in assessing a metabolic acidosis is calculating the AG, which will direct diagnosis and treatment (see Step 4 under Stepwise Approach for the Management of Acid-Base Disorders).

Etiology and Risk Factors[7–12,18–22]

Metabolic acidosis results from conditions, diseases, medications, or toxins that ultimately produce an acidic state. There are 2 classifications of metabolic acidosis, non-AG and AG metabolic acidosis. Non-AG metabolic acidosis is a result of the loss of HCO_3^- or retention of hydrogen ions. AG acidosis is the result of either an increase in the levels of acids normally present in the body or the introduction of exogenous acids.

1. Clinicians often use simple mnemonics to remember the major causes of non-AG and AG metabolic acidosis.

2. The commonly used mnemonic for non-AG metabolic acidosis is ACCRUED, where A = ammonium chloride, C = chronic renal failure,

C = carbonic anhydrase inhibitors, R = renal tubular acidosis, U = ureteroenterostomy (eg, ileal conduit), E = extra-alimentation (eg, excessive Cl^- supplementation in parenteral nutrition [PN] formulation) or endocrine disorders (eg, aldosterone deficiency), D = diarrhea/ gastrointestinal (GI) losses due to high output ostomies or GI fistula.

- Ammonium chloride is converted to urea and free hydrochloric acid, producing acidosis.
- Renal disorders reduce the amount of acid excreted or the amount of HCO_3^- reabsorbed (eg, renal failure, renal tubular acidosis)
- Carbonic anhydrase inhibitors (eg, acetazolamide) result in significant renal losses of HCO_3^-.
- Patients with a urinary diversion (eg, ileal conduit) following bladder resection can develop a hyperchloremic metabolic acidosis from ileal reabsorption of Cl^- and secretion of HCO_3^-.
- Excessive administration of chloride salts in PN or 0.9% NaCl infusions can lead to hyperchloremia.
- Aldosterone deficiency is associated with a hyperkalemic distal renal tubular acidosis.
- Excessive HCO_3^- loss from the GI tract can be seen with diarrhea and high output ostomy or fistula losses (> 1 L/d), leading to a positive balance of H^+ to HCO_3^-.

3. The commonly used mnemonic used for AG metabolic acidosis is GOLD MARK, where G = glycols (ethylene and propylene), O = oxoproline, L = lactate, D = D-lactate, M = methanol, A = aspirin (salicylates), R = renal failure, K = ketoacidosis.

- Suspected poisoning from substances such as salicylates, propylene, or ethylene glycol or from toxic alcohol (eg, methanol) overdose can lead to lactic acidosis with or without ketoacidosis.
- 5-Oxoprolinemia may result during therapeutic doses of acetaminophen in patients with sepsis, malnutrition, liver disease, pregnancy, or renal failure leading to depletion of glutathione stores and resultant accumulation of 5-oxoproline.
- Poor perfusion, circulatory failure, and sepsis leads to poor renal perfusion, disturbances in acid-base homeostasis, and tissue ischemia resulting in lactic acidosis.

- Thiamin is a cofactor for multiple steps in carbohydrate metabolism including the conversion of pyruvate to acetyl-coenzyme A for entry into the Krebs cycle. Dextrose administration during thiamin deficiency leads to conversion of pyruvate to lactate, resulting in lactic acidosis.

- Medications are known to cause lactic acidosis.

- D-Lactic acidosis is a rare complication in patients with blind intestinal loops and short bowel syndrome resulting from fermentation of unabsorbed dietary carbohydrate by luminal bacteria to D-lactic acid that is subsequently absorbed. Patients typically present with encephalopathy symptoms.

- Renal failure, both acute and chronic, can lead to retention of "unmeasured" anions in addition to reduced excretion of acids.

- Uncontrolled diabetes mellitus results in ketoacidosis due to the breakdown of fatty acid stores (eg, diabetic ketoacidosis) during insulin-deficient states.

- Ketosis in malnutrition and chronic alcohol abuse results from a lack of carbohydrate substrate leading to insulin deficiency, glucagon excess, and ultimately increased lipolysis. This leads to generation of free fatty acids that are subsequently converted in the liver to ketoacids.

- Alcoholism places patients at risk of developing ketoacidosis due to long-term malnutrition.

- Malnutrition or prolonged fasting can lead to ketoacidosis secondary to fatty acid metabolism.

4. Respiratory insufficiency or failure may lead to CO_2 retention resulting in impaired compensation.

5. Table 4-6 provides causes of non-AG and AG metabolic acidosis grouped by the underlying mechanism.

Clinical Presentation[7,10]

1. Patients with acute metabolic acidosis are typically symptomatic. Symptoms may include, but are not limited to hyperventilation, headache, nausea, vomiting, sweating, hypotension, ECG changes, arrhythmias, cyanosis, anxiety, lethargy, and altered mental status. Symptoms at presentation are highly dependent upon the underlying etiology.

2. Chronic metabolic acidosis leads to bone demineralization and fractures in adults and stunted growth and rickets in children.

Table 4-6. Causes of Metabolic Acidosis.

Non-Anion Gap	Anion Gap
Gastrointestinal loss of HCO_3^-	Acute and chronic renal failure
Cholestyramine	Ketoacidosis
Diarrhea	Diabetic ketoacidosis
High-output (> 1 L/d) ostomy	Alcohol ketoacidosis
Ileal conduit for urinary diversion	Starvation ketoacidosis
Pancreatic, biliary, or small bowel fistula	Lactic acidosis
Excessive ingestion of acidic/ chloride-based substances	Tissue hypoxia (shock, sepsis)
Ammonium chloride	Propofol (doses > 80 mcg/kg/min for > 48 h)
Overuse of chloride salts in parenteral nutriton	Metformin (use in renal failure)
Renal loss of HCO_3^-	Nitroprusside use
Carbonic anhydrase inhibitors (acetazolamide, zonisamide)	Nucleoside-analog reverse transcriptase inhibitors
Hyperparathyroidism	Carbon monoxide poisoning
Hypoaldosteronism	Liver disease
Renal tubular acidosis	Rhabdomyolysis
Spironolactone	Seizures
Amiloride	Thiamine deficiency
	Short bowel syndrome (D-lactic acid)
	5-Oxoprolinemia (acetaminophen)
	Toxins/overdoses
	Salicylates
	Propylene glycol (used also as a vehicle for intravenous lorazepam and phenobarbital solutions)
	Propyl alcohol
	Methanol
	Ethylene glycol

Diagnosis/Diagnostic Tests[23]

1. Complete a thorough patient history and physical, including a medication history upon presentation.

2. A toxicology panel may prove useful for patients with suspected drug or substance ingestion.

3. Obtain an ABG to determine the primary disorder and the presence of concomitant acid-base disorders.

Table 4-7. Determining Etiology of Hyperchloremic Metabolic Acidosis.

Urinary anion gap	Serum potassium	Urine pH	Diagnosis
Negative	Normal	< 5.5	Normal status
Negative	Normal, low	> 5.5	GI bicarbonate loss
Positive	Elevated	< 5.5	Selective aldosterone deficiency
Positive	Normal, low	> 5.5	Classic RTA
Positive	Elevated	> 5.5	Hyperkalemic distal RTA

GI, gastrointestinal; RTA, renal tubular acidosis.

4. Obtain serum chemistry to ascertain renal status and specific electrolyte abnormalities resulting from metabolic acidosis (eg, hyperkalemia).

5. In the setting of hyperchloremic metabolic acidosis, obtain urine chemistry (Na^+, K^+, and Cl^-) and pH to calculate the urine AG and identify specific renal tubular disorders.

   - Urine AG = (urine Na^+ + urine K^+) − urine Cl^-
   - Use urine AG, urine pH, and serum potassium to further delineate etiology (Table 4-7).

6. Radiographic imaging (eg, abdominal radiography, computed tomography, renal ultrasound) can identify hydronephrosis or gastrointestinal fistulas.

7. Use serum lactate and ketone levels to recognize lactic acidosis and ketoacidosis, respectively.

8. Use ECG to detect conduction abnormalities due to electrolyte abnormalities.

9. Obtain microbiology analysis (eg, blood, urine, sputum culture) in patients with suspected sepsis.

Goals of Therapy

The goals of therapy in metabolic acidosis are to normalize pH, treat and/or optimize therapy of the underlying condition, and prevent and/or relieve associated symptoms. In cases of severe acidemia, the initial goal should be to increase the pH to 7.1–7.2 to reduce the risk of arrhythmias and improve catecholamine responsiveness (eg, norepinephrine, epinephrine).

Management[7,8,11,12,17,19,20]

The management of metabolic acidosis depends on the severity of patient symptoms observed. Treat severe symptoms aggressively to safely restore acid-base homeostasis and prevent further patient decompensation. The presence of an AG determines which type of supportive care to provide to the patient. Correcting the underlying disorder or removing an offending agent is vital to ensure that recurrence of the metabolic disorder does not occur. Treatment and supportive care measures may include one or more of the following:

1. For non-AG metabolic acidosis
   - Discontinue offending medications.
   - Provide fluid replacement with isotonic solutions containing HCO_3^- or a bicarbonate precursor such as acetate or lactate to prevent hyperchloremia (eg, dextrose 5% with $NaHCO_3$ 150 mEq/L).
   - Use acetate salts in place of chloride salts in PN formulations to maintain acid-base homeostasis. $NaHCO_3$ is not compatible with PN formulations.
   - Use antidiarrheal agents (eg, loperamide, diphenoxylate/atropine, tincture of opium) to decrease GI losses of HCO_3^-.
2. For AG metabolic acidosis
   - Discontinue offending medications and/or remove toxins. Methods of removal may include gastric lavage, oral charcoal, and dialysis.
   - Use supportive care measures as appropriate.
   - IV fluid replacement is required in cases in which volume depletion is present. $NaHCO_3$-based IV fluids are not generally required except in cases of severe acidemia.
   - Provision of an insulin infusion, isotonic IV fluids, and electrolyte replacement (eg, hypokalemia, hypophosphatemia) are the primary therapies for diabetic ketoacidosis (see Chapter 5).
   - Initiate empiric antibiotics upon presentation for patients with suspected sepsis. Obtain cultures and sensitivities with de-escalation of antimicrobial agents to only those necessary for successful eradication of infection.
   - Thiamin should be supplemented to correct lactic acidosis in the setting of suspected thiamin deficiency (eg, malnutrition).

For treatment of alcoholic and starvation ketosis, administer dextrose to stimulate pancreatic insulin secretion, which in turn inhibits glucagon secretion and allows the use of dextrose as a primary energy source. Thiamin supplementation prior to dextrose administration and electrolyte supplementation is needed to prevent Wernicke's encephalopathy, Korsakoff's syndrome, and electrolyte depletion (eg, hypophosphatemia, hypokalemia, hypomagnesemia) due to refeeding syndrome (see Chapter 5).

- In cases of D-lactic acidosis, institute dietary restrictions of refined carbohydrate intake, thiamin supplementation if deficiency is suspected, and antibiotic therapy using agents such as metronidazole, neomycin, or vancomycin.

3. For severe metabolic acidosis (pH < 7.2), irrespective of AG, replace the HCO_3^- deficit promptly to restore acid-base homeostasis.

   - HCO_3^- supplementation (eg, $NaHCO_3$, acetate salts, lactate salts)

     - IV $NaHCO_3$, 2–5 mEq/kg infused over 4–8 hours
     - HCO_3^- deficit (mEq) = 0.5 L/kg × lean body weight (kg) × [desired serum HCO_3^- (mEq/L) – current serum HCO_3^- (mEq/L)]
     - Consider one-time bolus doses of $NaHCO_3^-$, 50–100 mEq via IV push, in severe cases of metabolic acidosis.
     - Infuse IV $NaHCO_3^-$ via a central line.

Monitoring

Base the frequency and extent of monitoring on clinical status and underlying causes of respiratory acidosis. Monitoring may include but is not limited to the following:

1. ABG and serum chemistries
2. Vital signs (blood pressure, heart rate, respiratory rate, continuous pulse oximetry)
3. Neurological assessments
4. ECG monitoring
5. Microbiology cultures
6. Radiologic imaging based on clinical condition or suspicion of disease

Metabolic Alkalosis[1,7,16]

1. Increased pH (> 7.4) as a result of a primary increase in serum HCO_3^- (> 24 mEq/L).

2. Respiratory compensation by hypoventilation may occur in response to metabolic alkalosis, resulting in increased PCO_2. Compensation may not be complete if concomitant pulmonary dysfunction is present.

3. The first step in assessing metabolic alkalosis is measurement of urine Cl^- concentration, which will determine if the disorder is either saline responsive or saline resistant. A spot urine check is sufficient for determining the urine chloride concentration.

    - Urine Cl^- < 10 mEq/L = saline responsive.

    - Urine Cl^- > 10 mEq/L = saline resistant.

Etiology and Risk Factors[7,8,10,16,22]

Metabolic alkalosis results from conditions, diseases, or medications ultimately producing an alkalotic state. There are 2 classifications of metabolic alkalosis, saline responsive and saline resistant. Saline-responsive metabolic alkalosis is a result of the loss of acidic fluids or volume depletion. Saline-resistant metabolic alkalosis results from having too much HCO_3^- in the body or a shift of hydrogen ions from the blood into the cells. Excessive $NaHCO_3$ supplementation or administration of bicarbonate precursors such as acetate, lactate, or citrate is an unclassified cause of metabolic alkalosis except during cases of excessive bicarbonate administration in patients with reduced renal function, which is consistent with saline-resistant metabolic alkalosis.

1. Clinicians often use simple mnemonics to remember the major causes for saline-responsive metabolic alkalosis.

2. The commonly used mnemonic for metabolic alkalosis is DAMPEN, where D = diuretics, A = adenoma of the colon, M = miscellaneous (eg, bulimia), P = post-hypercapnia, E = emesis, N = nasogastric tube output.

    - Thiazide and loop diuretics result in significant renal losses of Na^+ and K^+ primarily with Cl^-, secondary hyperaldosteronism due to intravascular volume depletion, and renal ammoniagenesis due to hypokalemia.

- Diarrhea associated with villous adenomas leads to losses of fluids high in Cl^- and low in HCO_3^-.

- Renal compensation during respiratory acidosis consists of increased HCO_3^- reabsorption. Rapid correction of hypercapnia (ie, reduction in elevated Pco_2 levels) through means of mechanical ventilation can lead to a period of elevated serum HCO_3^- until the kidneys are able to recompensate through excretion of excess HCO_3^-.

- Upper GI fluids are rich in H^+ and Cl^-. Excessive losses (eg, emesis, nasogastric tube output) facilitate an acid deficit relative to serum HCO_3^- levels, resulting in metabolic alkalosis. This process also occurs in bulimia patients who purge after eating.

- Intravascular volume depletion can alter the HCO_3^- balance between intracellular and extracellular fluid, leading to a contraction alkalosis.

3. The commonly used mnemonic for saline-resistant metabolic alkalosis is A BELCH, where A = alkali ingestion with reduced glomerular filtration rate, B = 11-β-hydroxylase deficiency, E = exogenous steroids, L = licorice ingestion, C = Cushing's syndrome, H = hyperaldosteronism.

   - Hypokalemia leads to increased renin activity and net acid excretion.

   - 11-β-Hydroxylase deficiency is a congenital adrenal hyperplasia and possesses features of androgen and mineralocorticoid excess leading to hypertension, hypokalemia, and metabolic alkalosis.

   - Exogenous steroids (eg, fludrocortisone, hydrocortisone) or conditions resulting in mineralocorticoid excess (eg, hyperaldosteronism, Cushing's syndrome) lead to significant renal H^+ and K^+ depletion.

   - Bartter's and Gitelman's syndromes have ion transporter defects impairing Na^+ and Cl^- reabsorption in the loop of Henle (Bartter's syndrome) and "diluting segment" of the distal tubule (Gitelman's syndrome) which leads to hypokalemia, secondary hyperaldosteronism, and metabolic alkalosis.

   - Licorice contains glycyrrhizic acid and upon excessive intake, results in a reversible inhibition of 11-β-hydroxysteroid dehydrogenase. This renal enzyme prevents the conversion of cortisol to cortisone and leads to excess mineralocorticoid production.

4. Table 4-8 provides causes of saline-responsive and saline-resistant metabolic alkalosis grouped by underlying mechanism.

Table 4-8. Causes of Metabolic Alkalosis.

Saline-Responsive (Urine Cl^- < 10 mEq/L)	Saline-Resistant (Urine Cl^- > 10 mEq/L)
Cystic fibrosis (loss of Cl^- in sweat)	Cushing's syndrome
Diuretic therapy	11-β-Hydroxylase deficiency
Loop diuretics (furosemide, bumetanide, torsemide, ethacrynic acid)	Excessive mineralcorticoid use
	Fludrocortisone
Thiazide diuretics (hydrochlorothiazide, chlorthalidone)	Hydrocortisone
Excessive HCO_3^- administration	Hyperaldosteronism
Sodium bicarbonate	Excessive licorice ingestion
Citrate	Renal artery stenosis
Antacids	Profound potassium depletion
Overuse of acetate salts in parenteral nutriton	Laxative abuse
Gastrointestinal losses	Clay ingestion
Vomiting	
Nasogastric suctioning	
Gastric fistula	
Villous adenoma	
Rapid correction of hypocapnia	

Clinical Presentation[7,10]

1. Patients with metabolic alkalosis present with symptoms that may include those associated with volume depletion (eg, fatigue, poor tissue turgor, dry mucus membranes, low blood pressure, tachycardia, and orthostasis) and/or hypokalemia (eg, muscle weakness, ECG changes, polyuria, polydipsia).

2. Severe cases may present with neuromuscular excitability, mental status changes, and vasoconstriction.

Diagnosis/Diagnostic Tests

1. Complete a thorough patient history and physical, including a medication history upon presentation.

2. Obtain an ABG to determine the primary disorder and the presence of concomitant acid-base disorders.

3. Obtain serum chemistry to ascertain renal status and identify electrolyte abnormalities.

4. Obtain urine Cl^- to determine etiology and treatment strategies.

5. Obtain plasma renin and aldosterone levels to identify hyperaldosteronism, and cortisol level to identify Cushing's syndrome, as appropriate.

6. Use ECG monitoring to identify arrhythmias due to hypokalemia.

Goals of Therapy

The goals of therapy in metabolic alkalosis are to normalize pH, treat and/or optimize therapy of underlying condition, and prevent and/or relieve associated symptoms.

Management[7,8,16,17,24,25]

The management of metabolic alkalosis depends on the severity of patient symptoms observed. Treat severe symptoms aggressively to safely restore acid-base homeostasis and prevent further patient decompensation. Correcting the underlying disorder or removing an offending agent is the primary focus of management and is vital to ensure that recurrence of the metabolic disorder does not occur. Supportive care measures may also be required to prevent or limit significant morbidity.

1. Saline-responsive metabolic alkalosis

    - Discontinue offending medications.

    - Use isotonic saline-based IV fluids to correct volume depletion (ie, 0.9% NaCl).

    - Use chloride salts in place of acetate salts in PN formulations to maintain acid-base homeostasis.

    - Use potassium supplements or potassium-sparing diuretics to correct potassium deficits (see Chapter 3).

    - Antiemetic medications (eg, promethazine, ondansetron) may decrease vomiting and loss of gastric fluids.

    - Acid suppression therapy using histamine-2 receptor blockers (eg, ranitidine, famotidine) or proton pump inhibitors (eg, omeprazole, esomeprazole, lansoprazole, pantoprazole) can decrease gastric hydrochloric acid production and acid losses.

- Use carbonic anhydrase inhibitors (eg, acetazolamide) to promote renal HCO_3^- excretion for diuretic-induced contraction alkalosis.
  - Acetazolamide 250–500 mg IV every 8 hours, with therapy duration depending on the degree of alkalosis and response to therapy

2. Saline-resistant metabolic alkalosis
   - Use potassium-sparing diuretics (eg, spironolactone, amiloride, triamterene) to treat primary mineralocorticoid excess and primary hyperaldosteronism.
   - Use potassium supplements or potassium-sparing diuretics to correct potassium deficits (see Chapter 3).
   - Consider corticosteroid replacement and antihypertensive agents as appropriate.
   - Surgical resections can be pursued for primary disorders caused by tumors or adenomas.
   - *Discontinue licorice intake.*
   - Adjust bicarbonate administration in patients with reduced glomerular filtration rate.

3. For severe cases of metabolic alkalosis ($pH > 7.6$), acidic solutions (eg, hydrochloric acid) or hemodialysis can restore acid-base homeostasis.
   - Hydrochloric acid (0.1 N)
     - Infusion only recommended through a central line and administered over 4–6 hours.
     - Hydrochloric acid dose (mEq or mmol) = weight (kg) × 0.5 L/kg × (observed HCO_3^- − desired HCO_3^-).
     - Evidence supporting the use of hydrochloric acid in correcting metabolic alkalosis is minimal, and it is not commonly used in clinical practice. Administer only under the supervision of an experienced clinician.
   - Hemodialysis using low HCO_3^- concentration
     - Reserved for patients with advanced renal failure or those resistant to acetazolamide.

Monitoring

Base the frequency and extent of monitoring on clinical status and underlying causes of respiratory acidosis. Monitoring may include but is not limited to the following:

1. ABG

2. Serum and urine chemistries

3. Vital signs (blood pressure, heart rate, respiratory rate, continuous pulse oximetry)

4. Neurological assessments

5. ECG monitoring

Patient Scenario 1

Carl is a 62-year-old man with a history of Crohn's disease. His disease course has included small bowel strictures resulting in multiple small bowel resections that ultimately required creation of an end-ileostomy. He was admitted to the hospital for weight loss and fatigue, high ostomy output, and volume depletion. Regular diet and IV fluids of 0.9% NaCl at 125 mL/h were initiated. The dietitian reports that Carl eats a regular diet without restrictions. On hospital day 3, he experiences shortness of breath, and an ABG is drawn.

Day	Weight, kg	Ileostomy output, mL
1	44	2550
2	43	4570
3	41.5	3220

Day	Na^+, mEq/L	K^+, mEq/L	Cl^-, mEq/L	HCO_3^-, mEq/L	BUN, mg/dL	Creatinine, mg/dL	Glucose, mg/dL
1	131	3.3	97	18	69	1.4	125
2	137	4.1	112	14	30	1.2	108
3	137	4.1	114	12	23	1.1	134

BUN, blood urea nitrogen.

	pH	PCO_2, mm Hg	PO_2, mm Hg	HCO_3^-, mEq/L	SO_2, %
Day 3	7.31	24	74	11	99

SO_2, oxygen saturation.

Steps in Assessment of ABGs

1. Assess pH—*acidemic*
   - pH < 7.4
2. Assess PCO_2—*respiratory alkalosis (since patient is acidemic, this is not the primary disorder)*
   - PCO_2 < 40 mm Hg
3. Assess HCO_3^-—*metabolic acidosis (since patient is acidemic, this is the primary disorder)*
   - HCO_3^- < 24 mEq/L
4. Calculate AG in metabolic acidosis—*non-AG metabolic acidosis*
   - $AG = Na^+ - (Cl^- + HCO_3^-) = 137 - (114 + 12) = 11$
5. Determine if the acid-base disorder is acute (< 48 hours) or chronic in nature (> 48 hours) and if compensation for the primary disorder is present—*metabolic acidosis*
   - It is not necessary to determine whether it is acute or chronic because it is a primary metabolic disorder.
   - Is the respiratory system compensating adequately?
     - Expected $PCO_2 = 1.5 \times HCO_3^- + (8 \pm 2) = 1.5 \times 11 + (8 \pm 2) =$ 22.5–26.5 mm Hg
     - Expected $PCO_2 \approx$ actual PC_0 – appropriate respiratory compensation
6. Diagnosis: Carl has a primary metabolic acidosis due to GI losses of HCO_3^- from his high-output ileostomy.

CHAPTER 4 Acid-Base Homeostasis and Disorders

7. Treatment options include the following:

- Provide patient education on consuming small frequent meals and avoiding disaccharides to reduce the osmotic load to the GI tract, maximize absorption, and minimize ostomy effluent.[26,27]

- Patients with ileostomies are at risk for acid-base disturbances due to GI losses of fluids and electrolytes. Management of high-output ileostomies (>1 L/d) should include fluid replacement that approximates the electrolyte composition of ileal fluid (see Table 1-5) and use of antidiarrheal agents as needed.

- If ileostomy continues to be high output and weight loss worsens, the patient may benefit from PN for the provision of nutrition support.

Patient Scenario 2

Andrea is a 60-year-old woman who reports to the emergency department (ED) with a 3-day history of nausea and vomiting, malaise, and generalized weakness. While in the ED, she becomes unarousable. Serum chemistries and ABG are drawn. Her past medical history is significant for hypertension. Home medications include amlodipine 5 mg by mouth daily and hydrochlorothiazide 25 mg by mouth daily.

	Na^+, mEq/L	K^+, mEq/L	Cl^-, mEq/L	HCO_3^-, mEq/L	BUN, mg/dL	Creatinine, mg/dL	Glucose, mg/dL
Day 1 (ED)	136	3	100	32	30	1.2	89

	pH	PCO_2, mm Hg	PO_2, mm Hg	HCO_3^-, mEq/L	SO_2, %
Day 1 (ED)	7.50	45	88	31	97

BUN, blood urea nitrogen; SO_2, oxygen saturation.

Steps in Assessment of ABGs

1. Assess pH—*alkalemic*

   - pH > 7.4

2. Assess PCO_2—*respiratory acidosis (since patient is alkalemic, this is not the primary disorder)*

   - PCO_2 > 40 mm Hg

3. Assess HCO_3^-—*metabolic alkalosis (since patient is alkalemic, this is the primary disorder)*

   - $HCO_3^- > 24$ mEq/L

4. Calculate AG in metabolic acidosis—*since this is a metabolic alkalosis, no need to calculate AG*

5. Determine if the acid-base disorder is acute (<48 hours) or chronic (> 48 hours) and if compensation for the primary disorder is present—*chronic metabolic alkalosis*

   - Metabolic alkalosis developed over >48 hours.

   - Is the respiratory system compensating adequately?

     - Expected $PCO_2 = 40 + [0.7 \times (\text{measured } HCO_3^- - 24)] = 40 + [0.7 \times (31 - 24)] = 44.9$ mm Hg

     - Expected $PCO_2 \approx$ actual PCO_2 – appropriate respiratory compensation

6. Diagnosis: Andrea has a primary metabolic alkalosis due to GI losses of H^+ and Cl^- from vomiting. In addition, she is also taking a diuretic, which can further potentiate metabolic alkalosis.

7. Treatment options include the following:

   - Provide saline-based IV fluids to replace her volume deficit and antiemetic therapy as needed for nausea and vomiting.

   - Hold diuretic therapy until fluid repletion is complete and AP is tolerating oral diet.

References

1. Adrogué HJ, Gennari FJ, Galla JH, Madias NE. Assessing acid-base disorders. *Kidney Int.* 2009;76(12):1239–1247.
2. Broughton JO. *Understanding Blood Gases.* Madison, WI: Ohio Medical Products; 1979:1–16. Form No. 456.
3. Gauthier PM, Szerlip HM. Metabolic acidosis in the intensive care unit. *Crit Care Clin.* 2002;18(2):289–308.
4. Jung B, Rimmele T, Le Goff C, et al; AzuRea Group. Severe metabolic or mixed acidemia on intensive care unit admission: incidence, prognosis and administration of buffer therapy. A prospective, multiple-center study. *Crit Care.* 2011;15(5):R238.
5. Kaplan LJ, Kellum JA. Initial pH, base deficit, lactate, anion gap, strong ion difference, and strong ion gap predict outcome from major vascular injury. *Crit Care Med.* 2004;32(5):1120–1124.
6. Maciel AT, Park M. Differences in acid-base behavior between intensive care unit survivors and nonsurvivors using both a physicochemical and a standard base excess approach: a prospective, observational study. *J Crit Care.* 2009;24(4):477–483.
7. Ayers P, Warrington L. Diagnosis and treatment of simple acid-base disorders. *Nutr Clin Pract.* 2008;23(2):122–127.
8. Ayers P, Dixon C. Simple acid-base tutorial. *JPEN J Parenter Enteral Nutr.* 2012;36(1):18–23.
9. Reddy P. Clinical utility of anion gap in deciphering acid-base disorders. *Intl J Clin Pract.* 2009;63(10):1516–1525.
10. Al-Jaghbeer M, Kellum JA. Acid-base disturbances in intensive care patients: etiology, pathophysiology, and treatment. *Nephrol Dial Transplant.* 2014;pii:gfu289.
11. Btaiche IF, Khalidi N. Metabolic complications of parenteral nutrition in adults, part 1. *Am J Health Syst Pharm.* 2004;61(18):1938–1949.
12. Androgue HJ, Madias N. Management of life-threatening acid-base disorders. Part 1. *N Engl J Med.* 1998;338:26–34.
13. Motley HL. Sodium bicarbonate in respiratory acidosis. *JAMA.* 1964;189(3):243.
14. Global Initiative for Chronic Obstructive Lung Disease. Global strategy for the diagnosis, management, and prevention of chronic obstructive pulmonary disease. https://goldcopd.org/gold-reports/. Updated January 2020. Accessed February, 2020.
15. National Heart, Lung, and Blood Institute, National Asthma Foundation and Prevention Program. Expert Panel Report 3: Guidelines for the diagnosis and management of asthma. http://www.nhlbi.nih.gov/health-pro/guidelines/current/asthma-guidelines. Published August 28, 2007. Accessed January, 2020.
16. Androgue HJ, Madias N. Management of life-threatening acid-base disorders. Second of two parts. *N Engl J Med.* 1998;338(2):107–111.
17. Btaiche IF, Khalidi N. Metabolic complications of parenteral nutrition in adults, part 2. *Am J Health Syst Pharm.* 2004;61(19):2050–2057.
18. Kang TM. Propofol infusion syndrome in critically ill patients. *Ann Pharmacother.* 2002;36(9):1453–1456.
19. Nightingale JM. Management of patients with a short bowel. *Nutrition.* 1999;15(7–8):633–637.
20. Wrenn KD, Slovis CM, Minion GE, Rutkowski R. The syndrome of alcoholic ketoacidosis. *Am J Med.* 1991;91(2):119–128.
21. Mehta AN, Emmett JB, Emmett M. GOLD MARK: an anion gap mnemonic for the 21st century. *Lancet* 2008;372(9642):892.

22. Kaplan LJ, Kellum JA. Fluids, pH, ions and electrolytes. *Curr Opin Crit Care.* 2010;16(4);323–331.

23. Batlle DC, Hizon M, Cohen E, Gutterman C, Gupta R. The use of the urinary anion gap in the diagnosis of hyperchloremic metabolic acidosis. *N Engl J Med.* 1988;318(10):594–599.

24. Mazur JE, Devlin JW, Peters MJ, Jankowski MA, Iannuzzi MC, Zarowitz BJ. Single versus multiple doses of acetazolamide for metabolic alkalosis in critically ill medical patients: a randomized, double-blind trial. *Crit Care Med.* 1999;27(7):1257–1261.

25. Wagner CW, Nesbit RR Jr, Mansberger AR Jr. The use of intravenous hydrochloric acid in the treatment of thirty-four patients with metabolic alkalosis. *Am Surg.* 1980;46(3):140–146.

26. Woolf GM, Miller C, Kurian R, Jeejeebhoy KN. Diet for patients with short bowel: high fat or high carbohydrate? *Gastroenterology.* 1983;84(4):823–828.

27. Matarese LE. Nutrition and fluid optimization for patients with short bowel syndrome. *JPEN J Parenter Enteral Nutr.* 2013;37(2):161–170.

CHAPTER 5

Common Clinically Applicable Situations

Numerous diseases and situations encountered in clinical practice affect fluid, electrolyte, and acid-base homeostasis. Clinicians must identify these situations, understand organ physiology and disease pathophysiology, and develop management strategies to prevent morbidity and mortality. This chapter will focus on renal, hepatic, and gastrointestinal (GI) disorders; hyperglycemic emergencies; refeeding syndrome; and adrenal insufficiency. It will also include each condition's effects on fluid, electrolyte, and acid-base homeostasis.

Renal Failure

Overview[1–3]

The kidneys play an integral part in many key functions in the body, including regulation of blood pressure, gluconeogenesis, hormone production, and vitamin D activation; removal of waste products, elimination of drugs, drug metabolites, and toxins; electrolyte homeostasis; and maintenance of acid-base and fluid balance. Each kidney's ability to perform many of its functions depends on intact filtration, reabsorption, and secretion.

Much of renal physiology occurs at the level of the nephron, the functional unit of the kidney. The kidney has approximately 1 million nephrons. Each section of the nephron is responsible for specific actions. Blood begins to be filtered at the glomerulus. As this filtrate travels through the nephron, certain substances are reabsorbed while others are secreted to maintain homeostasis (see Table 1-3). When renal injury occurs, abnormalities in fluid, electrolyte, and acid-base homeostasis can develop. These complications can be predicted and explained physiologically based on knowledge of the type and magnitude of renal injury or disease.

Disorders of the kidneys are classified according to the onset and length of renal impairment. The 2 major disorders include acute kidney injury (AKI) and chronic kidney disease (CKD).

Acute Kidney Injury[2,4–7]

- AKI is defined by a sudden decline in renal function occurring over a period of 48 hours to 7 days. AKI may be reversible if the offending condition is corrected or the causative agent is removed.

- AKI is reported to occur in up to 20% of hospitalized and 45% of critically ill patients. Morbidity and mortality are significantly higher in patients that develop AKI than in those without AKI, with an associated mortality rate ranging from 30% to 80%. The magnitude of renal injury directly correlates with mortality and the need for renal replacement therapy (RRT).

- The definition of AKI per the Kidney Disease: Improving Global Outcomes (KDIGO) is based on changes in serum creatinine (SCr) and/or urine output over time (Figure 5-1).

Figure 5-1. Kidney Disease: Improving Global Outcomes—Acute Kidney Injury Definition.

Must have at least 1 of the following parameters present:

Increase in SCr ≥ 0.3 mg/dL within 48 h
OR
Increase of ≥ 1.5 times baseline SCr within 7 d (known or presumed to have occurred during this time period)
OR
Urine output < 0.5 mL/kg/h for 6 h (oliguria)

SCr, serum creatinine.

Adapted with permission from Macmillan Publishers Ltd: Kidney Disease: Improving Global Outcomes (KDIGO) Work Group. KDIGO clinical practice guideline for acute kidney injury, section 2: AKI definition. *Kidney Int Suppl.* 2012;2(1):19–36.

Table 5-1. Kidney Disease: Improving Global Outcomes – Acute Kidney Injury Staging System.

Stage	Serum creatinine	Urine output
1	Increase of ≥ 0.3 mg/dL within 48 hours OR Increase of 1.5–1.9 times baseline SCr	< 0.5 mL/kg/hour for > 6 but < 12 hours
2	Increase of 2–2.9 times baseline SCr	< 0.5 mL/kg/hour for ≥ 12 hours
3	Increase of ≥ 3 times baseline SCr OR Increase in SCr to ≥ 4 mg/dL OR Need and use of renal replacement therapy	< 0.3 mL/kg/hour for ≥ 24 hours OR Anuria for ≥ 12 hours

SCr, serum creatinine.

Adapted with permission from Macmillan Publishers Ltd: *Kidney Int Suppl.* Kidney Disease: Improving Global Outcomes (KDIGO) Work Group. KDIGO clinical practice guideline for acute kidney injury, section 2: AKI definition. 2012;2(1):19–36.

- The KDIGO classification system can be used to stage AKI (Table 5-1). The system was created by merging 2 validated and widely used classification systems: the Risk, Injury, Failure, Loss, and End-stage Renal Disease (RIFLE) and the Acute Kidney Injury Network (AKIN). Similar to the way in which AKI is defined, severity staging is also based on changes in SCr and urine output over time. If the staging scores from SCr or urine output do not correlate, AKI staging should be based on the marker with the highest stage.

AKI Subtypes[2,4,5]

- Three subtypes of AKI have been described: prerenal, intrinsic, and postrenal AKI. Table 5-2 presents etiologies for each subtype.
    - Prerenal AKI is the most common presentation of AKI in outpatients. It results from decreased renal perfusion without structural renal damage. With prompt therapy directed at the underlying cause, prerenal AKI is reversible; however, if renal hypoperfusion is prolonged, irreversible damage will ensue.
    - Intrinsic (intrarenal) AKI is the most common type of AKI in inpatients, with 50% of cases due to renal ischemia. Damage to the kidney occurs with resultant reduction in the glomerular filtration rate (GFR). Intrinsic AKI is further divided into acute tubular necrosis, acute

Table 5-2. Etiology of Acute Kidney Injury Subtypes.[6,7]

AKI subtype	Etiology
Prerenal	Intravascular volume depletion Gastrointestinal, skin, or renal losses Hemorrhage Third spacing of fluid Decreased effective blood volume Sepsis Shock Cardiac failure Excessive or overdiuresis Alterations in intrarenal hemodynamics NSAIDs (eg, ibuprofen, ketorolac, naproxen), ACEIs (eg, lisinopril, captopril, enalapril), ARBs (eg, losartan, valsartan), calcineurin inhibitors (eg, tacrolimus, cyclosporine)
Intrinsic (intrarenal)	
Acute tubular necrosis	Ischemia Sepsis Hypotension Prolonged prerenal azotemia Cardiopulmonary arrest Rhabdomyolysis Nephrotoxic drugs Aminoglycosides (eg, gentamicin, tobramycin, amikacin), amphotericin B, vancomycin, cisplatin, pentamidine, cidofovir, foscarnet, radiocontrast agents
Acute interstitial nephritis	Renal infections Pyelonephritis Systemic diseases Systemic lupus erythematosus Sjögren's syndrome Sarcoidosis Drug-induced β-Lactam antibiotics (eg, penicillin, piperacillin/tazobactam, cefepime, ceftazidine, meropenem), sulfonamides (eg, sulfamethoxazole), rifampin, NSAIDs, diuretics (eg, furosemide, hydrochlorothiazide), antiepileptic agents (eg, phenytoin, valproic acid), proton pump inhibitors (eg, omeprazole), allopurinol, calcineurin inhibitors
Glomerulonephritis	Post-streptococcal infection Autoimmune diseases Goodpasture's syndrome Wegener's granulomatosis Systemic lupus erythematosus Drug induced (uncommon) NSAIDs, captopril, penicillamine, gold therapy
Renal vascular damage	Renal artery thrombosis Diffuse renal vasculitis

Table 5-2. *Continued.*

AKI subtype	Etiology
Postrenal	Ureteral obstruction Malignancy Inflammation Fibrosis Drug induced (crystal formation) Acyclovir, indinavir, methotrexate, sulfonamides, triamterene, foscarnet Bladder outflow obstruction Benign prostatic hypertrophy Malignancy Drug induced (anticholinergic effects) Diphenhydramine, doxylamine, promethazine

ACEI, angiotensin-converting enzyme inhibitor; AKI, acute kidney injury; ARB, angiotensin receptor blocker; NSAID, nonsteroidal anti-inflammatory drug.

interstitial nephritis, acute glomerulonephritis, and renal vascular damage.

- Acute tubular necrosis develops primarily as a result of ischemia or nephrotoxic agents. For patients without severe or permanent damage, large-volume diuresis and renal electrolyte losses frequently occur during the recovery phase and renal tubule cell regeneration.
- Acute interstitial nephritis results from infiltration of inflammatory cells in the interstitium. Drug-induced causes are common and manifest after drug exposure. Patients typically present with an allergic hypersensitivity response (ie, fever, rash, arthralgia, and rarely eosinophiluria).
- Acute glomerulonephritis is the third most common cause of CKD. It results from inflammation of the glomerular structure due to damage from immune complexes. This subtype includes nephritic and nephrotic syndrome.
- Renal vascular damage includes damage to or inflammation of the vascular structures of the kidney.

- Postrenal AKI results from obstruction of the urinary collection system.

Chronic Kidney Disease[2,8–10]

- An estimated 8% to 16% of the worldwide population has some degree of CKD. The actual value may be higher due to underdiagnosis of early stages of CKD. According to the 1999–2006 National Health and Nutrition Examination Survey, the prevalence of CKD in individuals ≥ 60 years of age is 39.4% and roughly 10% for those ages 20–59 years. This prevalence is consistent with aging of the population and an increased number of people with diabetes mellitus. Hypertension and diabetes mellitus are the major causes of CKD. Other causes include glomerulonephritis, polycystic kidney disease, and prolonged episodes of AKI.

- According to KDIGO, a diagnosis of CKD requires at least 1 structural or functional abnormality within the kidney to be present for > 3 months (Figure 5-2).

- CKD is staged based on cause, GFR (Table 5-3), and presence/degree of albuminuria (Table 5-4). Metabolic alterations increase with the severity of CKD. Similar to AKI, increases in morbidity and mortality occur with advanced CKD stages and the need for RRT.

Figure 5-2. Kidney Disease: Improving Global Outcomes—Chronic Kidney Disease Definition.

Must have <u>at least</u> 1 of the following parameters present for <u>at least</u> 3 months:

1. Albuminuria (AER of ≥ 30 mg/24 h or an ACR ≥ 30 mg/g)
2. Urine sediment abnormalities (eg, red blood cell, leukocytes, or other cellular casts)
3. Tubular disorders resulting in electrolyte or other abnormalities
4. Histological abnormalities (eg, fibrosis, sclerosis, amyloid deposits)
5. Structural abnormalities confirmed by imaging (eg, cysts, fibrosis, stones, renal asymmetry)
6. Previous renal transplantation
7. GFR < 60 mL/min/1.73 m^2

ACR, albumin-to-creatinine ratio (provided in approximate equivalent); AER, albumin excretion ratio; GFR, glomerular filtration rate.

Adapted with permission from Macmillan Publishers Ltd: Kidney Disease: Improving Global Outcomes (KDIGO) Work Group. KDIGO clinical practice guideline for the evaluation and management of chronic kidney disease: summary of recommendation statements. *Kidney Int Suppl.* 2013;3(1):5–14.

Table 5-3. Kidney Disease: Improving Global Outcomes—Chronic Kidney Disease Staging System Glomerular Filtration Rate Categories.

Category	GFR, mL/min/1.73 m^2	Description
G1	≥ 90	Normal or high
G2	60-89	Mildly decreased compared to young adult
G3a	49-59	Mildly to moderately decreased
G3b	30-44	Moderately to severely decreased
G4	15-29	Severely decreased
G5	< 15	Kidney failure or on dialysis

GFR, glomerular filtration rate.

Adapted with permission from Macmillan Publishers Ltd: Kidney Disease: Improving Global Outcomes (KDIGO) Work Group. KDIGO clinical practice guideline for the evaluation and management of chronic kidney disease: summary of recommendation statements. *Kidney Int Suppl.* 2013;3(1):5–14.

- Management is aimed at preventing CKD progression. Early intervention is vital because progression to later stages of CKD and the need for RRT increase mortality. Intervention occurs through optimization of blood pressure, glycemic control, reduction in cardiovascular risk factors and cardiovascular disease, and prevention of AKI. Angiotensin-converting enzyme inhibitors and angiotensin receptor blockers should be utilized in individuals who can tolerate therapy; however, close monitoring is necessary to prevent electrolyte abnormalities (eg, hyponatremia, hyperkalemia).

Table 5-4. Kidney Disease: Improving Global Outcomes—Chronic Kidney Disease Staging System Albuminuria Categories.

Category	AER, mg/24 h	ACR, mg/g	Description
A1	< 30	< 30	Normal to mildly increased
A2	30-300	30-300	Moderately increased compared to young adult
A3	> 300	> 300	Severely increased, includes nephrotic syndrome

ACR, albumin-to-creatinine ratio (provided in approximate equivalent); AER, albumin excretion ratio.

Adapted with permission from Macmillan Publishers Ltd: Kidney Disease: Improving Global Outcomes (KDIGO) Work Group. KDIGO clinical practice guideline for the evaluation and management of chronic kidney disease: summary of recommendation statements. *Kidney Int Suppl.* 2013;3(1):5–14.

Disorders Associated with AKI/CKD and Management Strategies[2,3,10–18]

- Disorders in fluid, electrolyte, and acid-base balance are common in patients with AKI and CKD.
- Nutrition support, urine output, RRT, and medications greatly influence the development of electrolyte and acid-base abnormalities and the need for management strategies to restore normal balance and prevent untoward complications.
    - Nutrition support
        - Initiation and advancement of nutrition support therapies in individuals with malnutrition or prolonged inadequate oral intake can lead to refeeding syndrome and consequent fluid retention and electrolyte abnormalities (see Refeeding Syndrome section).
    - Urine output
        - Oliguric and anuric AKI patients not receiving RRT generally have minimal requirements for fluid and electrolyte (K^+, Mg^{2+}, Ca^{2+}, PO_4) supplementation due to decreased elimination. Oliguria is referred to as < 400–500 mL urine production per day, and anuria is < 50 mL/d.
        - Conversely, AKI patients without oliguria and those in the recovery phase of acute tubular necrosis require close monitoring of urine output and serum electrolyte concentrations because increased electrolyte losses may occur along with the inability to conserve water.
    - RRT
        - Knowledge of the type, filter permeability, and dialysate solution is needed to determine electrolyte and acid-base management strategies because differences exist in fluid and micronutrient removal based on these factors. Care needs to be coordinated with the nephrology team to decrease the risk of potential complications related to electrolyte provision.
        - Peritoneal dialysis (PD) is a form of RRT utilized in 10%–15% of patients with stage 5 CKD, primarily in the ambulatory setting. Through a peritoneal catheter, dialysate solution is instilled into the peritoneal cavity where it is allowed to dwell for a set period of time. During this dwell time, solutes are removed from the blood

through the peritoneal membrane using diffusion and ultrafiltration. Dextrose or icodextrin in the dialysate solution provides the osmotic gradient for plasma water removal and absorption of dextrose via the peritoneal space can lead to worsening hyperglycemia. PD exchanges can be completed intermittently or continuously, using a manual technique or an automated device. Clearance of solute can be enhanced by increasing the number of dialysate exchanges per day, volume of dialysate instilled, and dwell time; however, adequacy can still prove problematic. Peritonitis, hyperglycemia, and malnutrition are complications associated with PD. Patient compliance and use of aseptic technique are vital to the success of PD use.

- Intermittent hemodialysis (IHD) is the most common type of RRT. It is used in both inpatient and outpatient settings and is done over a time period of 3–4 hours, 3 times a week to daily. Blood is removed from the patient via an intravenous (IV) catheter and run through a dialysis machine, which filters the blood against a dialysate solution to remove small molecules using diffusion. Filtered blood is then circulated back to the patient through a separate IV catheter lumen. The sodium, potassium, bicarbonate, and calcium content of the dialysate solution may vary; the solution does not contain phosphate. Hemodynamic stability is required because large fluid shifts may occur due to the rapid fluid removal, often 1–4 L per IHD session. IHD removes electrolytes effectively, with the exception of phosphorus because phosphate removal requires more time.

- Continuous RRT (CRRT) is preferred in the intensive care unit where hemodynamic compromise may not permit IHD use. CRRT requires a longer period of time but removes greater amounts of fluid and solutes (eg, electrolytes) compared with IHD and PD. Replacement fluids including electrolytes are generally required to prevent intravascular volume depletion, worsening renal function, and electrolyte deficiencies. Clotting may occur within the CRRT system, requiring the use of citrate anticoagulation to ensure adequate therapy and prevent interruptions. Hypocalcemia may develop with the use of 4% trisodium citrate anticoagulation, necessitating concomitant IV calcium replacement via intermittent dosing or continuous infusion.

- Dialysate solutions are fluids used during RRT to facilitate removal of wastes and electrolytes from the blood. They are either commercially available solutions or individualized, compounded formulations. Dialysate solutions are primarily composed of fluid, dextrose, sodium, potassium, calcium, magnesium, and bicarbonate. Dialysate solutions are chosen based on serum concentrations of electrolytes and acid-base status, as well as the type of RRT system utilized. The composition of dialysate solution can be adjusted to facilitate electrolyte and acid-base homeostasis. Supplementation via the oral, IV, and/or nutrition support route(s) can be added to help normalize serum electrolyte concentrations when the clinical situation dictates.

    - Medication therapy
        - A thorough medication review is essential for all patients with AKI and CKD because numerous medications affect electrolyte homeostasis. Chapter 3 presents comprehensive lists of these medications.
        - Use of medications predisposing patients to fluid retention (eg, corticosteroids, nonsteroidal anti-inflammatory drugs) should be minimized.

- Electrolyte dosing considerations exist for renal patients and should be employed to prevent untoward effects.
    - Fluid and electrolyte supplementation is largely based on weight, with dry weight preferred for patients with signs of fluid overload and ideal body weight recommended for obese patients. Actual weight should be used for all other patients.
    - In patients with AKI or grade 3–5 CKD, initial electrolyte supplementation dosing should not exceed 50% of the recommended dose for a normal patient unless patient condition and/or serum concentrations dictate otherwise. Subsequent bolus doses should be based on serum concentrations, underlying conditions and treatments, and medication therapy.
    - Recommendations for electrolyte provision in parenteral nutrition (PN) for adults with renal disorders can be found in Table 5-5.
- Management strategies are presented next according to specific disorder and type of renal injury or disease present.
    - Fluid and sodium
        - Fluid balance and serum sodium concentrations are tightly coupled (see sodium disorders in Chapter 3), with requirements dependent on renal function, urine output (nonoliguric, oliguric, anuric), and the need for and type of RRT utilized.

Table 5-5. Fluid and Electrolyte Requirements for Parenteral Nutrition in Renal Failure.

Nutrient	Parenteral Nutrition Content
Fluid	As tolerated or dictated by form of RRT
Sodium	35–75 mEq/L
Potassium	10–40 mEq/L
Magnesium	2–16 mEq/L
Calcium	5–10 mEq/L
Phosphate	3–15 mmol/L

Adapted with permission from Wolk R, Foulks C. Renal disease. In: Mueller CM, ed. *The A.S.P.E.N. Adult Nutrition Support Core Curriculum*. 2nd ed. Silver Spring, MD: American Society for Parenteral and Enteral Nutrition; 2012:491–510.

- Fluid restriction is required for predialysis, PD, and IHD when patients are oliguric or anuric (inpatients and outpatients) based on their fluid input and output, including fluid removed during IHD, where applicable. Use of concentrated enteral nutrition or PN formulations is necessary to restrict fluid input, especially for critically ill patients because adequate volume may be obtained from blood products or other IV medications. During CRRT, fluid intake as tolerated or liberal fluid intake is allowed because this therapy is more efficient at fluid removal; however, CRRT usually results in anuria.

- Sodium restriction is recommended, unless contraindicated. For patients receiving PN or IV fluids, solutions containing sodium at 35–75 mEq/L are preferred. Enteral nutrition products are formulated to meet this requirement.

- Loop diuretics (eg, furosemide, torsemide, bumetanide) administered with intermittent or continuous dosing may be utilized to aid in fluid removal for AKI or CKD patients who have maintained the ability to produce urine.

- Fluid-depleted patients presenting with AKI require IV fluid resuscitation with crystalloids (see Chapter 1) to restore fluid balance and hemodynamic stability and prevent further complications.

- Patients with nonoliguric AKI and those in the recovery phase of acute tubular necrosis should be monitored closely and administered hypotonic fluids (typically 0.45% NaCl) directed at replacement of renal fluid losses to prevent volume depletion and prerenal AKI.

- Additional strategies for fluid and sodium disorders can be found in Chapter 3 (sodium disorders section).

- Potassium
  - Ninety percent of potassium administered or taken in through the diet is eliminated by the kidney, which may present significant problems upon renal injury, impairment, or damage. Hyperkalemia is the most common potassium disorder observed in AKI and CKD.
  - Hyperkalemia develops due to reduced renal potassium excretion, release of intracellular potassium during tissue catabolism caused by acute or critical illness, and the presence of acidosis in AKI or grade 3–5 CKD.
  - Close monitoring of cardiac symptoms (electrocardiogram changes, palpitations, and arrhythmias) in hyperkalemic patients is warranted because IV administration of calcium salts is needed to stabilize the myocardium and prevent untoward events. Interventions should be undertaken to reduce or restrict potassium intake, assist in potassium removal (eg, loop diuretics, sodium polystyrene sulfonate, RRT), and/or facilitate extracellular-to-intracellular potassium shifts (eg, insulin, dextrose, sodium bicarbonate, inhaled albuterol) for all patients with hyperkalemia regardless of the presence or absence of cardiac symptoms.
  - Medications known to increase serum potassium (eg, potassium-sparing diuretics, such as spironolactone, eplerenone, triamterene, amiloride; tacrolimus; heparin; trimethoprim) should be identified and discontinued as deemed necessary.
  - Though much less common, hypokalemia may develop when potassium administration has been withheld, when intracellular shifts or potassium use during anabolism occur, and during CRRT. Treatment includes alterations in the potassium content of the dialysate solution, replacement fluid (CRRT), and/or modest potassium IV piggyback supplementation.
  - Agents, mechanisms, and doses for the treatment of hyperkalemia and hypokalemia can be found in Chapter 3 (potassium disorders section).

- Magnesium
  - As with potassium, magnesium is also tightly regulated by the kidneys, with alterations in serum magnesium concentrations being common.
  - Hypermagnesemia can occur in both AKI and CKD due to decreased renal excretion and release of magnesium arising from cellular catabolism during illness. Treatment includes administration of IV calcium salts if severe symptoms related to hypermagnesemia are present, restriction of magnesium intake and administration, therapies to enhance magnesium removal (eg, loop diuretics, RRT), and supportive care measures (eg, vasopressors, pacemaker, mechanical ventilation) if complications such as hypotension, cardiac arrhythmias, or respiratory failure occur.
  - Magnesium is readily removed during RRT, necessitating supplementation on an as-needed basis. CRRT removes a greater amount of magnesium compared to IHD and PD. Since magnesium is a cofactor in potassium retention and in the secretion of parathyroid hormone (PTH) affecting serum calcium, *close monitoring of serum magnesium* with supplementation is necessary for cases of refractory hypokalemia or symptomatic hypocalcemia. Magnesium IV should be used with RRT and those with nonfunctioning GI tracts. Oral magnesium supplements are also available, but they carry the risk of diarrhea and take a longer time to correct hypomagnesemia.
  - Refer to Chapter 3 (magnesium disorders section) for agents, mechanisms, and dosing strategies for treatment of hypermagnesemia and hypomagnesemia.
- Calcium and phosphorus
  - Calcium and phosphorus homeostasis are dependent on renal function, PTH, vitamin D status, and dietary intake. Hypocalcemia/hypercalcemia and hypophosphatemia/hyperphosphatemia occur in AKI and CKD. The corrected total calcium (see calcium disorders in Chapter 3) should be used when concomitant hypoalbuminemia is present and ionized calcium values are not readily obtainable. Complications related to calcium and phosphorus abnormalities vary based on whether they are acute (eg, hypotension and clotting disorders in AKI) or chronic (eg, bone mineral disorders and soft tissue calcifications in CKD).

- Inadequate dietary intake, decreased renal activation of vitamin D, and hyperphosphatemia often lead to hypocalcemia in renal disease, especially CKD. Intake of foods rich in calcium has decreased over time in the Western diet, replaced with protein and phosphate-rich foods. This situation emphasizes the importance of dietary education in CKD. Activation of vitamin D (1-α hydroxylation) occurs in the kidney, with impairment of this process during AKI and CKD resulting in decreased calcium absorption from the diet. Binding of excess phosphorus to calcium in the serum also decreases serum calcium levels and increases the risk of soft tissue and vascular calcifications. To limit these risks, the serum phosphorus should be maintained at ≤4.5 mg/dL through dietary limitation and use of phosphate-binding medications. Hypocalcemia and hyperphosphatemia stimulate PTH secretion, increasing calcium and phosphorus resorption from the bone and placing CKD patients at risk for bone demineralization. Strategies for managing hypocalcemia include the prevention and management of hyperphosphatemia (discussed next and in Chapter 3, phosphate disorders section), administration of vitamin D in individuals with documented deficiency (eg, calcitriol), dietary modifications, and/or calcium salt administration (limited to ≤ 2.5 g elemental calcium per day in CKD; see dosing recommendation in Chapter 3, calcium disorders section). Adjustments in calcium content of dialysate solutions may also be made during RRT.

- Hyperphosphatemia has been linked to progression of renal damage, bone disease, and increased mortality. Diets high in phosphate, decreased renal phosphorus excretion, and secondary hyperparathyroidism are associated underlying factors. Dietary phosphate restriction (800–1000 mg/d) is useful in stage 3–5 CKD including patients receiving RRT to normalize serum phosphorus levels. Education by a registered dietitian is required to prevent untoward effects on nutrition status based on dietary adjustments. Phosphate binders (eg, calcium carbonate, calcium acetate) may be required in addition to dietary modifications. When hypercalcemia is present, use of a non–calcium-based phosphate binder (eg, sevelamer, lanthanum) is indicated. IHD is not as effective as CRRT in removing excess phosphorus from the blood.

- Hypophosphatemia, while less likely to occur in renal disease, can become a potential problem during the initiation of nutrition support in malnourished patients as a consequence of refeeding syndrome and in patients receiving CRRT. Supplementation with phosphate salts should be guided by serum concentrations using conservative weight-based dosing (see phosphate disorders in Chapter 3).

- Acid-base homeostasis
  - Metabolic acidosis present during AKI and advanced stages of CKD is a result of increased acid production from nutrient metabolism or tissue catabolism during injury, impaired acid excretion, and bicarbonate loss or consumption.
  - IV sodium bicarbonate therapy may be utilized, but it is typically reserved for AKI patients with severe acidosis (dosing recommendations in Chapter 4). Close monitoring should be performed because fluid overload may potentially develop quickly due to the large sodium burden of this therapy.
  - Profound metabolic acidosis and fluid overload in AKI are indications for RRT.
  - During early stages of CKD, renal adaptation occurs to prevent acid-base disorders. As CKD progresses (GFR < 40 mL/min/1.73 m^2), this adaptation is no longer efficient. KDIGO guidelines recommend oral bicarbonate supplementation (using sodium bicarbonate, sodium citrate, or calcium carbonate) when serum bicarbonate concentrations are < 22 mEq/L to reduce or prevent complications of protein breakdown, loss of lean body mass, bone disease, cardiovascular dysfunction, and CKD progression. Monitoring of sodium balance is indicated to determine if reductions in dietary sodium intake should occur with concomitant use of sodium bicarbonate or citrate therapy. Adjustments in alkali supplementation should be based on serum bicarbonate concentrations to prevent metabolic alkalosis (serum bicarbonate > 32 mEq/L) and reduce mortality.

Monitoring

- General monitoring parameters include inputs and outputs, daily weights, vital signs, physical examination findings, serum electrolytes, blood urea nitrogen (BUN), and SCr. For CKD patients, serum PTH and vitamin D (25-hydroxy and 1,25-hydroxy) should be assessed.
- Clinicians should also monitor trends in laboratory values and examination findings because they are essential in designing a comprehensive, patient-centered plan.

Conclusion

Renal disorders predispose patients to numerous fluid, electrolyte, and acid-base disorders. Knowledge of the type and acuity of renal disorder present, concomitant therapies, and appropriate electrolyte management strategies help guide the clinician in developing safe and effective comprehensive treatment plans.

Hepatic Failure

The liver provides functions required to maintain homeostasis in the organism. To fulfill this role the liver synthesizes numerous, diverse essential molecules; extracts and metabolizes a plethora of nutrients and xenobiotics brought into the body through the GI tract (and substances entering by other routes), as well as worn-out molecules and cells; stores, exports, and/or excretes the metabolic products; and neutralizes numerous foreign antigens and microbes from the gut.

Fulminant Hepatic Failure

In 1970, Trey and Davidson[19] first used the term fulminant hepatic failure (FHF), which is also known as "acute liver failure," to refer to an uncommon but dramatic clinical syndrome characterized by rapid onset of severe hepatic dysfunction within 8 weeks of symptom appearance in the absence of preexisting liver disease. FHF is the culmination of severe liver cell injury from a variety of causes that leads to a relatively uniform clinical syndrome characterized by jaundice, encephalopathy, and coagulopathy. These hallmark features often arise from massive or submassive hepatic necrosis.[20] The causes of FHF encompass a wide variety of toxic, viral, metabolic, vascular, and autoimmune insults to the liver. Many patients with FHF develop a cascade of serious complications involving almost every organ system, and death is mostly due to multi-organ failure, hemorrhage, infection, and intracranial hypertension.

The syndrome has diverse etiologies, which vary by geography. In Africa and Asia, viral hepatitis is the predominant cause,[21] and in Europe and North America, toxic etiologies predominate.[22] In many cases, the cause of FHF cannot be established and remains indeterminate. Determination of etiology is important because specific therapies can be given once the diagnosis is established; additionally, knowing the etiology can provide a reasonably valid guide to predicting outcome.[23] The prognosis of patients with FHF is uniformly very poor, and without specialized intensive care management and the availability of liver transplantation, a diagnosis of FHF portends a poor outcome.

Clinical Manifestations of FHF

The clinical presentation of FHF is multifaceted, ranging from a slightly altered conscious level with profound coagulopathy to a catastrophic failure of multiple organs; hence, early diagnosis is crucial. The initial clinical features may be nonspecific and may include anorexia, fatigue, abdominal pain, and fever.[24] As the metabolic and detoxification functions of the liver become impaired, the signs of FHF emerge, including jaundice, encephalopathy, coagulopathy, hemodynamic instability, acute lung injury/acute respiratory distress syndrome, renal failure, sepsis, and metabolic disturbances (acidosis, alkalosis, hypoglycemia/hyperglycemia, and hyperlactatemia).[25] Meticulous clinical evaluation along with laboratory and imaging studies are helpful in the differential diagnosis of acutely decompensated chronic liver disease and sepsis from FHF. Based on the interval between development of jaundice and onset of encephalopathy, clinical manifestation can be stratified into 3 groups: hyperacute (< 7 days), acute (7–28 days), and subacute (4–26 weeks).[26]

- Hyperacute failure is most commonly caused by acetaminophen hepatotoxicity and is characterized by high aminotransferase level and low bilirubin levels.[27] Hepatic encephalopathy (HE) develops rapidly in this setting (0–7 days), sometimes preceding jaundice.
- Acute liver failure is most commonly caused by hepatitis B and medications. The interval from the time of onset, indicated by jaundice, to HE is 7–28 days. This subset less commonly has cerebral edema, and the spontaneous survival rate is < 50%.
- Subacute liver failure due to idiosyncratic medication toxicity presents as minimal encephalopathy with no cerebral edema, and it is usually associated with severe jaundice, renal dysfunction, and moderate coagulopathy.[28] Once diagnostic criteria are met, they are best managed in an intensive care unit, and transfer to a tertiary facility with a liver transplant program is urgent.

Hepatic Encephalopathy

- HE encompasses many neuropsychiatric disturbances, ranging from minor confusion and disorientation to frank coma and cerebral edema, with the latter resulting in intracranial hypertension (Table 5-6).[29,30]

Table 5-6. West Haven Criteria for Hepatic Encephalopathy.[30]

Stage	Consciousness	Intellect and Behavior	Neurological Findings
0	Normal	Normal	Normal
1	Mild lack of awareness	Shortened attention span; impaired attention or subtraction	Mild asterixis or tremor
2	Lethargic	Disoriented, inappropriate behavior	Obvious asterixis; slurred speech
3	Somnolent but arousable	Gross disorientation; bizarre behavior	Muscular rigidity and clonus; hyperreflexia
4	Coma	No response to pain stimuli	Decerebrate posturing

- Intracranial hypertension is rare among patients with grade I or II HE, while its incidence is 25%–35% with grade III, and as high as 65%–75% with grade IV HE.[20]

- A high index of suspicion is needed because patients may not exhibit classic features including headache, vomiting, bradycardia, hypertension, blurred vision, papilledema, brisk reflexes, and decerebrate rigidity. The speed with which HE develops has differential prognostic importance.

- In patients presenting with subacute liver failure, even low-grade HE indicates an extremely poor prognosis, whereas in hyperacute disease, high grades of HE clearly indicate a poor prognosis. Therefore, patients with FHF who develop altered mental status should be urgently transferred to a facility where liver transplant is available.

Pathogenesis

- The pathogenesis of HE in FHF is only partly understood, but clinical and experimental evidence suggests an important role for hyperammonemia.[31]

- Ammonia is converted in the astrocytes to osmotically active glutamine, producing cerebral edema. Albrecht and Norenberg[32] proposed a "Trojan horse hypothesis" in which glutamine executes its toxic effects in astrocytes, causing mitochondrial dysfunction and oxidative stress, which in turn results in cytotoxicity and cellular edema.

- An arterial ammonia level > 200 mcg/dL in humans is strongly associated with cerebral herniation.[33]

Treatment

- In the early stages of HE, lactulose may be used either orally or rectally to effect a bowel purge. Patients who progress to high-grade HE (grade III or IV) should undergo endotracheal intubation.[34]

- Lactulose is a nonabsorbable disaccharide that inhibits intestinal ammonia production through a number of mechanisms. The conversion of lactulose to organic acids (such as lactic and acetic acid) by colonic bacteria results in acidification of the gut lumen, which inhibits ammoniagenic coliform bacteria, leading to increased levels of nonammoniagenic lactobacilli.

- Acidification of the gut lumen also reduces the absorption of ammonia by non-ionic diffusion and favors the movement of ammonia from blood into the gut lumen. Lactulose also increases the osmotic pressure in the intestinal lumen and has a laxative effect, reducing the colonic bacterial load.

- As an osmotic cathartic, however, lactulose may cause fecal water loss in excess of sodium, resulting in contraction of extracellular fluid volume. In these settings, water is lost in excess of sodium plus potassium, resulting in a reduction of total body water without commensurate reduction in sodium and potassium, thus leading to hypernatremia. In a series of 113 hypernatremic patients, the contribution of lactulose in the development of hypernatremia was 7.7%.[35] Such patients need to be closely monitored while holding the lactulose and managed with free water supplementation orally or in severe cases with IV 5% dextrose in water or 0.45% sodium chloride.

Acute Renal Failure In FHF

- The incidence of acute renal failure is as high as 50%–80%.[36]

- Acute renal failure is a frequent complication in patients with FHF and may be due to hemodynamic alterations (functional renal failure similar to the hepatorenal syndrome [HRS] in patients with cirrhosis) or acute tubular necrosis.[36]

- Acute renal failure resembling HRS is multifactorial in the setting of FHF,[37] which may be even greater with drug nephrotoxicity (ie, acetaminophen overdose, trimethoprim-sulfamethoxazole) and acute tubular necrosis due to ischemia from hypotension.

- Other causes include development of abdominal compartment syndrome due to ascites, intra-abdominal hemorrhage, or severe abdominal and gut wall edema.

Treatment Modalities

- Early targeted volume replacement with an IV fluid challenge (crystalloid [eg, 0.9% sodium chloride or lactated Ringer's]; 1–1.5 L) is recommended to exclude prerenal azotemia, but large volumes of dextrose-containing solutions should be avoided in consideration of the risk of hyperglycemia and hyponatremia.

- If the initial fluid challenge causes no result, then consider IV albumin (colloid) at a dose of 1 g/kg body weight up to a maximum of 100 g to expand intravascular volume. IV albumin is preferred over saline (eg, 0.9% sodium chloride) solution as a volume expander because sodium load is significantly lower with albumin, and it will not worsen fluid retention.

- Vasoactive agents, such as IV norepinephrine or vasopressin, are essential to avoid arterial hypotension and ensure adequate renal perfusion.

- When dialysis is needed, continuous modes of RRT should be used because they result in improved stability in cardiovascular and intracranial parameters compared with intermittent modes of hemodialysis, which can cause transient hypotension.[38]

Metabolic Abnormalities in FHF

- Alkalosis and acidosis may both occur and are best managed by identifying and treating the underlying cause.

- In the setting of extensive hepatocyte necrosis, patients are prone to developing hypoglycemia because of glycogen depletion and defective glycogenolysis and gluconeogenesis.

- Rapid hypoglycemia should be managed with continuous dextrose infusions. IV dextrose infusion (1.5–2 g/kg/d) is recommended in patients who develop hypoglycemia because symptoms may be obscured in the presence of HE.

- Hyperglycemia should also be avoided because it may contribute to poor intracranial pressure control.

- Profound hypotension and poor systemic microcirculation result in accumulation of lactate, a complication that may be accentuated by the lack of the lactate metabolism in the failing liver.[25] Correction of hyperlactatemia is important because the disorder can affect circulatory function and aggravate cerebral hyperemia.

Chronic Liver Disease With Cirrhosis and Hepatic Decompensation

- Chronic liver diseases are characterized by unrelenting progression of liver inflammation and fibrosis over a prolonged period of time, which may eventually lead to cirrhosis.

- Advanced cirrhosis leads to a complex syndrome of chronic liver failure, which involves many different organs besides the liver, including the brain, heart and systemic circulation, adrenal glands, lungs, and kidneys.[39,40]

- The high morbidity and mortality secondary to chronic liver failure is due to complications related to the dysfunction of these organs, either alone or more frequently in combination.

Understanding Temporal Relationship Between Renal and Circulatory Dysfunction in Cirrhosis

- In the setting of decompensated liver disease, arterial pressure decreases, which leads to an increase in antidiuretic hormone (ADH) and ADH receptor activity, increase in plasma catecholamine levels, and activation of the renin-angiotensin system. As a result, aldosterone levels increase, causing sodium and water retention.[41]

- Sodium retention, an impairment of free water excretion, and a reduction in the GFR are the most relevant renal abnormalities in cirrhosis. Their main consequences are ascites, dilutional hyponatremia, and HRS.[42]

Ascites

- The occurrence of ascites in patients with chronic liver disease is related to the development of portal hypertension and is associated with worsening prognosis. If left untreated, nearly 60% of patients with compensated cirrhosis develop ascites within 10 years.[43]

The probability of survival 5 years after the appearance of ascites has been estimated to be 30%–40%.[44]

- Uncomplicated ascites is defined as ascites that is not infected and is not associated with refractoriness to conventional medical treatment, development of hyponatremia, spontaneous bacterial peritonitis, or HRS.

- The goal of treatment of cirrhotic ascites is to achieve a negative sodium balance by 2 means: (1) moderate restriction of sodium intake and (2) enhancement of renal sodium excretion by diuretics.

- The current leading opinion is that in patients with cirrhosis who need diuretics to achieve a negative sodium balance, dietary salt intake should be moderately restricted (90 mEq/d of sodium, which is equivalent to approximately 2 g/d of NaCl).[45]

- A sequential diuretic treatment should be preferred in patients who have their first episode of ascites, starting with an anti-aldosterone drug (eg, spironolactone 100–200 mg/d). A loop diuretic (eg, furosemide) should be added only in nonresponders receiving up to 400 mg/d of spironolactone. Combination therapy from the beginning of treatment is advised in patients with recurrent ascites, starting with 40 mg/d of furosemide and 100–200 mg/d of spironolactone.[46]

- In nonresponders, the dose of diuretics should be increased stepwise in either a sequential or combination treatment, every 4–5 days to a maximum of 400 mg/d of spironolactone and 160 mg/d of furosemide.

- In either sequential or combined diuretic therapy, an insufficient diuretic response is defined by a weight loss of < 1 kg in the first week or 2 kg every week thereafter, until ascites is adequately controlled.

- The safe upper limit of the rate of weight loss is contentious, but most experts agree that the diuretic dosage should be adjusted to achieve a weight loss rate of < 0.5 kg/d in patients without peripheral edema or 1 kg/d in patients with edema.[47]

- Diuretics can induce electrolyte imbalances; furosemide can induce hypokalemia and hypomagnesemia, spironolactone can induce hyperkalemia because of its potassium-sparing effect, and both can induce hyponatremia. Therefore, furosemide should be discontinued if serum potassium is < 3 mEq/L, and spironolactone should be stopped if serum potassium is ≥ 6 mEq/L. If the serum sodium is < 120 mEq/L, no diuretic should be given. Diuretics should also be discontinued if other diuretic-induced complications occur, such as renal failure, worsening HE, or severe muscle cramps.

- In treating large-volume or refractory ascites, therapeutic paracentesis combined with the infusion of 25% albumin is more effective than standard diuretic treatment in patients with cirrhosis.[48]

- Therapeutic paracentesis can induce postparacentesis-induced circulatory dysfunction (PICD), which is defined as an increase of ≥ 50% of plasma renin activity 1 week after the procedure. PICD is irreversible and is associated with lower survival.[49] The administration of IV albumin, at a dose of 8 g per liter of ascites removed, is the most effective measure to prevent PICD.

Hepatorenal Syndrome

- HRS is a unique form of functional renal failure due to diminished renal blood flow, which occurs typically in kidneys that are histologically normal.

- It is a severe complication of advanced liver disease and characteristically affects patients with cirrhosis and ascites. Peripheral arterial vasodilation is the most widely accepted explanation for the pathophysiology of HRS. This theory proposes that the splanchnic vasodilation that occurs as a consequence of portal hypertension with cirrhosis incites the development of HRS.

- Due to the absence of recognized biomarkers, the diagnosis of HRS relies on a combination of clinical and laboratory criteria.

- HRS is diagnosed on the basis of a SCr > 1.5 mg/dL, which is not reduced after > 2 days with diuretic withdrawal and volume expansion with IV albumin; absence of shock; absence of parenchymal kidney disease as indicated by proteinuria > 500 mg/d; > 50 red cells per high-power field; or abnormal kidneys on ultrasonography.[50]

- The 2 types of HRS correspond to the severity and progression of kidney failure (Table 5-7).[51]

Table 5-7. Classification of Hepatorenal Syndrome.[50]

Type	Characteristics
1	Rapidly progressive decrease in kidney function (defined as a 100% increase in the serum creatinine level to a final value > 2.5 mg/dL in 2 wk). The clinical presentation is usually that of acute kidney failure. The median survival is only 2 wk if not treated.
2	Stable or slowly progressive decrease in kidney function that does not meet the criteria for type 1 hepatorenal syndrome. The typical clinical presentation is that of refractory ascites. The median survival is approximately 6 mo.

Treatment Goals

- The main goal in the management of patients with HRS, particularly those awaiting liver transplantation, is the reversal of kidney failure in order to provide a successful bridge to transplantation.
- Treatment options in patients who are refractory to medical treatment include RRT—mainly hemodialysis in the management of patients with type 1 HRS and especially candidates for liver transplantation in an attempt to keep patients alive until transplantation is performed.
- Liver transplantation is the treatment of choice for both type 1 and type 2 HRS.[52]

Acid-Base Disorders[53]

Acid-base disorders in the setting of liver disease are frequent and complex. Mixed acid-base disturbances are common due to the underlying disease process and the therapy used to treat it.

- Metabolic acidosis: Increased anion gap (AG) metabolic acidosis may be seen in 10%–20% of patients with chronic stable and compensated liver disease, often as a result of type B lactic acidosis. However, patients with decompensated liver disease in the setting of sepsis or hemorrhage may have increased blood lactic acid levels and present as having type A lactic acidosis (ie, due to hypoperfusion and hypoxia).
- Hyperchloremic metabolic acidosis: Non-AG metabolic acidosis in patients with liver diseases also can be the result of diarrhea, particularly in patients on lactulose therapy for HE or those with renal tubular acidosis.
- Respiratory acidosis: Respiratory acidosis may also occur, but this situation is rare except when the patient is exposed to sedatives or in the context of associated lung disease.
- Respiratory alkalosis: Respiratory alkalosis is thought to be the most common acid-base derangement found in patients with liver disease as a result of hyperventilation and an increase in blood ammonia levels. Proposed causative factors for respiratory alkalosis include hypoxemia in the setting of massive ascites, anemia, hepatopulmonary syndrome, hepatic hydrothorax, or bacterial infection.
- Metabolic alkalosis: Metabolic alkalosis is another common acid-base disorder found in patients with liver disease, often as a result of therapy with loop diuretics (eg, furosemide). This disorder occurs due

to increased urinary hydrogen loss from enhanced distal renal tubule hydrogen secretion. High aldosterone levels and hypokalemia further increase distal renal tubule hydrogen secretion.

Hyponatremia

- Hyponatremia in the setting of cirrhosis has been arbitrarily defined as a serum sodium level ≤ 130 mEq/L, and it has been found to occur in 22% of patients with cirrhosis and ascites.[54] These patients can have 2 types of hyponatremia: hypovolemic hyponatremia or hypervolemic hyponatremia.
  - Hypovolemic hyponatremia is a result of fluid losses either from the kidneys secondary to diuretic use or from the GI tract (ie, diarrhea) secondary to lactulose usage for HE.
  - In contrast, the majority of patients with cirrhosis present with hypervolemic hyponatremia that is characterized by a pronounced deficit of free water excretion and leads to inappropriate water retention in comparison with the sodium concentration. Patients with hypervolemic hyponatremia usually have ascites and/or edema and may have concurrent kidney injury.[55]
  - Early determination of the volume status is critical for the management of hyponatremia in patients with cirrhosis.
  - Patients with hypovolemic hyponatremia must be treated with saline solutions (eg, 0.9% sodium chloride) aimed at increasing intravascular volume and normalizing the low total body sodium along with the removal of the precipitating factor (usually diuretics).
  - Conversely, hypervolemic hyponatremia should be managed by restricting water ingestion, by increasing renal excretion of solute-free water with diuretics, and ultimately by correcting the systemic and splanchnic vasodilatation to decrease effective arterial blood volume.
  - V2 receptor antagonists (also known as vaptans—conivaptan, tolvaptan) increase serum sodium levels in the short term, but without an effect on ascites or mortality. Therefore, vaptans could be considered for hospitalized patients with hyponatremia who are high on the liver transplantation waiting list.[56]

Conclusion

This section presents an overview of common metabolic derangements and fluid and electrolyte abnormalities in the management of patients with FHF or cirrhosis with and without decompensation. Correct classification of hepatic disorders and knowledge of necessary supportive care measures are important for the clinician to manage these patients in a safe and effective manner.

Gastrointestinal Disorders

Overview[57–63]

Patients with GI fluid losses are at risk of developing severe fluid, electrolyte, and acid-base abnormalities. These abnormalities can be associated with significant morbidity, increased hospital readmissions due to dehydration and electrolyte abnormalities, and increased mortality.

- Increased risk of morbidity in these patients is likely associated with several factors, including the following:
  - Location of any intestinal loss/resection, length of residual bowel and its functionality, duration of time since intestinal resection, and degree of adaptation
  - Absence of the colon and/or ileocecal valve
  - Underlying disease states (eg, pancreatic exocrine insufficiency)
  - Presence/characteristics of GI fistula or ostomy
  - High volume (> 2 L/d) of GI fluid loss
- Certain patients are at risk for development of fluid, electrolyte, and acid-base abnormalities related to GI alterations/disorders. Sources of fluid loss and underlying conditions placing individuals at risk may include:
  - Vomiting, nasogastric suctioning or drainage
  - Surgically placed GI drains
  - Enterocutaneous fistula > 400 mL/d

- Mucous fistula due to bowel in discontinuity
- End jejunostomy
- Ileostomy (end ileostomy, loop ileostomy)
- Colostomy (primarily ascending or transverse)
- Uretero-enteric conduit (ileal conduit)
- Intestinal insufficiency: intestinal failure due to malabsorption, short bowel syndrome, or inflammatory bowel disease
- Diarrhea

Physiology[16,64]

Fluids throughout the GI tract are rich in electrolytes, chloride, hydrogen ions, and bicarbonate, with lesser amounts of potassium and magnesium. The volume of fluid and electrolyte content of GI secretions varies based on the location within the GI tract. The approximate volume and composition of GI secretions can be found in Table 1-6. Losses of GI secretions and resulting consequences can be related to decreased absorption, increased secretion, osmotic losses, and/or increased intestinal transit time.

Fluid, Electrolyte, and Acid-Base Disorders Associated With GI Losses[16,59,60,62,63,65–70]

Due to the differences in fluid composition throughout the GI tract, identifying the origin and type of GI secretion losses is necessary to determine the appropriate therapy recommendations. Measuring the electrolyte content of GI fluids being lost is beneficial to aid in the treatment or prevention of abnormalities. Pharmacologic therapies may be considered to decrease GI fluid and electrolyte losses in patients with short bowel syndrome, high-output jejunostomy or ileostomy, and severe diarrhea. For specific electrolyte replacement recommendations, please refer to Chapter 3.

Saliva and Gastric Losses

- Saliva and gastric fluid losses can represent a significant source of fluid and electrolyte loss, especially in hospitalized surgical patients who require nasogastric drainage or patients with significant vomiting.

- The composition of gastric fluid, in particular the sodium and hydrogen ion content, may be affected by acid-suppressing medications such as histamine-2 receptor antagonists and proton pump inhibitors or by medical conditions such as achlorhydria.
    - Higher acid secretion results in lower gastric pH and sodium content.
    - Lower acid secretion results in higher gastric pH and sodium content.
- Fluid, electrolyte, and acid-base abnormalities may arise from the following:
    - Hypovolemia due to abnormal fluid loss
    - Hyponatremia secondary to increased sodium losses, increased ADH production, and thirst-mediated water retention
        - Hypovolemia increases ADH production and thirst-mediated water retention potentially resulting in hyponatremia.
    - Hypokalemia associated with direct potassium loss, increased aldosterone production, and/or alkalemia from hydrogen ion losses
        - During hypovolemia, increased aldosterone production occurs, resulting in increased renal potassium excretion and renal sodium retention.
        - The presence of alkalemia from hydrogen ion losses increases the extracellular to intracellular shift in potassium, thus lowering serum potassium concentrations.
    - Hypomagnesemia due to increased GI losses
    - Hypochloremic metabolic alkalosis as a result of excessive loss of GI secretions high in chloride and resultant increased renal bicarbonate reabsorption as a means for compensation of hypovolemia
- Management strategies include the following:
    - Fluid replacement solutions with 77 mEq NaCl/L mimic the sodium and chloride content of gastric fluid under normal conditions. Solutions include 0.45% NaCl or 5% dextrose + 0.45% NaCl. The addition of potassium chloride 10–20 mEq/L may be appropriate to prevent the development of concomitant hypokalemia.
    - Determination of fluid replacement dosing is dependent upon the amount of additional fluids administered (eg, maintenance IV fluids, concomitant medications), cardiac function, and

clinical status. The goal should be to keep the patient at neutral or slightly net positive fluid balance depending on volume status. In general, administering 0.5–1 mL of fluid replacement solutions for every 1 mL of GI fluid lost is appropriate. Monitoring of inputs and outputs, vital signs, and serum electrolytes should be done to avoid untoward complications.

- Patients receiving PN may require increased fluid, sodium, and potassium in their PN formulations. Prior to PN being ordered, fluid replacement solutions, volume status, serum electrolytes, and organ function should be considered. Increased supplementation using chloride salts (either as sodium or potassium) may be required to offset chloride losses and maintain normal acid-base balance.

Proximal Small Bowel/Pancreatic/Biliary Losses

- Proximal small bowel or pancreatic fluid losses can occur as a result of several conditions, including GI fistulas, intestinal failure, surgically placed GI drains, and bowel discontinuity.
- Relative to gastric secretions, these fluids are higher in sodium and bicarbonate and may contain magnesium (1–6 mEq/L).
- Fluid, electrolyte, and acid-base abnormalities include the following:
  - Hypovolemia due to abnormal fluid loss
  - Hyponatremia secondary to increased sodium losses, increased ADH production, and thirst-mediated water retention
  - Hypokalemia associated with direct potassium loss and increased aldosterone production
  - Hypomagnesemia due to increased GI losses
  - Non-AG metabolic acidosis (hyperchloremic) arising from significant GI bicarbonate losses
  - Hypocalcemia in patients with acute pancreatitis due to sequestration of calcium into fat necrosis, hypoalbuminemia, and reduction in PTH secretion
- Management strategies include the following:
  - Fluid replacement solutions containing sodium at 130–154 mEq/L mimic the sodium content of small bowel fluid under normal conditions. Solutions include lactated Ringer's, 5% dextrose + lactated Ringer's, 0.9% NaCl, or 5% dextrose + 0.9% NaCl. The addition of potassium chloride 10–20 mEq/L may also be appropriate to prevent the development of concomitant hypokalemia.

- Patients with excessive pancreatic or biliary losses as a result of high-output duodenal, pancreatic, or biliary fistula may require a replacement fluid containing bicarbonate or acetate in the setting of metabolic acidosis. Bicarbonate is preferred to acetate salts in patients with significant hepatic dysfunction because acetate must be converted in the liver to bicarbonate.

- Determination of fluid replacement dosing is dependent upon the amount of additional fluids administered (eg, maintenance IV fluids, concomitant medications), cardiac function, and clinical status. The goal should be to keep the patient at neutral or slightly net positive fluid balance depending on volume status. In general, administering 0.5–1 mL of fluid replacement solutions for every 1 mL of GI fluid lost is appropriate. Monitoring of inputs and outputs, vital signs, and serum electrolytes should be done to avoid untoward complications.

- Patients receiving PN may require increased fluids, sodium, potassium, and magnesium in their PN formulations. Prior to PN being ordered, fluid replacement solutions, volume status, serum electrolytes, and organ function should be considered. Increased supplementation using acetate salts (either as sodium or potassium) may be required to offset bicarbonate losses and maintain normal acid-base balance.

Distal Small Bowel/Ileal Losses

- Distal small bowel and ileal fluid losses can arise from several conditions, including intestinal failure, end jejunostomy, proximal ileostomy, GI fistulas, intestinal infections (eg, small bowel bacterial overgrowth), malabsorption, surgical GI drains, and bowel discontinuity.

- Relative to gastric secretions, these fluids contain similar amounts of sodium and chloride, but higher amounts of bicarbonate and magnesium.

- Fluid, electrolyte and acid-base abnormalities include the following:

  - Hypovolemia due to abnormal fluid loss

  - Hyponatremia secondary to increased sodium losses, increased ADH production, and thirst-mediated water retention

  - Hypokalemia associated with direct potassium loss and increased aldosterone production

- Hypomagnesemia due to increased GI losses
    - Hypomagnesemia may lead to hypokalemia refractory to supplementation due to impairment in Na^+-K^+-ATPase pump activity and increased renal potassium wasting.
- Non-AG metabolic acidosis (hyperchloremic) due to bicarbonate losses found in distal small bowel and ileal fluid losses
    - Patients with uretero-enteric conduits are at risk for this type of acid-base disorder.

- Management strategies include the following:
    - In cases of diarrhea, determination of the cause is necessary because management strategies distinctly differ between diarrhea types.
    - Fluid replacement solutions containing sodium at 130–154 mEq/L mimic the sodium content of small bowel fluid under normal conditions. Solutions include lactated Ringer's, 5% dextrose + lactated Ringer's, 0.9% NaCl, or 5% dextrose + 0.9% NaCl. The addition of potassium chloride at 10–20 mEq/L may also be appropriate to prevent the development of concomitant hypokalemia.
    - Patients with high-output distal small bowel losses such as with end jejunostomy or ileostomy or high-output ileal fistula may require a replacement fluid containing bicarbonate or acetate in the setting of metabolic acidosis. Bicarbonate is preferred to acetate salts in patients with significant hepatic dysfunction because acetate must be converted in the liver to bicarbonate.
    - Determination of fluid replacement dosing is dependent upon the amount of additional fluids administered (eg, maintenance IV fluids, concomitant medications), cardiac function, and clinical status. The goal should be to keep the patient at neutral or slightly net positive fluid balance depending on volume status. In general, administering 0.5–1 mL of fluid replacement solutions for every 1 mL of GI fluid lost is appropriate. Monitoring of inputs and outputs, vital signs, and serum electrolytes should be done to avoid untoward complications.
    - IV magnesium replacement strategies should be instituted in patients with refractory hypokalemia prior to potassium supplementation to decrease renal potassium excretion and restore potassium homeostasis.

- Patients receiving PN may require increased fluids, sodium, potassium, and magnesium in their PN formulations. Prior to PN being ordered, fluid replacement solutions, volume status, serum electrolytes, and organ function should be considered. Increased supplementation with acetate salts (either as sodium or potassium) may be required to offset bicarbonate losses and maintain normal acid-base status.

Colon Losses

- Large bowel fluid losses can result from several causes, such as osmotic diarrhea, secretory diarrhea, infectious diarrhea, or steatorrhea.
- Relative to gastric secretions, these fluids contain similar amounts of sodium, lower amounts of chloride, and higher amounts of potassium and magnesium.
- Fluid, electrolyte, and acid-base abnormalities include the following:
    - Hypovolemia due to abnormal fluid loss
    - Hyponatremia secondary to increased sodium losses, increased ADH production, and thirst-mediated water retention
    - Hypokalemia associated with direct potassium loss and increased aldosterone production
    - Hypomagnesemia due to increased GI losses.
        - Hypomagnesemia may lead to hypokalemia refractory to supplementation. This is due to impairment in Na^+-K^+-ATPase pump activity and increased renal potassium wasting.
- Management strategies include the following:
    - In cases of diarrhea, determination of the cause is necessary because management strategies distinctly differ between diarrhea types.
    - Fluid replacement solutions containing NaCl at 77 mEq/L mimic the sodium content of large bowel fluid under normal conditions. IV solutions include 0.45% NaCl or 5% dextrose + 0.45% NaCl. The addition of potassium chloride at 20 mEq/L and magnesium sulfate at 8–16 mEq/L may also be appropriate to prevent hypokalemia and hypomagnesemia.
    - IV magnesium replacement strategies should be instituted in patients with refractory hypokalemia prior to potassium supplementation to decrease renal potassium excretion and restore potassium homeostasis.

- Patients receiving PN may require increased fluids, sodium, potassium, and magnesium in their PN formulations. Prior to PN being ordered, fluid replacement solutions, volume status, serum electrolytes, and organ function should be considered.

Other Considerations[71]

- Patients with impaired renal function due to AKI or CKD are at risk for fluid overload and accumulation of electrolytes. Metabolic acidosis often occurs due to reduced renal acid excretion and bicarbonate reabsorption. The extent of these metabolic disorders varies depending on the patient's underlying renal function, the type of renal insult, and the use or type of RRT.

- As the patient's GI condition improves with adaptation (ie, natural hypertrophy of remnant bowel to increase nutrient processing surface area during the 2–3 years after resection) and abnormal GI secretion output/losses decrease, doses of replacement fluids and supplemental electrolytes need to be reassessed. This reassessment is especially important in patients receiving teduglutide, a degradation-resistant human recombinant enzyme analogue of glucagon-like peptide 2, because it is a GI trophic hormone involved in the normal growth and maintenance of the GI intestinal epithelium. These effects are predominantly apparent through the patient's gradual weight gain and increased urine output despite stable doses of parenteral nutrition or other IV fluids containing electrolytes. Teduglutide effects can be seen within 8 weeks of treatment.

Conclusion

Conditions and diseases leading to increased GI losses can significantly affect fluid, electrolyte, and acid-base status. Knowledge of the underlying cause and composition of GI secretions lost are important in providing appropriate treatment recommendations and preventing unwanted complications.

Hyperglycemic Emergencies

Hyperglycemic emergencies are life-threatening conditions classified as diabetic ketoacidosis (DKA) and hyperosmolar hyperglycemic state. These conditions are responsible for an estimated 170,000 emergency department visits and 2400 deaths per year. Proper management is important to prevent morbidity and mortality.

Diabetic Ketoacidosis

Overview[72-75]

DKA is a hyperglycemic crisis that occurs in patients with uncontrolled diabetes mellitus. Although it occurs most commonly in type 1 diabetes mellitus, it also may occur in type 2 diabetes mellitus as a result of acute illness or surgery. The incidence of DKA is increasing in the United States. The number of hospital discharges with DKA listed as the first diagnosis has increased from 80,000 discharges in 1988 to 140,000 in 2009. Overall mortality in adult patients is low at < 1%; however, mortality can increase to > 5% in the elderly and individuals with life-threatening illnesses. DKA is characterized by a serum glucose > 250 mg/dL, ketonemia, and an AG metabolic acidosis. These disorders result from insulin deficiency and/or resistance and elevations in the counterregulatory hormones glucagon, cortisol, growth hormone, and catecholamines.

Etiology[72,73,75]

- DKA is caused by many different conditions and factors (Table 5-8).
- Infection remains the most common predisposing factor for the development of DKA.
- Numerous medications are associated with DKA, warranting a comprehensive medication review upon presentation.

Pathogenesis[72,73,75,76]

- Lack of insulin causes hyperglycemia to develop through 3 mechanisms: increased gluconeogenesis, glycogenolysis, and decreased glucose uptake by muscle and peripheral tissues.

Table 5-8. Causes of Diabetic Ketoacidosis.[73]

• Newly diagnosed type 1 diabetes mellitus	• Acute pancreatitis
• Infection (pneumonia, urinary tract infection, etc.)	• Inadequate insulin therapy
• Surgery	• Corticosteroids
• Myocardial infarction	• Thiazide diuretics
• Cerebrovascular accident	• Pentamidine
• Sympathomimetics	• Cocaine
• Atypical antipsychotics	• Alcohol

- Gluconeogenesis is stimulated by glucagon, catecholamines, and cortisol, with the latter also causing increased glucagon activity.
- Since carbohydrates cannot be utilized, energy is obtained through fatty acid metabolism.
- Increased free fatty acids in the circulation increase the formation of ketone bodies (acetone, acetoacetate, and β-3-hydroxybutyrate).
- Ketone bodies produced begin to appear in the urine, leading to AG metabolic acidosis.
- Osmotic diuresis and dehydration also occur as a result of hyperglycemia, glucosuria, decreased oral intake, and GI losses.
- Figure 5-3 provides a schematic describing the pathophysiology of DKA.

Figure 5-3. Pathophysiology of Diabetic Ketoacidosis.

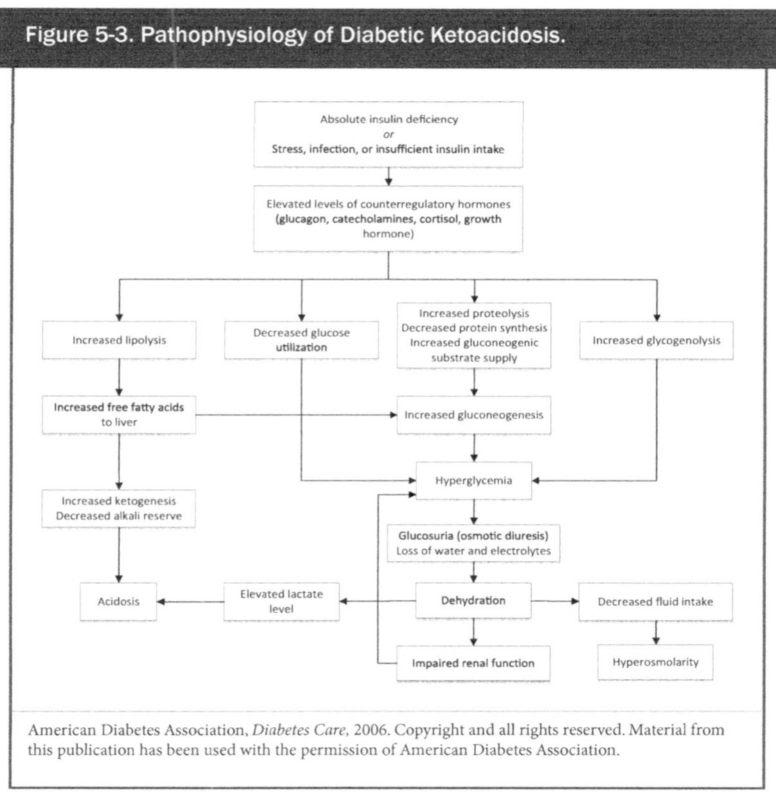

American Diabetes Association, *Diabetes Care*, 2006. Copyright and all rights reserved. Material from this publication has been used with the permission of American Diabetes Association.

CHAPTER 5 Common Clinically Applicable Situations

Table 5-9. Diagnostic Criteria for Diabetic Ketoacidosis.

Variable	Mild	Moderate	Severe
Plasma glucose, mg/dL	> 250	> 250	> 250
pH	7.25–7.3	7–7.24	< 7
Serum bicarbonate, mEq/L	15–18	10–15	< 10
Ketones, urine or serum	Positive	Positive	Positive
Anion gap	> 10	> 12	> 12
Osmolality, mOsm/kg	Variable	Variable	Variable
Mental status	Alert	Alert/drowsy	Stupor/coma

Patient Presentation and Laboratory Abnormalities[72,75]

- Patients in DKA will generally present with complaints of fatigue, abdominal pain, nausea, and vomiting.
- Classic findings of hyperglycemia (polyuria, polydipsia, weight loss) are also seen.
- Patients may exhibit deep breathing, known as Kussmaul respirations, to compensate for metabolic acidosis.
- Fruity breath odor is often present, caused by ketone body exhalation.
- Neurologic status varies upon presentation, ranging from normal to comatose (severe DKA).
- DKA may be classified as mild, moderate, or severe, based on several diagnostic criteria (Table 5-9).
- Serum sodium is decreased due to the movement of water into the extracellular space as a result of the hyperosmolar state. Serum sodium correction due to hyperglycemia should be performed (Table 5-10) to estimate the true serum sodium concentration. Failure to do this can lead to inappropriate therapy and subsequent adverse neurological consequences.
- Serum potassium may appear elevated at presentation, often due to metabolic acidosis despite a total body potassium deficit. Serum potassium should be closely monitored once insulin therapy is initiated because extracellular to intracellular shifts occur, leading in some

Table 5-10. Useful Formulas in Diabetic Ketoacidosis.	
Measurement	**Equation**
Corrected serum sodium	Measured Na (mEq/L) + [0.016 × (Glucose (mg/dL) − 100)]
Anion gap	Na (mEq/L) − [Cl (mEq/L) + HCO_3 (mEq/L)]
Serum osmolality	[2 × measured Na (mEq/L)] + [glucose (mg/dL)/18] + [BUN (mg/dL)/2.8]

BUN, blood urea nitrogen; Cl, chloride; HCO_3, bicarbonate; Na, sodium.

cases to profound hypokalemia. Consequences of moderate to severe hypokalemia include nausea, vomiting, cardiac arrhythmias, and muscle weakness.

- Serum phosphorus levels are often elevated initially due to an extracellular shift during insulin deficiency, but they will decrease once insulin therapy is initiated in the same manner as potassium. Respiratory muscle dysfunction, cardiac arrhythmias, hemolysis, and altered mental status can occur as a result of serum phosphorus levels < 1 mg/dL.

- Serum bicarbonate is typically < 18 mEq/L in DKA, and a decrease to < 10 mEq/L classifies the patient as having severe DKA.

- Elevated AG metabolic acidosis is characteristic of DKA and used to estimate the amount of ketone bodies present in the serum. The formula to calculate AG metabolic acidosis can be found in Table 5-10 (see also Chapter 4).

- Serum osmolality is an indicator of neurologic impairment and can be calculated using the formula in Table 5-10.

- Leukocytosis may also be present, even in the absence of infection. White blood cell counts may range from 10,000 to 15,000 cells/mm^3; however, if the counts are > 25,000 cells/mm^3, infection should be strongly suspected.

Treatment[72,73,75]

Proper management of DKA should concentrate on restoring fluid balance, correcting hyperglycemia, and responding to electrolyte abnormalities. The following section will describe how to effectively manage patients with DKA. In conjunction with the treatment recommendations below, the underlying cause of DKA should be identified and treated accordingly.

Fluid Replacement

- Use of IV fluids is recommended over oral fluid replacement.
- IV fluid administration should begin immediately with 0.9% NaCl infused at a rate of 15–20 mL/kg (or 1 L/h) during the first hour. Balanced electrolyte solutions such as lactated Ringer's or Normosol-R (contains sodium 140 mEq/L; potassium 5 mEq/L; magnesium 3 mEq/L; chloride 98 mEq/L; acetate 27 mEq/L; gluconate 23 mEq/L) may be substituted for 0.9% NaCl during fluid resuscitation to help prevent hyperchloremic metabolic acidosis. If hyperkalemia (K > 5.5 mEq/L) is present, these balanced electrolyte solutions should be used cautiously with frequent monitoring since lactated Ringer's and Normosol-R contain small amounts of potassium.
- After the first hour, if the corrected serum sodium is elevated or normal, 0.45% NaCl may be infused at a rate of 250–500 mL/h in the absence of any symptoms of fluid overload.
- If the corrected serum sodium remains low after the first hour, 0.9% NaCl may continue to be used at an infusion rate of 250–500 mL/h in the absence of any symptoms of fluid overload.
- The goal of fluid replacement is to correct deficits within the first 24 hours.
- Once serum glucose is < 200 mg/dL, 5% dextrose + 0.45% NaCl should begin to be infused at a rate of 150–250 mL/h to avoid hypoglycemia during IV insulin therapy.
- Additional information concerning fluid replacement can be found in Chapter 2.

Insulin

- Regular insulin therapy using a continuous IV insulin infusion should begin after fluid replacement is initiated with dosing adjustments guided by hourly glucose assessments.
- Subcutaneous (SC) insulin administration is not recommended during DKA because absorption is not reliable with volume depletion.
- Regular insulin should be administered as a bolus IV dose of 0.1 units kg followed by a continuous IV infusion of 0.1 units kg/h.
- Alternatively, a continuous IV infusion of 0.14 units kg/h may be used without a bolus dose.

- Within the first hour, the serum glucose should decrease by 10%. If this 10% decrease does not occur, a bolus IV dose of 0.14 units kg of regular insulin should be given in addition to the continuous IV insulin infusion.

- The optimal rate of serum glucose decrease should be 50–75 mg/dL/h. If the serum glucose decrease is not adequate, the rate of insulin infusion should be increased to ensure a steady glucose decline. Prevention of hypoglycemia is imperative to prevent rebound ketosis.

- Once the serum glucose level reaches 200 mg/dL, the rate of IV insulin infusion should decrease to 0.02–0.05 units kg/h. Although not commonly used, an alternative regimen it to provide 0.1 units kg of rapid-acting insulin SC (eg, insulin lispro) every 2 hours. Discontinuation of insulin therapy at this time should not occur.

- Serum glucose should be maintained between 150 and 200 mg/dL until DKA has resolved.

Potassium

- Serum potassium levels may be falsely normal or high initially due to metabolic acidosis, despite a total body deficit of potassium.

- The goal of potassium repletion is to maintain serum levels between 4 and 5 mEq/L. Potassium replacement should begin once the serum potassium falls to < 5 mEq/L.

- If serum potassium is > 5 mEq/L, no replacement is necessary, and measurement should be repeated within 1 hour.

    - If repeat serum potassium is 4–5 mEq/L, add 10–20 mEq/L KCl to IV fluids and infuse at rates of up to 10 mEq/h for potassium.

    - If repeat serum potassium is 3.5–3.9 mEq/L, add 20–40 mEq/L KCl to IV fluids and infuse at rates of up to 20 mEq/h for potassium.

    - If repeat serum potassium is < 3.5 mEq/L, do not administer insulin, add 20–80 mEq/L KCl to IV fluids, and attach a continuous cardiac monitor to the patient with serum potassium repeated within 1–2 hours because rates of potassium infusion may require 40 mEq/h for correction.

    - Additional information concerning potassium replacement can be found in Chapter 3.

Bicarbonate

- Currently no role exists for the use of IV bicarbonate in DKA, although IV bicarbonate therapy may be used in cases of profound acidosis.

- Risks of IV bicarbonate administration include hypokalemia, rebound metabolic alkalosis, decreased tissue oxygen uptake, cerebral edema, and a delay in improvement of hyperosmolarity and ketosis.

  - If serum pH < 6.9, administer 100 mEq (2 × 50-mL vials) of IV sodium bicarbonate in 400 mL of sterile water for injection with 20 mEq KCl administered intravenously at 200 mL/h for 2 hours. Repeat this infusion every 2 hours until serum pH > 7.

  - Alternatively, sodium bicarbonate provided as 150 mEq in 1000 mL of sterile water for injection (or dextrose 5% in water depending on serum glucose) can be continuously administered intravenously at 200 mL/h until serum pH > 7.

Phosphorus

- Similar to potassium, serum phosphorus is often normal or high and can decrease abruptly once DKA treatment with regular insulin is initiated.

- Phosphate replacement therapy is indicated in hypophosphatemic patients with cardiac dysfunction, anemia, or respiratory depression/failure, or when serum phosphorus concentration is < 1 mg/dL.

- Phosphate at 15–30 mmol/L as potassium phosphate can be added to IV fluids at a maximum rate of 7.5 mmol/h for phosphate (resulting in 10 mEq/h for potassium). Use of IV sodium phosphate is preferred when concomitant hyperkalemia is present.

- Additional phosphate replacement recommendations can be found in Chapter 3.

Monitoring[72,76]

- Serum electrolytes, BUN, SCr, glucose, ketones (eg, acetoacetate, β-hydroxybutyrate), and venous pH should be monitored every 2–4 hours during DKA treatment until stable. Laboratory assessment for BUN and SCr may be less frequent at provider discretion if values are not initially abnormal.

  - If a urinalysis is done, note it only measures the ketones, acetone, and acetoacetate, not β-hydroxybutyrate, the primary ketone in DKA.

- Neurologic assessments and hemodynamic parameters should be performed based on the patient's clinical status.

Resolution of DKA[72]

- Continuous IV regular insulin infusion should be maintained until DKA has resolved.
- A serum glucose < 200 mg/dL and 2 of the following criteria are needed to determine if resolution of DKA has occurred:
  - Serum bicarbonate ≥ 15 mEq/L
  - Venous pH > 7.3
  - AG metabolic acidosis ≤ 12 mEq/L
  - Serum ketone—negative
- Once resolution has occurred, the patient can be transitioned to SC insulin therapy.
- Continuous IV infusion of insulin should be continued for 1–2 hours after initiating SC insulin therapy to ensure appropriate concentrations of insulin are achieved/maintained.
- Patients receiving insulin before the episode of DKA may resume their previous insulin doses.
- Those naïve to insulin therapy may be initiated on SC insulin 0.5–0.8 units kg/d administered as neutral protamine Hagedorn plus regular insulin or as a basal-bolus regimen with basal (glargine or detemir) plus bolus (lispro, aspart, or glulisine) insulin.
- Education of patients and/or caregivers about the signs and symptoms of DKA and the importance of glucose monitoring including medication compliance should be done to prevent future DKA episodes.

Complications[72,75]

The most common complications of DKA result from aggressive management of hyperglycemia. These include hypoglycemia and hypokalemia. Less commonly, cerebral edema, volume overload, acute respiratory distress syndrome, and pulmonary edema may occur. Patients should be closely monitored for development of these complications.

Hyperosmolar Hyperglycemic State

Overview[72,74]

Hyperosmolar hyperglycemic state (HHS) is a hyperglycemic emergency similar to DKA, but with several key differences. HHS is characterized by greater degrees of hyperglycemia, hyperosmolality, osmotic diuresis, and dehydration *without* ketoacidosis. Patients presenting with HHS are most commonly elderly patients with type 2 diabetes mellitus. The exact incidence of HHS is unknown, but it has been estimated as < 1% of hospital admissions in patients with diabetes. The mortality rate in HHS is approximately 10%–20%, which is 10 times higher than for DKA. HHS may also be referred to as hyperglycemic nonketotic dehydration syndrome, hyperosmolar hyperglycemic nonketotic syndrome, hyperosmolar nonketotic coma, and nonketotic hyperosmolar coma. For the purposes of this section, this condition is referred to as HHS.

Etiology[72,75,77]

- Causes of HHS are similar to those of DKA (Table 5-9), although patients with HHS are more likely to have decreased fluid intake due to reduced water intake.
- The most common cause of HHS is infection.

Pathogenesis[72,75,77]

- Insulin deficiency, increased gluconeogenesis, increased counterregulatory hormones, and increased glycogenolysis cause extreme hyperglycemia in HHS.
- As the serum glucose concentration increases, water is drawn out of cells into the extracellular fluid to compensate for increased osmolality.
- Glomerular filtration is increased, causing glucosuria and osmotic diuresis.
- In contrast to DKA, patients in HHS typically have enough pancreatic insulin production to inhibit lipolysis and subsequent development of ketoacidosis.
- HHS develops over a much longer period of time, usually days to weeks, compared to < 24 hours in DKA.

Table 5-11. Diagnostic Criteria for Hyperosmolar Hyperglycemic State.

Variable	HHS
Serum glucose, mg/dL	> 600
pH	> 7.3
Serum bicarbonate, mEq/L	> 18
Ketones, urine or serum	Minimal or negative
Anion gap	Variable
Osmolality, mOsm/kg	> 320
Mental status	Stupor/coma

HHS, hyperosmolar hyperglycemic state.

Patient Presentation and Laboratory Abnormalities[72,75,77]

- Patients in HHS will present with signs and symptoms of hyperglycemia. Serum glucose concentrations are typically > 600 mg/dL.
- Serum osmolality is elevated (> 320 mOsm/kg) in HHS.
- Fatigue, lethargy, dry mucous membranes, and poor skin turgor are often present due to volume depletion.
- The presence of neurologic abnormality is necessary to make a diagnosis of HHS. Neurologic abnormalities ranging from limb weakness to seizures or coma may be present upon presentation. Neurologic abnormalities are caused by severe dehydration and hyperosmolality.
- Laboratory abnormalities characteristic of DKA (AG metabolic acidosis, presence of ketones, low pH) are absent in HHS.
- The diagnostic criteria for HHS are listed in Table 5-11.

Table 5-12 provides a comparison of HHS to DKA relative to patient risk factors, presenting symptoms, and laboratory abnormalities.

Table 5-12. Comparison of Hyperosmolar Hyperglycemic State and Diabetic Ketoacidosis.[65]

Variable	HHS	DKA
Patient characteristics		
Mortality	High mortality rate	High recovery rate with lower mortality
Diabetes	Type 2, with or without insulin treatment	Type 1
Age	> 40 y	< 40 y
Symptom onset	Subtle	Rapid
Patient presentation		
Polyuria	2 d to 2 wk before clinical symptoms	1–3 d prior to symptoms
Thirst	Failure of thirst mechanisms resulting in inadequate water intake	Polydipsia for 1–3 d
Neurologic symptoms	Present (disorientation, seizures, coma)	Variable
Ventilation	Normal	Hyperventilation with Kussmaul respirations
Breath odor	None	Fruity
Hydration/Volume Status	Dehydration, hypovolemia	Dehydration, hypovolemia
Gastrointestinal symptoms	Occasional	Abdominal pain, nausea, vomiting, diarrhea
Laboratory tests		
Serum glucose, mg/dL	600–2400	300–1000
Serum sodium	Hypernatremia	Mild hyponatremia
Serum osmolality	High, > 320 mOsm/kg	High
Renal function	Slightly altered	Impaired
Serum pH	Normal	Moderate to severe acidosis (pH < 7.3)
Serum HCO_3, mEq/L	> 20	< 15
Anion gap, mEq/L	< 7	> 7
Serum potassium	Usually normal	Normal or elevated
Serum ketones	Absent	Present

DKA, diabetic ketoacidosis; HHS, hyperosmolar hyperglycemic state.

Treatment[72,75,77]

The management of HHS is very similar to DKA, and includes treatments to reverse hypovolemia, hyperglycemia, and electrolyte abnormalities. Patients with HHS should be managed using the treatment algorithm discussed in the DKA section, with the following important differences.

- Dextrose 5% should be added to the IV fluids once serum glucose reaches 300 mg/dL.
- The rate of continuous IV insulin infusion should be reduced to 0.02–0.05 units kg/h once serum glucose reaches 300 mg/dL.
- The goal serum glucose range is between 200 and 300 mg/dL until the patient is mentally alert.
- The role of potassium and phosphate replacement in HHS should be based upon laboratory monitoring of serum electrolytes.
- No role exists for IV sodium bicarbonate administration in HHS.

Monitoring[72,76]

- Serum electrolytes, BUN, SCr, glucose, ketones (only initially), osmolality, and possibly venous pH should be monitored every 2–4 hours during HHS treatment until they are stable. Laboratory assessment for BUN, SCr, osmolality, and venous pH may be less frequent at provider discretion.
- Routine neurologic assessments should be performed hourly until resolution of HHS.

Resolution of HHS[73]

- Resolution of HHS has occurred once serum osmolality has normalized and mental status has returned to baseline.
- At this time, patients may be transitioned to SC insulin therapy, with an overlap of 1–2 hours of the continuous IV insulin infusion to ensure adequate insulin concentrations.
- Education of patients and/or caregivers about the importance of glucose monitoring, hydration, and medication compliance should be done to prevent future HHS episodes.

Conclusion

DKA and HHS both lead to significant abnormalities in fluid, electrolyte, and acid-base homeostasis. Management of these disorders centers on IV fluid repletion, hyperglycemia management with insulin, electrolyte replacement, and treatment of the underlying cause. Understanding of the pathophysiology of DKA and HHS along with appropriate supportive care is vital in the prevention of untoward morbidity and mortality.

Refeeding Syndrome

Overview[78–93]

Refeeding syndrome describes the spectrum of metabolic alterations that occur during nutrition repletion of underweight, severely malnourished, or chronically starved individuals. The hallmark sign of refeeding syndrome is hypophosphatemia and its associated complications (including, but not limited to, somnolence, mental status changes, encephalopathy, respiratory failure, impaired cardiac function, paresthesias, weakness, infections, seizures, coma, and death); however, it can encompass a constellation of fluid and electrolyte abnormalities including hypokalemia, hypomagnesemia, and possibly hyponatremia and fluid overload. These derangements can affect multiple organ systems, including neurological, cardiac, hematological, neuromuscular, and pulmonary function. Reports in the literature describe severe electrolyte abnormalities and severe adverse effects associated with refeeding syndrome, including cardiac failure, arrhythmias, respiratory failure, encephalopathy, seizures, coma, and death. If severe malnutrition is present, refeeding syndrome can be life threatening and even fatal if appropriate supportive care is not provided.

Physiology[78-81]

- During the initial stages of starvation (24–72 hours), blood glucose levels fall and the liver utilizes noncarbohydrate sources for glucose production (eg, liver glycogen); specifically, glycogen stores are used for energy, and skeletal muscles are catabolized to amino acids for gluconeogenesis. Maintaining blood glucose levels is vital for glucose-dependent tissues such as the brain, erythrocytes, and renal medulla.

- After 72 hours, glycogen stores are depleted and metabolic pathways shift to obtain energy from ketone production from free fatty acid oxidation and anaerobic metabolism.

- Additionally, depletion of potassium, phosphate, and magnesium occurs. The body adapts to maintain extracellular concentrations of these electrolytes by using intracellular stores. Serum levels may remain normal despite marked reduction in total body stores.
- Reintroduction of nutrition in starved or nutritionally depleted patients results in a rapid shift back to aerobic metabolism using carbohydrates as a fuel source. Insulin is secreted in response to carbohydrate introduction, gluconeogenesis declines rapidly, and potassium, phosphate, and magnesium are shifted to the intracellular compartment. Preexisting total body depletion and a large intracellular to extracellular concentration gradient result in a rapid fall of extracellular concentrations of potassium, phosphorus, and magnesium.
- To maintain serum osmolality within a normal range, sodium and water are retained, resulting in the expansion of the extracellular fluid compartment and hyponatremia. This sodium and water retention can result in cardiac and pulmonary symptoms of volume overload.
- Thiamin is a cofactor required for carbohydrate-dependent metabolic pathways. Once nutrition is reintroduced, the demand for thiamin is increased in malnourished patients with decreased baseline stores. If thiamin deficiency is present, glucose is metabolized to pyruvate but is unable to enter the Krebs cycle, and lactate is produced leading to a refractory lactic acidosis.

Definition[78]

- No internationally agreed-upon definition exists for refeeding syndrome. In general, refeeding syndrome describes a collection of metabolic derangements that occur as a result of nutrition initiation to severely malnourished or chronically starved individuals.

Prevalence and Mortality[93]

- With no strict definition for refeeding syndrome, ascertaining the overall incidence in the general population is difficult. In one study of critically ill patients, 52% developed hypophosphatemia within 24 hours, 92% developed it within 48 hours, and 100% developed it within 72 hours of starting nutrition support.
- While the majority of patients experience only mild clinical manifestations of refeeding syndrome, it can be life threatening or even fatal when symptoms are severe.

Table 5-13. Risk Factors for Developing Refeeding Syndrome.

Unintentional Weight Loss	Low Nutrient Intake	Increased Nutrient Losses/ Decreased Nutrient Absorption
Loss of > 5% of body weight in 1 mo	Hypocaloric or no oral intake for > 7 d	Significant vomiting or diarrhea
Loss of > 7.5% of body weight in 3 mo	Anorexia nervosa	Dysfunction or inflammation of the GI tract (short bowel syndrome, inflammatory bowel disease, motility disorders, malabsorption)
Loss of > 10% of body weight in 6 mo	Chronic alcoholism	Chronic pancreatitis
	Depression	Chronic antacid use
	Cancer/chemotherapy/radiation	Chronic high-dose diuretic use
	Chronic infectious disease (AIDS, tuberculosis)	Bariatric surgery
	Chronic disease (cirrhosis, CKD)	Pregnancy
	Convalescence from catabolic illness	
	Dysphagia	
	Postoperative patients	
	Diabetic hyperosmolar states (ie, DKA, HHS)	
	Morbid obesity with profound weight loss	
	Homelessness, social deprivation	
	Idiosyncratic/eccentric diets	

AIDS, acquired immune deficiency syndrome; CKD, chronic kidney disease; DKA, diabetic ketoacidosis; GI, gastrointestinal; HHS, hyperglycemia hyperosmolar state.

Etiology/Pathophysiology[78-81,85,88,91,94]

- Several patient characteristics may lead to underlying malnutrition and increase the risk of developing refeeding syndrome. These characteristics include unintentional weight loss, low nutrient intake, and increased nutrient losses or decreased nutrient absorption (see Table 5-13).

- While many case reports describe refeeding syndrome associated with PN since the risk of refeeding syndrome may be greater with PN, it has also been associated with oral or enteral nutrition.

- Clinical manifestations of refeeding syndrome are described in Table 5-14.

Table 5-14. Clinical Manifestations of Refeeding Syndrome.

Hypophosphatemia	Hypokalemia	Hypomagnesemia	Vitamin/Thiamin Deficiency	Sodium Retention
Impaired oxygen transport and delivery, hypoxia	Nausea	Weakness	Encephalopathy (eg, Wernicke-Korsakoff encephalopathy)	Fluid overload
Impaired cardiac function	Vomiting	Muscle twitching	Lactic acidosis	Pulmonary edema
Impaired diaphragm contractility	Constipation	Tremor	Death	Cardiac decompensation
Respiratory failure	Weakness	Altered mental status		
Paresthesias	Paralysis	Anorexia		
Weakness	Respiratory compromise	Nausea		
Lethargy	Rhabdomyolysis	Vomiting		
Somnolence	Alterations in myocardial contraction	Diarrhea		
Confusion	Electrocardiograph changes	Refractory hypokalemia and hypocalcemia		
Disorientation	ST-segment depression	Electrocardiograph changes		
Restlessness	T-wave flattening	Prolonged PR		
Encephalopathy	T-wave inversion	Widened QRS		
Areflexic paralysis	Presence of U-waves	Prolonged QT		
Seizures	Cardiac arrhythmias	ST depression		
Coma	Atrial tachycardia	Peaked T-wave		
Death	Bradycardia	T-wave flattening		
	Atrioventricular block	Cardiac arrhythmias		
	Premature ventricular contractions	Atrial fibrillation		
	Ventricular tachycardia	Torsade de pointes		
	Ventricular fibrillation	Ventricular arrhythmias		
	Sudden death	Ventricular tachycardia		
		Tetany		
		Seizures		
		Coma		
		Death		

Reprinted with permission from Kraft MD, Btaiche IF, Sacks GS. Review of the refeeding syndrome. *Nutr Clin Pract*. 2005;20(6):625–633.

Management[79-81,92,93]

- Correct underlying electrolyte abnormalities *before* initiating nutrition support, especially hypophosphatemia, hypokalemia, and hypomagnesemia (refer to Chapter 3 for dosing recommendations).

- Nutrition support should not be used as a way to treat underlying electrolyte and acid-base abnormalities; rather, adjustments can be made to more appropriately meet maintenance needs and avoid or minimize exacerbating abnormalities.

- In an effort to prevent refeeding syndrome, remember to "start low and go slow." Initiate nutrition support at a maximum of 480 kcal/d for 2 days. Next, provide 960 kcal/d for 1 day, 1440 kcal/d for 1 day, and 80% of calculated energy goals for another day, before finally reaching 100% of goal intake. If hypophosphatemia reoccurs when more than 480 kcal/d are provided, reducing to a lower intake for 1–2 days is advised, followed by resuming advancement if hypophosphatemia resolves. Increasing over 4–10 days has also been suggested.

- For all electrolyte and acid-base disorders, considerations are listed below:

  - Patients at risk for refeeding syndrome may require approximately 20%–50% higher maintenance doses (eg, phosphate, potassium, magnesium) when initiating nutrition support and for the first 3–7 days, depending on clinical response.

  - Maintenance needs for electrolytes can vary depending on renal function, underlying disease states, and any abnormal losses (eg, GI losses). Dosing recommendations given in the following points are for patients with normal renal function and without abnormal losses (eg, GI losses).

  - Oral dosage forms of phosphate, potassium, and magnesium can be associated with adverse GI effects, and IV therapy is often needed in severe cases:

    - Phosphate = diarrhea, poor oral absorption

    - Potassium = nausea, vomiting, diarrhea, discomfort

    - Magnesium = diarrhea, poor oral absorption

- Patients at risk for refeeding syndrome may have other vitamin or micronutrient deficiencies and should be assessed for these prior to nutrition initiation. Providing empiric supplemental thiamin (eg, 100 mg/d) and folic acid (eg, 1 mg/d) for the first 3–7 days of nutrition support is reasonable.

- Patients at risk for refeeding syndrome will likely require increased frequency of monitoring in the first 5–7 days of nutrition support (eg, monitoring serum electrolytes 2–3 times a day rather than once daily, monitoring specifically for signs/symptoms of refeeding syndrome).

- Thiamin deficiency is also a potential factor and can lead to severe sequelae including lactic acidosis and Wernicke's encephalopathy.

- Refeeding syndrome generally manifests within the first 24–72 hours of initiating nutrition support in patients at risk, although it may occur later in some cases. Prevention of refeeding syndrome is essential, and the first step is to identify patients at risk.

Fluid, Acid-Base, and Electrolyte Disorders Associated with Refeeding[78–81,83,95]

Maintaining electrolyte homeostasis (especially phosphorus, potassium, and magnesium, possibly sodium/fluid) is a key component of the plan to prevent or treat refeeding syndrome. Below are suggestions for electrolyte management and dosing in patients at risk for refeeding syndrome.

Phosphorus

- Well-nourished, nonstressed adults with normal renal function typically require maintenance doses of 10–15 mmol of phosphorus (provided as phosphate) per 1000 kcal per day, or about 20–40 mmol/d. As stated above, patients at risk for refeeding syndrome will likely have higher requirements initially and may require repletion before initiating nutrition support.

- When PN admixtures are prescribed and compounded, an initial reduction in calcium dosing in PN may be required to accommodate increased doses of phosphate (due to calcium-phosphate solubility limits).

- One needs to be aware of the sodium and potassium content of phosphate dosage forms and consider it when determining total daily electrolyte doses:

    - 1 mmol IV potassium phosphate = 1.47 mEq potassium

    - 1 mmol IV sodium phosphate = 1.33 mEq sodium

- To simplify the prescription and reduce aluminum exposure for patients receiving PN, and if clinically appropriate, a limitation to 1 phosphate salt form, provided as sodium phosphate, should be considered since it contains approximately 3 times less aluminum than potassium phosphate.

Potassium

- Well-nourished adults with normal renal function typically require 1–2 mEq/kg/d of potassium to meet maintenance needs.

- IV potassium can be provided as chloride, acetate, and phosphate salts, with chloride and acetate doses adjusted based on acid-base status, and phosphate salt as described above.

- To simplify the prescription and help reduce aluminum content for patients receiving PN, and if clinically appropriate, providing potassium as one salt form (eg, potassium chloride) should be considered. Phosphate can be provided as sodium phosphate, and sodium as sodium chloride and sodium acetate (and adjust chloride to acetate ratio with these salts).

Magnesium

- Well-nourished adults require approximately 8–20 mEq/d of magnesium, or usually in the range of 0.1–0.4 mEq/kg/d to meet maintenance needs.

- IV magnesium is usually provided as magnesium sulfate (1 g of magnesium sulfate contains 8.12 mEq of magnesium).

Sodium/Fluid

- Well-nourished adults require 1–2 mEq/kg/d of sodium to meet maintenance needs.

- Patients at risk for refeeding syndrome, especially those with severe malnutrition, may have impaired cardiac and/or pulmonary function due to muscle loss and may accumulate sodium and fluid during refeeding with resulting symptomatic volume overload.

- In patients at risk for fluid overload, limiting sodium to < 2 mEq/kg/d and fluid to 20–25 mL/kg/d should be considered when initiating nutrition support.

Acid/Base

- Patients at risk for refeeding syndrome can have underlying acid-base disturbances, which require complete evaluation.
- While nutrition support should not be used to treat underlying acid-base disorders (and is not an effective means of treating the underlying disorder), adjustments to PN can be made to minimize exacerbating underlying disorders:
  - Normal chloride to acetate ratio of 1:1 to 1.5:1 (since commercially available amino acids contain predominately acetate)
  - For patients at risk for metabolic acidosis (eg, AKI, CKD, significant small intestine/GI bicarbonate losses), increase acetate, decrease chloride (eg, chloride to acetate ratio of ~1:2 or lower)
  - For patients at risk for metabolic alkalosis (eg, volume contraction, large gastric volume losses or vomiting), increase chloride and decrease acetate (eg, chloride to acetate ratio 2:1 or higher)

Other Considerations

- Patients with impaired renal function may ultimately require restriction of phosphate, potassium, and/or magnesium, but may have higher requirements when initiating nutrition support. Assess their underlying renal function and the presence of any forms of RRT and individualize dosing.
- Once patients have reached their goal intake of nutrition support and their serum electrolyte concentrations have stabilized, they may require a reduction in maintenance doses of phosphate, potassium, and magnesium (back to "normal" maintenance doses) and adjustment of sodium and/or fluid dosing.

Conclusion

Refeeding syndrome is a serious complication associated with initiation of nutrition support in malnourished or chronically starved individuals. It has been associated with significant morbidity and even mortality. Refeeding syndrome is preventable by following some key steps:

- Identify patients at risk.
- Correct electrolyte abnormalities before initiating nutrition support.

- "Start low and go slow"—initiate nutrition support at 480 kcal/d for at least 2 days, then advance over the next 3–5 days to goal nutrient requirements.

- Increase maintenance doses of phosphate, potassium, and magnesium (in patients with normal renal function), and adjust doses based on response and renal function.

- Consider sodium and fluid restriction for the first few days if appropriate.

- Provide supplemental thiamin 100 mg/d and folic acid 1 mg/d for 3–7 days.

- Monitor at least daily for the first 5–7 days.

- Once electrolytes are at goal and stabilized, consider reducing electrolyte doses back to "standard" maintenance doses (again depending on response and renal function).

Adrenal Insufficiency

Overview

Acute adrenal insufficiency (AI), also referred to as adrenal crisis or Addisonian crisis, is a deficiency in the production or action of glucocorticoids, namely cortisol, with or without a deficiency in the production of mineralocorticoids or adrenal androgens. It can be a life-threatening emergency. Both primary and central AI can contribute to electrolyte abnormalities, alterations in the renal excretion of water, hypoglycemia, and/or metabolic acidosis. An understanding of the metabolic consequences of AI is important for nutrition support practitioners to recognize fluid, electrolyte, and acid-base abnormalities commonly associated with AI.

Adrenal Gland Physiology[96-98]

- The adrenal gland consists of 2 layers, the cortex and the medulla.
  - The adrenal cortex is the outermost layer of the adrenal gland and consists of 3 zones, the zona glomerulosa, zona fasciculata, and zona reticularis. Mineralocorticoids, glucocorticoids, and adrenal androgens are synthesized and secreted by the adrenal cortex (Figure 5-4).
    - The zona glomerulosa is the outermost layer of the adrenal cortex and is responsible for synthesis of mineralocorticoids, namely aldosterone. Aldosterone secretion causes renal sodium and water retention, resulting in an increase in effective blood volume and

Figure 5-4. Physiology of the adrenal gland.

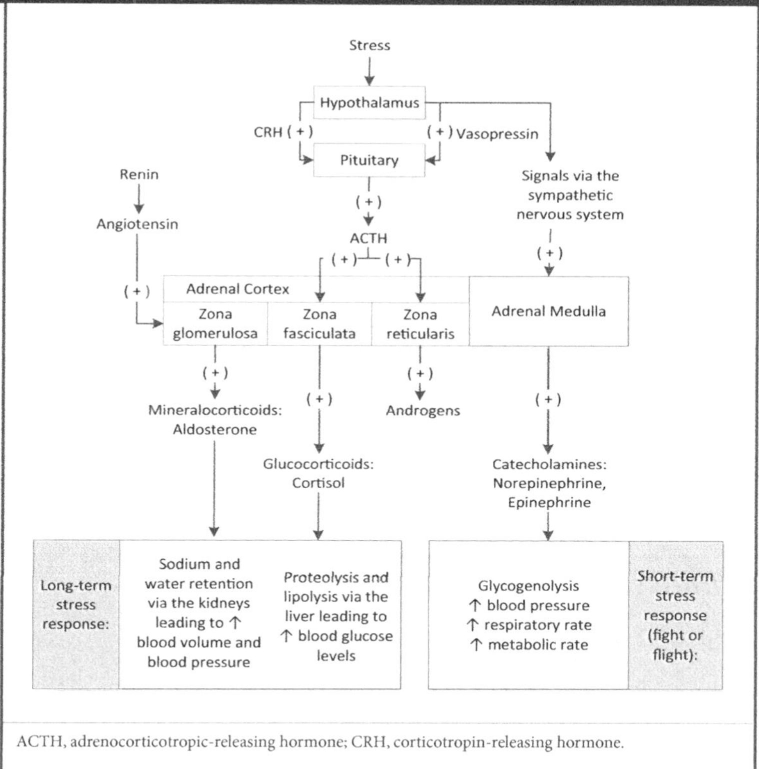

ACTH, adrenocorticotropic-releasing hormone; CRH, corticotropin-releasing hormone.

blood pressure (see Chapter 1). Aldosterone also causes renal potassium excretion.

- The zona fasciculata is the middle layer of the adrenal cortex and is responsible for synthesis of glucocorticoids, namely cortisol. The function of cortisol is to raise blood glucose levels by increasing hepatic glucose output by stimulating the catabolism of lipids and protein for gluconeogenesis. Additional effects of corticosteroids are summarized in Table 5-15.

- The zona reticularis is the innermost layer of the adrenal cortex and is responsible for synthesis of adrenal androgens.

- The adrenal medulla is the innermost layer. The catecholamines epinephrine and norepinephrine are synthesized and secreted by the adrenal medulla and are vital to the “flight or fight” phenomenon.

Table 5-15. Systemic Effects of Cortisol.[99]

Target	Effect
Cardiovascular system	Increases effective blood volume via renal sodium and water retention
	Increases peripheral vascular tone
Immune system	Immunosuppression
	Anti-inflammatory
Lipids	Increases lipolysis
Liver	Increases gluconeogenesis
	Increases glycogen synthesis and storage
	Increases blood glucose levels
Kidneys	Increases glomerular filtration rate
Muscle	Decreases glucose uptake
	Decreases protein synthesis
	Increases catabolism

Primary AI[98,99]

Definition

- Primary AI, also known as Addison's disease, results from the progressive destruction/dysfunction of the adrenal cortex either by autoimmune disease, infectious pathogens, inflammation, medications, trauma, or genetic mutations leading to a reduction in circulating glucocorticoids, mineralocorticoids, and adrenal androgens.

Prevalence

- Prevalence of primary AI in the Western world ranges from 39 to 60 cases per million population.

- Severe AI can manifest as a life-threatening emergency. This typically occurs as the initial presentation of undiagnosed Addison's disease, or it can be precipitated with known Addison's disease in response to physiological stress, such as surgery, trauma, or infection.

Etiology/Pathophysiology

- The most common cause of primary AI in developed countries is autoimmune adrenalitis, characterized by destruction of the adrenal cortex by cell-mediated immune mechanisms.

Table 5-16. Medications That Can Cause Primary Adrenal Insufficiency.[96-99]

Medications	Mechanism
Anticoagulants (apixaban, argatroban, bivalirudin, dabigatran, dalteparin, enoxaparin, fondaparinux, heparin, rivaroxaban, warfarin)	Bilateral adrenal hemorrhage
Phenobarbital, phenytoin, rifampin	Increases cortisol metabolism through induction of cytochrome P450 enzymes
Aminoglutethimide, ketoconazole, fluconazole, etomidate	Inhibits the production of cortisol by inhibiting cytochrome P450 enzymes
Ipilimumab	Hypophysitis

- Infectious adrenalitis resulting in primary AI can be seen with tuberculosis, acquired immune deficiency syndrome, syphilis, and fungal infections.
- Trauma or malignancy involving bilateral adrenal glands can lead to primary AI.
- Medications can cause primary AI (see Table 5-16).
- Clinical manifestations of primary AI result from a deficiency in all adrenocortical hormones (cortisol, aldosterone, and androgens) (Figure 5-5).

Management

- For women, decreased adrenal androgen production results in clinical symptoms because the adrenal cortex is the primary location for synthesis of these androgens, as compared to males, who synthesize and secrete androgens via the male reproductive organs in addition to the adrenal glands. These clinical manifestations include a decreased sexual libido and the loss of axillary and pubic hair due to a decrease in testosterone production.
- Treatment of primary AI focuses on glucocorticoid and mineralocorticoid replacement and supportive care. Hydrocortisone and/or fludrocortisone are typically used to treat primary AI. Androgen replacement may be considered in female patients who continue to have diminished mood or quality of life despite adequate glucocorticoid and mineralocorticoid replacement.

Figure 5-5. Clinical Manifestations of Primary and Secondary Adrenal Insufficiency. ACTH, Adrenocorticotropic-Releasing Hormone; SIAD, Syndrome of Inappropriate Diuresis.

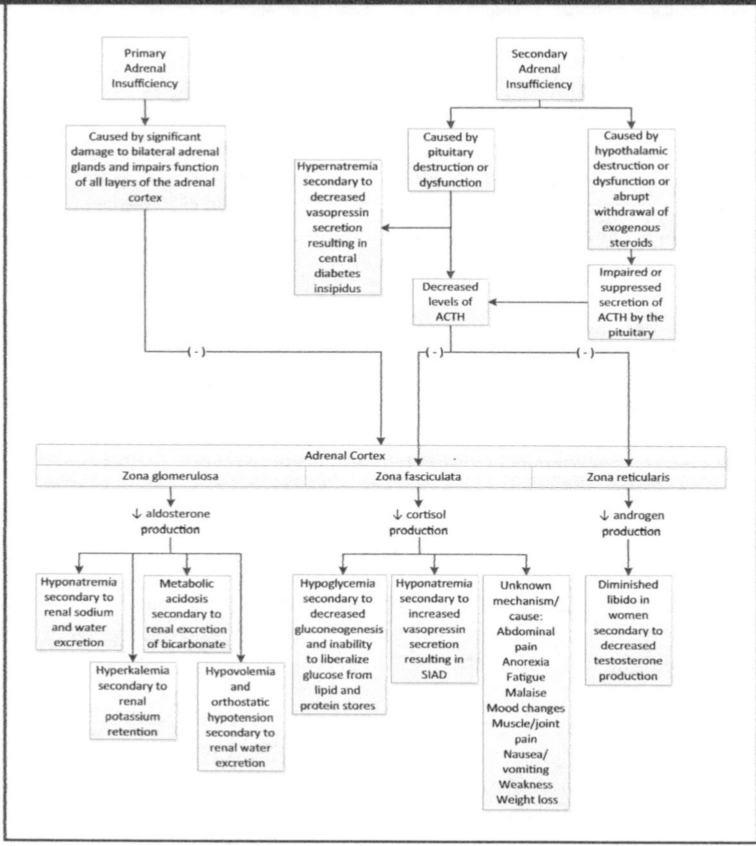

Fluid, Electrolyte, and Acid-Base Disorders Associated With Primary AI

- Decreased aldosterone from the zona glomerulosa results in electrolyte, fluid, and acid-base disorders.
    - Hyponatremia manifests secondary to an increase in both renal sodium and water excretion. The increase in renal water excretion also results in hypovolemia, prerenal azotemia, and orthostatic hypotension. Salt craving is reported in approximately 20% of patients with primary AI. See the sodium disorders section in Chapter 3 for management of hyponatremia secondary to hypoaldosteronism.

- Hyperkalemia is a result of decreased renal potassium excretion.
- Metabolic acidosis occurs secondary to increased renal excretion of bicarbonate. Depending on its severity, metabolic acidosis may also worsen hyperkalemia.

- Decreased cortisol production from the zona fasciculata results in electrolyte and glucose disorders.
  - Hypoglycemia results from a decrease in hepatic gluconeogenesis and inability of the body to liberalize glucose production from lipid and protein stores.
  - Hyponatremia may occur due to the increase in ADH (ie, vasopressin) from the posterior pituitary gland resulting in syndrome of inappropriate diuresis (SIAD). See the sodium disorders section in Chapter 3.
  - Other clinical manifestations include abdominal pain, anorexia, fatigue, malaise, mood changes, muscle/joint pain, nausea and vomiting, weakness, and weight loss, but the exact cause and mechanisms behind these manifestations are not well understood.

Secondary AI[98]

Definition

- Secondary AI most commonly results from adrenocorticotropic hormone (ACTH) deficiency caused by chronic exogenous glucocorticoid therapy (eg, asthma, rheumatoid arthritis, ulcerative colitis).
- It may less commonly result from the destruction or dysfunction of the pituitary gland impairing the production of ACTH or as a result of hypothalamic destruction, dysfunction, or suppression. Hypothalamic corticotropin-releasing hormone (CRH) production is impaired or suppressed leading to decreased secretion of ACTH.
  - Secondary AI results in the decreased production of glucocorticoids, while mineralocorticoid production is not affected because aldosterone secretion is regulated by the renin-angiotensin system and serum (extracellular) potassium concentration.

Prevalence[97]

- The estimated prevalence of secondary AI ranges from 150 to 280 cases per million population.
- Severe AI can manifest in secondary AI and is most commonly seen in patients with chronic corticosteroid use. Abrupt withdrawal of corticosteroids may precipitate adrenal crisis, which can be life threatening.

Etiology/Pathophysiology

- Secondary AI can be caused by pituitary tumors, irradiation or surgery involving the pituitary, infections or infiltrative processes (eg, amyloidosis, sarcoidosis, hemochromatosis), or genetic disorders inhibiting pituitary development.
  - Long-term hypothalamic suppression of CRH by exogenous corticosteroid administration is the most common cause of secondary AI (Figure 5-5).

Management

- Clinical manifestations of secondary AI result from glucocorticoid deficiency only because the secretion of aldosterone and androgens are largely preserved.
- Treatment of secondary AI focuses on glucocorticoid replacement with hydrocortisone. In patients with central AI caused by long-term suppression of glucocorticoid production due to exogenous corticosteroids, a cautious, slow taper of exogenous glucocorticoids is necessary to prevent symptoms of AI, including adrenal crisis.

Fluid, Electrolyte and Acid-Base Disorders Associated with Secondary AI

- Hyponatremia results from increased secretion of ADH (ie, vasopressin) resulting in renal water retention and volume expansion from SIAD (see sodium disorders in Chapter 3).
- Hypoglycemia results from a decrease in hepatic gluconeogenesis and inability of the body to liberalize glucose production from lipid and protein stores. Exogenous carbohydrate or even IV dextrose may need to be administered to maintain adequate blood glucose levels.

Conclusion

Both primary and secondary AI can contribute to electrolyte abnormalities, alterations in the renal excretion of water, hypoglycemia, and/or metabolic acidosis. Management of AI includes replacement of corticosteroids, mineralocorticoids, and/or adrenal androgens. An understanding of the pathophysiology of AI and appropriate supportive care is vital in the management of fluid, electrolyte, and acid-base disorders related to AI.

References

1. Neilson S, Kwon TH, Fenton RA, Praetorious J. Anatomy of the kidney. In: Taal MW, Chertow GM, Marsden PA, Skorecki K, Yu AS, Brenner BM, eds. *Brenner and Rector's The Kidney.* 9th ed. Philadelphia, PA: Elsevier Saunders; 2012:611–632.
2. Wolk R, Foulks C. Renal disease. In: Mueller CM, ed. *The A.S.P.E.N. Adult Nutrition Support Core Curriculum.* 2nd ed. Silver Spring, MD: A.S.P.E.N.; 2012:491–510.
3. Gervasio JM, Garmon WP, Holowatyj MR. Nutrition support in acute kidney injury. *Nutr Clin Pract.* 2011;26(4):374–381.
4. Li PK, Burdmann EA, Mehta RL. Acute kidney injury: global health alert. *Curr Opin Nephrol Hypertens.* 2013;22(2):253–258.
5. Kidney Disease: Improving Global Outcomes (KDIGO) Acute Kidney Injury Work Group. KDIGO clinical practice guideline for acute kidney injury. *Kidney Int Suppl.* 2012;2(1):1–138.
6. Halilovic Maker J, Dager W. Acute kidney injury. In: DiPiro JT, Talbert RL, Yee GC, Matzke GR, Wells BG, Posey LM, Ellingrod VL, Haines ST, Nolin TD, eds. *Pharmacotherapy: A Pathophysiologic Approach.* 10th ed. New York, NY: McGraw-Hill Education; 2017:589–608.
7. Pannu N, Nadim MK. An overview of drug-induced acute kidney injury. *Crit Care Med.* 2008;36(4 suppl):S216–S223.
8. Jha V, Garcia-Garcia G, Iseki K, et al. Chronic kidney disease: global dimension and perspectives. *Lancet.* 2013;382(9888):260–272.
9. Centers for Disease Control. Prevalence of chronic kidney disease and associated risk factors—United States, 1999-2004. *MMWR Morb Mortal Wkly Rep.* 2007;56(8):161–165.
10. Kidney Disease: Improving Global Outcomes (KDIGO) CKD Workgroup. KDIGO 2017 clinical practice guideline update for the diagnosis, evaluation, prevention and treatment of chronic kidney disease-mineral and bone disorder (CKD-MBD). *Kidney Int Suppl.* 2017;7(1):1–59.
11. Murray P, Hall J. Renal replacement therapy for acute renal failure. *Am J Respir Crit Care Med.* 2000;162(3 pt 1):777–781.
12. Maursetter L, Kight CE, Mennig J, Hofmann RM. Review of the mechanism and nutrition recommendations for patients undergoing continuous renal replacement therapy. *Nutr Clin Pract.* 2011;26(4):382–390.
13. Kraft MD, Btaiche IF, Sacks GS, Kudsk KA. Treatment of electrolyte disorders in adult patients in the intensive care unit. *Am J Health-Syst Pharm.* 2005;62(16):1663–1682.
14. Kent PS. Integrating clinical nutrition practice guidelines in chronic kidney disease. *Nutr Clin Pract.* 2005;20(2):213–217.
15. Moore LW. Implications for nutrition practice in the mineral-bone disorder of chronic kidney disease. *Nutr Clin Pract.* 2011;26(4):391–400.
16. Canada TW, Lord LM. Fluid, electrolytes, and acid-base disorders. In: Mueller CM, Lord LM, Marian M, McClave SA, Miller SJ, eds. *The A.S.P.E.N. Adult Nutrition Support Core Curriculum.* 3rd ed. Silver Spring, MD: A.S.P.E.N.; 2017:113–137.
17. Oreopoulos DG, Ossareh S, Thodis E. Peritoneal dialysis. Past, present and future. *Iran J Kidney Dis.* 2008;2(4):171–182.
18. Bieber SD, Burkart J, Golper TA, *et al.* Comparative outcomes between continuous ambulatory and automated peritoneal dialysis: a narrative review. *Am J Kidney Dis.* 2014;63(6):1027–1037.
19. Trey C, Davidson CS. The management of fulminant hepatic failure. *Prog Liver Dis.* 1970;3:282–298.

20. Polson J, Lee WM. AASLD position paper: the management of acute liver failure. *Hepatology.* 2005;41(5):1179–1197.

21. Sugawara K, Nakayama N, Mochida S. Acute liver failure in Japan: definition, classification, and prediction of the outcome. *J Gastroenterol.* 2012;47(8):849–861.

22. Murray KF, Hadzic N, Wirth S, Bassett M, Kelly D. Drug-related hepatotoxicity and acute liver failure. *J Pediatr Gastroenterol Nutr.* 2008;47(4):395–405.

23. Du WB, Pan XP, Li LJ. Prognostic models for acute liver failure. *Hepatobiliary Pancreat Dis Int.* 2010;9(2):122–128.

24. Shakil AO, Kramer D, Mazariegos GV, Fung JJ, Rakela J. Acute liver failure: clinical features, outcome analysis, and applicability of prognostic criteria. *Liver Transpl.* 2000;6(2):163–169.

25. Wang DW, Yin YM, Yao YM. Advances in the management of acute liver failure. *World J Gastroenterol.* 2013;19(41):7069–7077.

26. Lee WM. Recent developments in acute liver failure. *Best Pract Res Clin Gastroenterol.* 2012;26(1):3–16.

27. Rumack BH, Bateman DN. Acetaminophen and acetylcysteine dose and duration: past, present and future. *Clin Toxicol (Phila).* 2012;50(2):91–98.

28. Lat I, Foster DR, Erstad B. Drug-induced acute liver failure and gastrointestinal complications. *Crit Care Med.* 2010. 38(6 suppl):S175–S187.

29. Bernal W, Auzinger G, Dhawan A, Wendon J. Acute liver failure. *Lancet.* 2010;376(9736): 190–201.

30. Weissenborn K. Hepatic encephalopathy: definition, clinical grading and diagnostic principles. *Drugs.* 2019;79(Suppl 1):S5–S9.

31. Bjerring PN, Eefsen M, Hansen BA, Larsen FS. The brain in acute liver failure. A tortuous path from hyperammonemia to cerebral edema. *Metab Brain Dis.* 2009;4(1):5–14.

32. Albrecht J, Norenberg MD. Glutamine: a Trojan horse in ammonia neurotoxicity. *Hepatology.* 2006;44(4):788–794.

33. Clemmesen JO, Larsen FS, Kondrup J, Hansen BA, Ott P. Cerebral herniation in patients with acute liver failure is correlated with arterial ammonia concentration. *Hepatology.* 1999;29(3):648–653.

34. Vilstrup H, Amodio P, Bajaj J, et al. Hepatic encephalopathy in chronic liver disease: 2014 Practice Guideline by the American Association for the Study of Liver Diseases and the European Association for the Study of the Liver. *Hepatology.* 2014;60(2): 715–735.

35. Liamis G, Tsimihodimos V, Doumas M, Spyrou A, Bairaktari E, Elisaf M. Clinical and laboratory characteristics of hypernatraemia in an internal medicine clinic. *Nephrol Dial Transplant.* 2008;23(1):136–143.

36. Jain S, Pendyala P, Varma S, Sharma N, Joshi K, Chawla Y. Effect of renal dysfunction in fulminant hepatic failure. *Trop Gastroenterol.* 2000;21(3):118–120.

37. Munoz SJ. The hepatorenal syndrome. *Med Clin North Am.* 2008;92(4):813–837, viii-ix.

38. Devauchelle P, Page M, Brun P, et al. Continuous haemodialysis with citrate anticoagulation in patients with liver failure: three cases [in French]. *Ann Fr Anesth Reanim.* 2012;31(6):543–546.

39. Schuppan D, Afdhal NH. Liver cirrhosis. *Lancet.* 2008;371(9615):838–851.

40. Sen S, Williams R, Jalan R. The pathophysiological basis of acute-on-chronic liver failure. *Liver.* 2002;22(suppl 2):5–13.

41. Cardenas A, Arroyo V. Mechanisms of water and sodium retention in cirrhosis and the pathogenesis of ascites. *Best Pract Res Clin Endocrinol Metab.* 2003;17(4):607–622.

42. Arroyo V, Ginès P, Gerbes AL, et al. Definition and diagnostic criteria of refractory ascites and hepatorenal syndrome in cirrhosis. International Ascites Club. *Hepatology.* 1996;23(1):164–176.

43. Angeli P. Current management of uncomplicated ascites. *Clin Liver Dis.* 2013;2(3): 125–127.

44. European Association for the Study of the Liver. EASL clinical practice guidelines on the management of ascites, spontaneous bacterial peritonitis, and hepatorenal syndrome in cirrhosis. *J Hepatol.* 2010;53(3):397–417.

45. Moore KP, Wong F, Gines P, et al. The management of ascites in cirrhosis: report on the consensus conference of the International Ascites Club. *Hepatology.* 2003;38(1):258–266.

46. Angeli P, Fasolato S, Mazza E, et al. Combined versus sequential diuretic treatment of ascites in non-azotaemic patients with cirrhosis: results of an open randomised clinical trial. *Gut.* 2010;59(1):98–104.

47. Shear L, Ching S, Gabuzda GJ. Compartmentalization of ascites and edema in patients with hepatic cirrhosis. *N Engl J Med.* 1970;282(25):1391–1396.

48. Ginés P, Arroyo V, Quintero E, et al. Comparison of paracentesis and diuretics in the treatment of cirrhotics with tense ascites. Results of a randomized study. *Gastroenterology.* 1987;93(2):234–241.

49. Ginès A, Fernández-Esparrach G, Monescillo A, et al., Randomized trial comparing albumin, dextran 70, and polygeline in cirrhotic patients with ascites treated by paracentesis. *Gastroenterology.* 1996;111(4):1002–1010.

50. Salerno F, Gerbes A, Ginès P, Wong F, Arroyo V. Diagnosis, prevention and treatment of hepatorenal syndrome in cirrhosis. *Gut.* 2007;56(9):1310–1318.

51. Sola E, Ginès P. Renal and circulatory dysfunction in cirrhosis: current management and future perspectives. *J Hepatol.* 2010;53(6):1135–1145.

52. Fagundes C, Ginès P. Hepatorenal syndrome: a severe, but treatable, cause of kidney failure in cirrhosis. *Am J Kidney Dis.* 2012;59(6):874–885.

53. Ahya SN, José Soler M, Levitsky J, Batlle D. Acid-base and potassium disorders in liver disease. *Semin Nephrol.* 2006;26(6):466–470.

54. Angeli P, Wong F, Watson H, Ginès P; CAPPS Investigators. Hyponatremia in cirrhosis: results of a patient population survey. *Hepatology.* 2006;44(6):1535–1542.

55. Ginès P, Guevara M. Hyponatremia in cirrhosis: pathogenesis, clinical significance, and management. *Hepatology.* 2008;48(3):1002–1010.

56. Fortune BE, Garcia-Tsao G. Hypervolemic hyponatremia: clinical significance and management. *Clin Liver Dis.* 2013;2(3):109–112.

57. Jeppesen PB. Spectrum of short bowel syndrome in adults: intestinal insufficiency to intestinal failure. *JPEN J Parenter Enteral Nutr.* 2014;38(1 suppl):8S-13S.

58. O'Keefe SJD, Buchman AL, Fishbein TM, Jeejeebhoy KN, Jeppesen PB, Shaffer J. Short bowel syndrome and intestinal failure: consensus definitions and overview. *Clin Gastroenterol Hepatol.* 2006;4(1):6–10.

59. Weise WJ, Serrano FA, Fought J, Gennari FJ. Acute electrolyte and acid-base disorders in patients with ileostomies: a case series. *Am J Kidney Dis.* 2008;52(3):494–500.

60. Hayden DM, Mora Pinzon MC, Francescatti AB, et al. Hospital readmission for fluid and electrolyte abnormalities following ileostomy construction: preventable or unpredictable? *J Gastrointest Surg.* 2013;17(2):298–303.

61. Soeters PB, Ebeid AM, Fischer JE. Review of 404 patients with gastrointestinal fistulas: impact of parenteral nutrition. *Ann Surg.* 1979;190(2):189–202.

62. Matarese LE. Nutrition and fluid optimization for patients with short bowel syndrome. *JPEN J Parenter Enteral Nutr.* 2013;37(2):161–170.

63. Evenson AR, Fischer JE. Current management of enterocutaneous fistula. *J Gastrointest Surg.* 2006;10(3):455–464.

64. Keely SJ, Montrose MH, Barrett KE. Electrolyte secretion and absorption: small intestine and colon. In: Yamada T, Alpers DH, Kalloo AN, et al., eds. *Textbook of Gastroenterology.* 5th ed. Hoboken, NJ: Wiley-Blackwell; 2009:330–367.

65. Kumpf VJ. Pharmacologic management of diarrhea in patients with short bowel syndrome. *JPEN J Parenter Enteral Nutr.* 2014;38(1 suppl):38S-44S.

66. Btaiche IF, Khalidi N. Metabolic complications of parenteral nutrition in adults, part 2. *Am J Health-Syst Pharm.* 2004;61(19):2050–2059.

67. Tong GM, Rude RK. Magnesium deficiency in critical illness. *J Intensive Care Med.* 2005;20(1):3–17.

68. Williams RN, Hemingway D, Miller AS. Enteral *Clostridium difficile*, an emerging cause for high-output ileostomy. *J Clin Pathol.* 2009;62(10):951–953.

69. al-Ghamdi SM, Cameron EC, Sutton RA. Magnesium deficiency: pathophysiologic and clinical overview. *Am J Kidney Dis.* 1994;24(5):737–752.

70. Hamill-Ruth RJ, McGory R. Magnesium repletion and its effect on potassium homeostasis in critically ill patients: results of a double-blind, randomized, controlled trial. *Crit Care Med.* 1996;24(1):38–45.

71. Seidner DL, Schwartz LK, Winkler MF, et al. Increased intestinal absorption in the era of teduglutide and its impact on management strategies in patients with short bowel syndrome-associated failure. *JPEN J Parenter Enteral Nutr.* 2013;37(2):201–211.

72. Kitabchi AE, Umpierrez GE, Miles JM, Fisher JN. Hyperglycemic crises in adult patients with diabetes. *Diabetes Care.* 2009;32(7):1335–1343.

73. Fayfman M, Pasquel FJ, Umpierrez GE. Management of hyperglycemic crises: diabetic ketoacidosis and hyperglycemic hyperosmolar state. *Med Clin North Am.* 2017;101(3):587–606.

74. Centers for Disease Control and Prevention. National hospital discharge survey. http://www.cdc.gov/nchs/nhds.htm. Accessed December 10, 2019.

75. Corwell B, Knight B, Olivieri L, Willis G. Current diagnosis and treatment of hyperglycemic emergencies. *Emerg Med Clin N Am.* 2014;32(2):437–452.

76. Westerberg DP. Diabetic ketoacidosis: evaluation and treatment. *Am Fam Physician.* 2013;87(5):337–346.

77. Pasquel F, Umpierrez G. Hyperosmolar hyperglycemic state: a historic review of the clinical presentation, diagnosis, and treatment. *Diabetes Care.* 2014;37(11):3124–3131.

78. Kraft MD, Btaiche IF, Sacks GS. Review of the refeeding syndrome. *Nutr Clin Pract.* 2005;20(6):625–633.

79. Stanga Z, Brunner A, Leuenberger M, et al. Nutrition in clinical practice—the refeeding syndrome: illustrative cases and guidelines for prevention and treatment. *Eur J Clin Nutr.* 2008;62(6):687–694.

80. Boateng AA, Sriram K, Meguid MM, Crook M. Refeeding syndrome: treatment considerations based on collective analysis of literature case reports. *Nutrition.* 2010;26(2):156–167.

81. Skipper A. Refeeding syndrome or refeeding hypophosphatemia. *Nutr Clin Pract.* 2012;27(1):34–40.

82. Weinsier RL, Krumdieck CL. Death resulting from overzealous total parenteral nutrition: the refeeding syndrome revisited. *Am J Clin Nutr.* 1980;34(3):393–399.

83. Sheldon GF, Grzyb S. Phosphate depletion and repletion: relation to parenteral nutrition and oxygen transport. *Ann Surg.* 1975;182(6):683–689.

84. Silvis SE, Paragas PD. Paresthesias, weakness, seizures, and hypophosphatemia in patients receiving hyperalimentation. *Gastroenterology*. 1972;62(4):513–520.

85. Silvis SE, DiBartolomeo AG, Aaker HM. Hypophosphatemia and neurological changes secondary to oral caloric intake. *Am J Gastroentenerol.* 1980;73(3):215–222.

86. Furlan AJ, Hanson M, Cooperman A, Farmer RG. Acute areflexic paralysis: association with hyperalimentation and hypophosphatemia. *Arch Neurol.* 1975;32(10):706–707.

87. Youssef HAE. Hypophosphatemic respiratory failure complicating total parenteral nutrition—an iatrogenic potentially lethal hazard. *Anesthesiology.* 1982;57(3):246.

88. Hayek ME, Eisenberg PG. Severe hypophosphatemia following the institution of enteral feedings. *Arch Surg*. 1989;124(11):1325–1328.

89. Vanneste J, Hage J. Acute severe hypophosphatemia mimicking Wernicke's encephalopathy. *Lancet.* 1986;1(8471):44.

90. Newman JH, Neff TA, Ziporin P. Acute respiratory failure associated with hypophosphatemia. *N Engl J Med*. 1977;296(19):1101–1103.

91. Patel U, Sriram K. Acute respiratory failure due to refeeding syndrome and hypophosphatemia induced by hypocaloric enteral nutrition. *Nutrition*. 2009;25(3): 364–367.

92. Chadda K, Raynard B, Antoun S, Thyrault N, Nitenberg G. Acute lactic acidosis with Wernicke's encephalopathy due to acute thiamine deficiency. *Intensive Care Med.* 2002;28(10):1499.

93. Doig GS, Simpson F, Heighes PT, et al. Restricted versus continued standard caloric intake during the management of refeeding syndrome in critically ill adults: a randomised, parallel-group, multicentre, single-blind controlled trial. *Lancet Resp Med.* 2015;3(12):943–952.

94. Craddock PR, Yawata Y, VanSanten L, Gilberstadt S, Silvis S, Jacob HS. Acquired phagocyte dysfunction. A complication of the hypophosphatemia of parenteral hyperalimentation. *N Engl J Med.* 1974;290(25):1403–1407.

95. Mirtallo J, Canada T, Johnson D, et al. Safe practices for parenteral nutrition. *JPEN J Parenter Enteral Nutr.* 2004;28(6):S39–S70.

96. Charmandari E, Nicolaides NC, Chrousos GP. Adrenal insufficiency. *Lancet.* 2014;383(9935):2152–2167.

97. Else T, Hammer GD. Disorders of the adrenal cortex. In: Hammer GD, McPhee SJ, eds. *Pathophysiology of Disease: An Introduction to Clinical Medicine*. 8th ed. https://accessmedicine.mhmedical.com/content.aspx?bookid=2468§ionid=198224279. Accessed December 21, 2019.

98. Navoa P, Vela ET, Garcia NP, Rodriguez MM, Guerras IS, Santamaria MA. Guidelines for diagnosis and treatment of adrenal insufficiency in adults. *Endocrinol Nutr.* 2014;61(suppl 1):1–34.

99. Rushworth RL, Torpy DJ, Falhammar H. Adrenal crisis. *N Engl J Med.* 2019;381(9): 852–861.

CHAPTER 6

Pediatric Considerations for Fluids, Electrolytes, and Acid-Base Disorders

Fluid, electrolyte, and acid-base management in the pediatric patient continues to be a challenge for many practitioners. Chapters 1–5 provide an excellent framework for the diagnosis and treatment of fluid, electrolyte, and acid-base disorders; however, pediatric patients require special considerations. This chapter will cover considerations for fluids, electrolytes, and acid-base disorders specific to the pediatric patient population, which includes premature neonates (gestational age < 37 weeks), infants (birth to 12 months of age), toddlers (1–3 years), children (4–13 years), and adolescents (14–18 years).

Fluids Status and Requirements

The diversity of the pediatric population results in a corresponding variability in fluid requirements. As the patient ages, the percentage of total body water (TBW) decreases from 85% in the preterm neonate to 60% in the adolescent patient. As the TBW decreases, a corresponding decrease in fluid volume per body weight is seen.[1-3] Patients with higher TBW also tend to develop fluid/electrolyte imbalances more frequently than patients with lower TBW.

Table 6-1. Calculating Estimated Fluid Requirements (Holliday-Segar Formula).[4]

Body Weight, kg	Daily Fluid Requirement (Holliday-Segar)	Fluid Requirements (4:2:1 Short Cut)
1–10	100 mL/kg	4 mL/kg/h[a]
11–20	1000 mL + 50 mL/kg for each kilogram over 10 kg	40 mL/h + 2 mL/kg for each kilogram over 10 kg
>20	1500 mL + 20 mL/kg for each kilogram over 20 kg	60 mL/h + 1 mL/kg for each kilogram over 20 kg

[a]This may underestimate fluid requirements by about 5% in young children. To avoid this underestimation, 5 mL/kg/h is often used.

Daily fluid requirements can be estimated in a variety of ways. One of the most common ways, the Holliday-Segar Formula, is a weight-based method (Table 6-1).[4] Based on this formula, a child weighing 27 kg would require a minimum of 1640 mL of fluid per day.

100 mL/kg for first 10 kg =	100 × 10 =	1000 mL
50 mL/kg for next 10 kg =	50 × 10 =	500 mL
20 mL/kg for weight > 20 kg =	20 × 7 =	140 mL
Total		1640 mL

This formula, however, does not address fluid requirements in patients with disease states, such as kidney failure or congestive heart failure, that alter fluid accumulation.[4–6]

Fluid Disorders

Hypovolemia is a condition in which TBW is decreased significantly enough to cause signs and symptoms such as dry mucous membranes, tachycardia, and, if conditions worsen, hypotension and orthostasis. The causes and treatment of hypovolemia in adult patients are covered in Chapter 2. In addition to the causes for hypovolemia seen in adult patients, those more specific to pediatric patients include vomiting, diarrhea, excessive sweating, and inadequate fluid intake over a significant period of time. Treatment of hypovolemia in the pediatric patient is based on weight loss, and in order to treat the patient appropriately, the practitioner must classify the patient's level of dehydration.

- Mild dehydration is distinguished by the presence of dry mucous membranes but normal hemodynamic parameters. It corresponds to a weight loss of about 5% in infants and about 3% in children and adolescents.
- Moderate dehydration is defined by changes in hemodynamic parameters that suggest intravascular depletion such as tachycardia, mild hypotension, and orthostasis. The corresponding weight loss for moderate dehydration is about 10% in infants and about 5% in children and adolescents.
- With severe dehydration, the hemodynamic parameters are more pronounced, resulting in moderate to severe hypotension, tachycardia, and poor perfusion. A 15% weight loss in infants and a 7% weight loss in children and adolescents would be expected.

If pre-illness weights are known, the percent dehydration can be calculated by using the following equation:

$$\frac{\text{Pre-illness weight} - \text{illness weight}}{\text{Pre-illness weight} \times 100} \times 100$$

If pre-illness weights are not available, weight loss can be estimated based on the degree of dehydration (mild, moderate, or severe). Treatment must include replacement of the fluid deficit and provision of maintenance fluids. The amount of fluid to be administered in milliliters per kilogram is then determined based on the severity of dehydration or percentage of weight loss. Infants, children, and adolescents would receive an initial bolus of 20 mL/kg of isotonic fluid given over 1 hour. Fifty percent of the remaining deficit would then be administered over the next 8 hours along with regular maintenance fluids. The remaining 50% of the deficit would be administered over the next 16 hours along with regular maintenance fluids. Usual amounts of maintenance fluids for co-administration with deficit replacement can be found in Table 6-1.

- Example: A 10-kg infant with a 10% weight loss has a 1000-mL fluid deficit. Given the deficit (10%), a bolus of 20 mL/kg or 2% of the patient's body weight, or 200 mL, would be indicated initially. After the initial bolus is given over 1 hour, 50% of the remaining deficit (400 mL, or 4%) would be given over the next 8 hours, and then the final 400 mL (4%) would be given over 16 hours.

- If the patient is severely volume depleted, more than 1 fluid bolus of 20 mL/kg may be necessary. Once tachycardia and hypotension have been resolved, the fluid deficit and maintenance requirements can be calculated. In adolescents, the fluid deficit is about 50% of that of an infant based on the degree of dehydration (mild, moderate, or severe); therefore, the initial bolus would be 10 mL/kg.[7–9]

- Hypertonic dehydration is treated more conservatively due to the hyperosmolar state of the blood. The deficit volume should be replaced over 48 hours to prevent significant osmotic fluid shifts, which can result in cerebral edema and convulsions.

- If the patient is hemodynamically compromised (hypotension, severe tachycardia), then a bolus of 10–20 mL/kg of an isotonic fluid is necessary to restore hemodynamic stability. Serum sodium should be corrected no faster than 0.5 mEq/L/h or no more than 10 mEq/L/d. Serum sodium concentrations should be checked every 4–6 hours to ensure rehydration is not occurring too rapidly.[7,8,10]

Several conditions require adjustments in fluid intake for providing optimal care. These conditions include birth, prematurity, and congenital anomalies.

- After birth, a contraction of the extracellular compartment occurs due to the loss of interstitial fluid. This results in a 5%–10% weight loss in healthy neonates and possibly up to 15% in preterm neonates due to the higher TBW. This loss is a normal physiologic process, and fluid intake should be restricted for the first 1–2 days to allow the process to complete. Attempts to replace these losses to prevent weight loss will result in fluid overload and poorer outcomes.[3,7,11,12]

- Insensible losses play a large role in fluid balance in the premature neonate. Skin immaturity, radiant warmers, and phototherapy often increase insensible losses by as much as 20–40 mL/kg. Insensible losses are high during the first few weeks of life. Up to 200 mL/kg/d of fluid may be needed to maintain normal fluid balance in the preterm neonate. Table 6-2 summarizes fluid requirements for neonates based on birth weight.[1,2] The decrease in insensible losses is due mainly to the thickening of the skin, which reduces fluid losses.

- Congenital defects can have a variable effect on fluid requirements. Conditions such as gastroschisis and omphalocele increase fluid requirements by increasing insensible water losses. Conditions that may require fluid restriction include kidney and lung dysfunction and congenital heart defects resulting in heart failure.[7,13,14]

Table 6-2. Estimated Insensible Losses and Fluid Requirements for Neonates Based on Birth Weight.

Birth weight, g	Insensible Losses, mL/kg	Fluid Requirements, mL/kg	
		Days 1–2	Days 3–7
<750	100-200	100-200	150-200
750-1000	60-80	80-150	100-150
1000-1500	30-60	60-120	100-150
>1500	20	60-80	90-150

Electrolyte Balance

Prior to any electrolyte correction, the validity of the laboratory value should be assessed to make sure the serum values are correct and not just an error in collection or assessment. Once the result is validated, the process for altering electrolytes can begin. Figure 6-1 shows an algorithm for laboratory assessment.[15] When electrolyte abnormalities are being corrected, a stepwise process should be followed.

1. Determine the cause of the electrolyte abnormality.

2. Determine if the abnormality is an acute or a chronic issue.

3. Determine if a supplemental infusion or adjustments in maintenance fluids are necessary. Acute electrolyte abnormalities are typically corrected using supplemental infusions, whereas chronic electrolyte abnormalities are usually treated with maintenance solutions.

4. Determine the relative therapeutic window of the electrolyte to be corrected. Electrolytes such as phosphate and magnesium have a relatively wide therapeutic window and therefore have significantly fewer complications if overcorrection occurs. Potassium has a relatively narrow therapeutic window, and an overcorrection of potassium can have serious consequences. For electrolytes with a relatively narrow therapeutic window, 2 smaller supplements may be better than 1 large supplement.

5. Determine if the serum level is critical or life threatening. If the serum electrolyte is critical or life threatening, acute treatment should begin immediately, and then if appropriate, changes in maintenance electrolytes can be made. An electrolyte replacement assessment algorithm is presented in Figure 6-2.[15]

Figure 6-1. Laboratory Assessment.

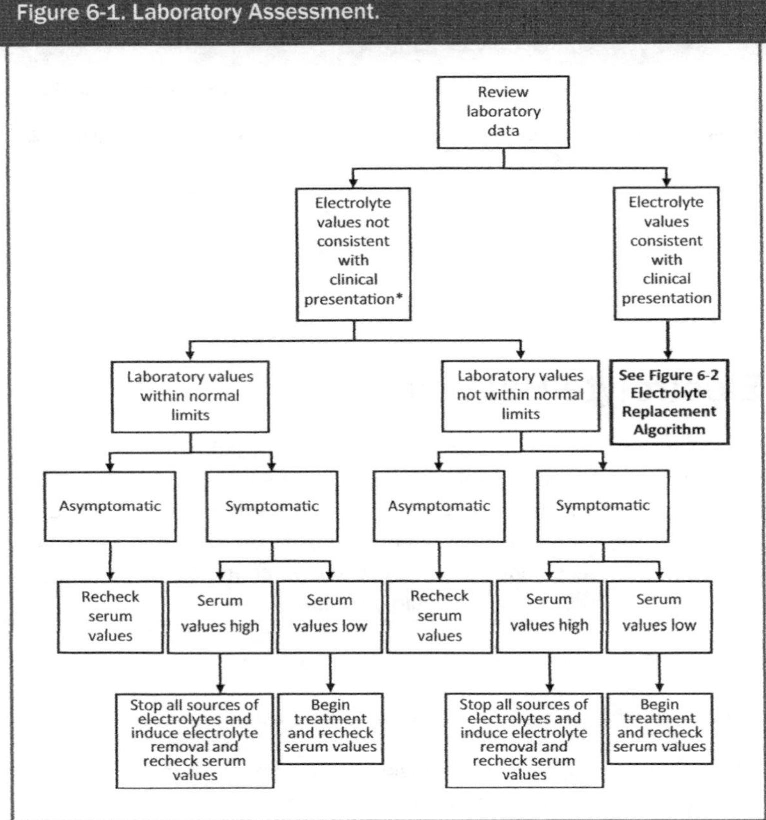

Reprinted with permission from Schmidt GL. Fluids and electrolytes. In: Corkins MR, ed. *The A.S.P.E.N. Pediatric Nutrition Support Core Curriculum*. 2nd ed. Silver Spring, MD: American Society for Parenteral and Enteral Nutrition; 2015:107–128.

*Send for repeat labs on serum electrolytes.

Electrolyte Function and Requirements

In some instances, electrolyte needs in the pediatric population are altered due to differences in TBW, metabolic rate, and immature organ systems (ie, prematurity). Reference values for normal serum concentrations of common electrolytes based on age are available below.[15] An algorithm for adjusting maintenance electrolyte requirements can be found in Figure 6-3,[15,16] and oral daily electrolyte requirements based on age can be found in Table 6-3.[15]

Please note the following reference values are for comparative purposes only and may not reflect normal reference values for an individual institution. Practitioners should use reference values listed at their individual institutions to make adjustments in electrolyte therapy.

Figure 6-2. Electrolyte Replacement Assessment Algorithm.

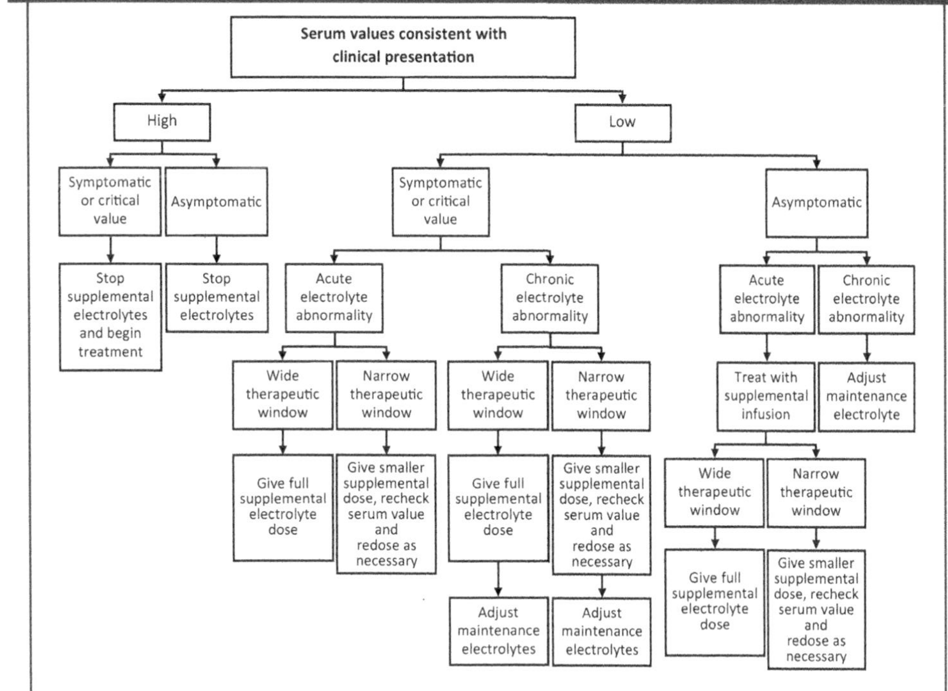

Reprinted with permission from Schmidt GL. Fluids and electrolytes. In: Corkins MR, ed. *The A.S.P.E.N. Pediatric Nutrition Support Core Curriculum*. 2nd ed. Silver Spring, MD: American Society for Parenteral and Enteral Nutrition; 2015:107–128.

Figure 6-3. Maintenance Electrolyte Replacement Flow Chart.

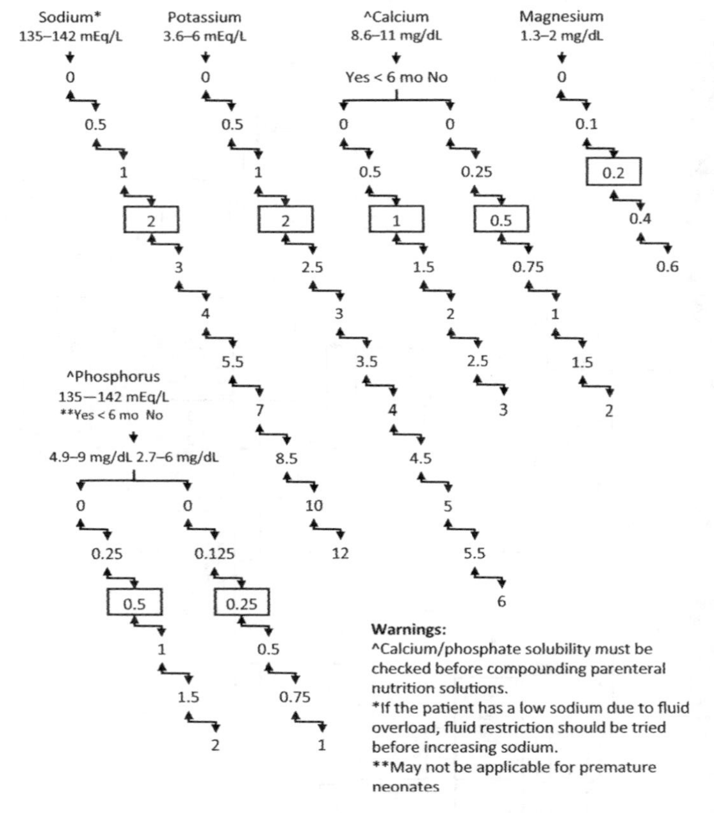

Reprinted with permission from Schmidt GL. Fluids and electrolytes. In: Corkins MR, ed. *The A.S.P.E.N. Pediatric Nutrition Support Core Curriculum*. 2nd ed. Silver Spring, MD: American Society for Parenteral and Enteral Nutrition; 2015:107–128.

Table 6-3. Daily Oral Electrolyte Requirements by Age.

<table>
<tr><th rowspan="2">Age, y</th><th colspan="2">Sodium</th><th colspan="2">Potassium</th><th colspan="2">Magnesium</th><th colspan="2">Calcium</th><th colspan="2">Phosphorus</th></tr>
<tr><th>mg</th><th>mEq</th><th>mg</th><th>mEq</th><th>mg</th><th>mEq</th><th>mg</th><th>mEq</th><th>mg</th><th>mmol</th></tr>
<tr><td>0 to <0.5</td><td>120</td><td>11</td><td>500</td><td>26</td><td>302</td><td>2.5</td><td>210</td><td>10.5</td><td>100</td><td>3</td></tr>
<tr><td>0.5 to <1</td><td>200</td><td>18</td><td>700</td><td>37</td><td>75</td><td>6</td><td>270</td><td>13.5</td><td>275</td><td>9</td></tr>
<tr><td>1 to <2</td><td>225</td><td>20</td><td>1000</td><td>53</td><td rowspan="3">80</td><td rowspan="3">7</td><td rowspan="3">500</td><td rowspan="3">25</td><td rowspan="3">460</td><td rowspan="3">15</td></tr>
<tr><td>2 to <3</td><td rowspan="4">300</td><td rowspan="4">27</td><td rowspan="4">1400</td><td rowspan="4">74</td></tr>
<tr><td>3 to <4</td></tr>
<tr><td>4 to <5</td><td rowspan="5">130</td><td rowspan="5">11</td><td rowspan="4">500</td><td rowspan="4">25</td><td rowspan="4">500</td><td rowspan="4">16</td></tr>
<tr><td>5 to <6</td></tr>
<tr><td>6 to <7</td><td rowspan="4">400</td><td rowspan="4">36</td><td rowspan="4">1600</td><td rowspan="4">89</td></tr>
<tr><td>7 to <8</td></tr>
<tr><td>8 to <9</td><td rowspan="6">1300</td><td rowspan="6">65</td><td rowspan="6">1250</td><td rowspan="6">40</td></tr>
<tr><td>9 to <10</td><td rowspan="4">240</td><td rowspan="4">20</td></tr>
<tr><td>10 to <11</td><td rowspan="4">500</td><td rowspan="4">45</td><td rowspan="4">2000</td><td rowspan="4">111</td></tr>
<tr><td>11 to <12</td></tr>
<tr><td>12 to <13</td></tr>
<tr><td>≥13 (M)
≥13 (F)</td><td>400
360</td><td>30
33</td></tr>
</table>

F, female; M, male.

Reprinted with permission from Schmidt GL. Fluids and electrolytes. In: Corkins MR, ed. *The A.S.P.E.N. Pediatric Nutrition Support Core Curriculum.* 2nd ed. Silver Spring, MD: American Society for Parenteral and Enteral Nutrition; 2015:107–128.

Sodium

- Preterm neonate — 130–140 mEq/L
- Term neonate — 133–146 mEq/L
- Children/adolescents — 135–145 mEq/L

Sodium is the most abundant extracellular cation in the body. Sodium has two primary functions, maintaining fluid balance and maintaining membrane potential. Pediatric reference values for sodium are within 1–2 mEq/L of the adult reference values, except for premature neonates, who have reference values 3–5 mEq/L lower. Sodium requirements in adult patients and pediatric patients are very similar, except for three conditions specific to the pediatric population that alter sodium requirements: being newborn, prematurity, and rapid growth. Daily

Table 6-4. Estimated Electrolyte Requirements for Pediatric Patients Based on Birth Weight and Age.

	Term/ Preterm	Preterm	Term				
Electrolyte	**Days 1–2**	**>2 d**	**>2 d**	**1–3 y**	**4–6 y**	**7–10 y**	**11–18 y**
Sodium, mEq/kg	0	2-6	2-4	2-4	2-4	2-4	2-4
Potassium, mEq/kg	0	2-4	2-4	2-4	2-4	2-4	2-4
Magnesium, mEq/kg	0	0.5-1	0.25-1	0.25-0.5	0.25-0.5	0.25-0.5	0.2-0.4
Calcium, mEq/kg	0-2	2-4	1-2	0.5-1	0.5-1	0.5-1	0.25-0.5
Phosphorus, mmol/kg	0-1.5	1-1.5	1-1.5	0.5-1.5	0.5-1.5	0.5-1.5	0.2-0.6
Chloride, mEq/kg	0	2-4	2-4	2-4	2-4	2-4	2-4

sodium requirements for patients based on birth weight and age can be found in Table 6-4.

- Term newborn neonates: The extracellular fluid contraction seen at birth causes a 5%–10% weight loss in term newborn neonates, which also affects sodium requirements. Sodium and water restrictions are recommended in newborn neonates for the first 1–2 days of life or until the serum sodium concentration drops below 133 mEq/L. Afterward, 2–3 mEq/kg/d of sodium is recommended for maintenance.

- Preterm newborn neonates: The extracellular fluid contraction seen at birth causes up to a 15% weight loss in preterm newborn neonates, which also affects sodium requirements. Sodium and water restrictions are recommended in newborn preterm neonates for the first 1–2 days or until the serum sodium concentrations drop below 130 mEq/L. Afterward, a maintenance dose of 2–4 mEq/kg/d of sodium is recommended for days 3–7 of life. Sodium requirements may be as high as 4–6 mEq/kg/d in the preterm neonate (<28 weeks) due to the inability to concentrate the urine; in some cases patients may require up to 12 mEq/kg/d of sodium to maintain normal serum sodium concentrations.[1,3,11]

- Rapid growth: Sodium is an integral component in the growth process, and patients undergoing rapid growth require additional sodium (3–4 mEq/kg/d).[3]

The treatment of hyponatremia with hypertonic saline (3%) is usually reserved for patients who have acute hyponatremia with serum sodium concentrations < 120 mEq/L or patients exhibiting signs and symptoms of hyponatremia.[7,17] An approximation of the sodium deficit can be calculated with the following equation[18]:

$$\text{Sodium deficit (mEq)} = \text{TBW} \times \text{wt (kg)} \times (\text{Na}_{desired} - \text{Na}_{actual})$$

TBW = 0.8 in premature infants; 0.7 in term infants to ≤6 months of age; and 0.6 in infants > 6 months of age.

- Example: An 8-kg infant with a serum sodium of 125 mEq/L and a desired serum sodium of 135 mEq/L would have a sodium deficit of 48 mEq:

$$(135 - 125) \times 8 \text{ (kg)} \times 0.6 = 48$$

Potassium

- Newborns 3.7–5.9 mEq/L
- Infants 4.1–5.3 mEq/L
- Children/adolescents 3.4–4.7 mEq/L

Potassium is the primary intracellular fluid cation. It is essential for cell metabolism and maintenance of resting membrane potential. Reference values for potassium are higher in the pediatric population than the adult population. This increase is related to the higher metabolic rate in pediatric patients and the subsequent need to have potassium available for normal metabolic functions. Potassium requirements in adults are very similar to those in pediatric patients, except for the 1–2 days after birth. Potassium requirements for patients based on birth weight and age can be found in Table 6-4.

In term and preterm newborn neonates, serum potassium levels increase even in the absence of renal dysfunction. This increase appears to be due to a shift of potassium from the intracellular to the extracellular spaces. The retention of potassium seems to correlate with the degree of immaturity; therefore, potassium is withheld for the first 1–2 days of life or until serum potassium levels normalize for the term newborn neonate and for the first 2–3 days or until serum potassium levels normalize for the preterm newborn neonate. Once serum potassium levels normalize, 2 mEq/kg/d of potassium is recommended.[1,3,7,11] Heel stick samples are at increased risk for hemolyzation, which needs to be factored into the evaluation of laboratory results.

Magnesium

- All age groups 1.5–2.3 mg/dL

Magnesium is an essential cofactor in more than 300 enzymatic reactions, including those involved in glucose metabolism, fatty acid synthesis and breakdown, and DNA and protein metabolism. Magnesium plays a critical role in the functioning of the Na^{+}-K^{+}-ATPase pump, thus affecting neuromuscular transmission, cardiovascular excitability, vasomotor tone, and muscle contraction. Magnesium is also an integral component of bone and parathyroid hormone secretion. Pediatric reference values for magnesium are very similar to adult reference values. Based on magnesium's role in metabolism and bone formation, one would expect requirements to be higher in pediatric patients than in the adult population; however, intravenous (IV) requirements for magnesium are virtually the same in children and adults, at 0.2–0.4 mEq/kg/d.[19] IV magnesium requirements based on age can be found in Table 6-4. It is important to acknowledge the interrelationships between electrolytes (ie, potassium and magnesium), and a discussion of these interactions is available in Chapter 3.

For term and preterm neonates, magnesium is typically withheld for the first 1–2 days after birth or until serum levels normalize. Once the serum levels normalize, 0.2–0.4 mEq/kg/d is recommended. Further restriction may be necessary in patients whose mothers received magnesium as a tocolytic. Magnesium passes through the placenta resulting in hypermagnesemia. Serum levels typically return to normal within 72 hours without treatment.[20] Supplementation with magnesium can begin once levels return to normal.

Calcium

Age Group	Total Calcium
Preterm neonate	6.2–11 mg/dL
Full-term neonate	7.6–10.4 mg/dL
10 d to 2 y	9–11 mg/dL
2–12 y	8.8–10.8 mg/dL
>12 y	8.6–10 mg/dL

Age Group	Ionized, SI Units
Preterm	1.75–2 mmol/L
Full term, <36 h	1.05–1.37 mmol/L
Full term, 36–84 h	1.1–1.42 mmol/L
>84 h	1.2–1.38 mmol/L

Calcium is one of the most abundant ions in the body. It is necessary for many physiologic functions including, but not limited to, neuromuscular activity, regulation of endocrine secretory activities, and bone metabolism. Reference values for calcium are based on age. Reference values are highest in the 10-day to 2-year age group and drop as the patient ages. Prematurity, rickets, and growth are the most prominent factors that affect calcium requirements. Calcium requirements are higher in the pediatric population secondary to bone formation and growth, and they range from 1 to 4 mEq/kg based on age.[21] Ionized calcium concentrations provide the most accurate laboratory test for assessing physiologically active calcium. A serum calcium level measures both bound and free calcium. Therefore, if the serum albumin level is low, the serum calcium concentration will also be low. An equation for correcting calcium due to hypoalbuminemia is listed here; however, it is not completely reliable in critically ill patients:

$$\text{Corrected calcium} = \text{measured total calcium (mg/dL)} + 0.8 \times [4 - \text{albumin (g/dL)}]$$

IV calcium requirements based on age are presented in Table 6-4.

Premature neonates have higher calcium requirements due to the increased need for bone formation and the inability of the kidney to retain calcium due to immaturity and medications such as L-cysteine. That, coupled with the limited solubility of calcium and phosphate in parenteral nutrition (PN) solutions and potentially inadequate vitamin D intake, can lead to rickets in the premature neonate.[22-24]

Phosphorus

- Newborn 4.5–9 mg/dL
- 10 days to 2 years 4.5–6.7 mg/dL
- 2–12 years 4.5–5.5 mg/dL
- >12 years 2.7–4.5 mg/dL

Phosphorus, mainly in the form of phosphate, is the primary intracellular anion in the body. It has many functions including bone and cell membrane composition, maintenance of normal pH, provision of energy-rich bonds (ATP), glucose utilization, glycolysis, 2,3-diphosphoglycerate synthesis, and neurologic and muscle function. Reference values are highest in the newborn and decrease with age. Phosphate requirements are higher in the pediatric population than the adult population due to a higher metabolic rate as well as bone formation. The primary factors specific to the pediatric population that affect phosphorus are prematurity, bone formation, and growth. IV phosphate requirements based on birth weight and age can be found in Table 6-4.

Premature neonates have higher phosphorus requirements due to increased bone formation. Phosphate is typically provided within 1–2 days, and supplementation begins at 1–2.5 mmol/kg in preterm neonates.[1,24,26] Inadequate supplementation of phosphorus, whether due to limited calcium/phosphate solubility in PN solutions or due to inadequate intake can cause rickets in the premature neonate. Severe hypophosphatemia can also cause hypercalcemia in neonates.[27]

Electrolyte Disorders

Electrolyte disorders in pediatric patients are similar to those in adults; please refer to Chapters 1–5 for considerations. In addition to electrolyte maintenance requirements, patients with acute disturbances or critical serum electrolyte abnormalities may require acute replacement. Recommendations for acute electrolyte replacement are presented in Table 6-5.[18,28-34]

Table 6-5. Acute Electrolyte Replacement.

Electrolyte	Condition	Dose	Max dose	Infusion time
Calcium	Tetany	0.5–1 mEq/kg	10 mEq	10–30 min
	Asymptomatic hypocalcemia			1 h
Magnesium	Torsades de pointes	0.2–0.4 mEq/kg	16 mEq	10–20 min
	Symptomatic hypomagnesemia			1–2 h
	Asymptomatic hypomagnesemia			2–4 h
Phosphorus	Mild hypophosphatemia, 2.3–3 mg/dL	0.5 mmol/kg		4 h
	Moderate hypophosphatemia, 1.6–2.2 mg/dL	0.75 mmol/kg		6 h
	Severe hypophosphatemia, ≤1.5 mg/dL	1 mmol/kg		8 h
Potassium	Oral replacement	2–5 mEq/kg in divided doses	1–2 mEq/kg per dose	N/A
	Intravenous replacement	0.5–1 mEq/kg	40 mEq	0.25–0.5 mEq/kg/h

N/A, not applicable.

Acid-Base Homeostasis: Chloride and Bicarbonate

When chloride and bicarbonate are assessed for electrolyte management, it is usually in response to acid-base issues. Chloride requirements for all age groups are from 1 to 4 mEq/kg. No defined requirements for bicarbonate exist. Bicarbonate is not compatible with PN solutions, so acetate, which is converted to bicarbonate via the liver, is adjusted in conjunction with chloride to mitigate acid-base disturbances. Reference values can be found below.

Chloride

• All age groups	98–108 mEq/L

Bicarbonate

• Newborn	17–24 mEq/L
• Infant	19–24 mEq/L
• 2 months to 2 years	16–24 mEq/L
• >2 years	22–26 mEq/L

For simplicity, when chloride or acetate is being adjusted in IV solutions, an equal split of chloride and acetate is recommended for patients with normal pH. If the patient becomes acidotic then moving to one-third chloride and two-thirds acetate is suggested, then all acetate and no chloride if the acidosis progresses. For patients with metabolic alkalosis, a two-thirds chloride and one-third acetate split is recommended, then all chloride and no acetate if the alkalosis progresses.

Acid-Base Disorders

Acute renal failure affects 1%–24% of newborns in the neonatal intensive care unit, and metabolic acidosis can be a common finding in this population. Premature newborns and infants generally have a low capacity for renal acid excretion due to the functional and anatomical immaturity of their kidneys, which cannot fully help to maintain the acid-base balance in the body. The low renal acid excretion capacity in addition to a low bicarbonate reabsorption threshold puts preterm infants at an increased risk of metabolic acidosis and acid-base disturbances.[35-39] Additionally, regardless of gestational age, all newborns have a low glomerular filtration rate and immature renal tubular transport mechanisms that limit functional adaptation to stress.[36,40]

Preterm infants are also more vulnerable to acid-base disturbances associated with feeding.[41] Late metabolic acidosis of prematurity occurs when hydrogen ion intake exceeds renal acid excretion due to immature kidney function, and it may occur with administration of PN. High chloride intake is also associated with metabolic acidosis. In addition to chloride in the PN solution, patients may be receiving other sources of sodium chloride, including medications and IV and arterial line flushes. Replacement of some of the chloride in the PN solution or IV solutions with acetate has been proposed as a way to correct metabolic acidosis in this patient population due to the decrease in chloride intake as well as the metabolism of acetate to bicarbonate. Acetate does not contribute to the hydrogen ion load because the hydrogen ions that are released are consumed during conversion of acetate to bicarbonate.[41-44] Newborns with acute renal failure may have increased sodium bicarbonate requirements, however, and persistent acidosis may require dialysis.[44]

Additional Considerations

Aluminum is a contaminant found in IV solutions used to make PN solutions. Aluminum is normally eliminated in the urine; however, adult patients with renal failure as well as neonates are at risk for developing toxicity from the aluminum present in PN solutions. Impaired bone growth and delayed mental development are complications associated with aluminum toxicity. The U.S. Food and Drug Administration has set a limit of no more than 25 mcg/L of aluminum in large-volume PN solutions and requires that all small-volume parenteral solutions list the maximum amount of aluminum in the solution. The label should also include a warning that patients with impaired renal function (including premature neonates) who receive > 4–5 mcg/kg/d of aluminum may experience central nervous system and bone toxicity. Table 6-6 lists common small-volume parenteral solutions used to make PN solutions and the aluminum levels found in the product. Please note only one product in each category was selected and concentrations of aluminum vary from manufacturer to manufacturer. Thus, small-volume parenteral solutions used at individual institutions should be referenced to determine the actual aluminum load.[45]

Table 6-6. Aluminum Concentrations in Small-Volume Parenteral Solutions.[a]

Small-Volume Parenteral	Manufacturer	Vial Size, mL	Max. Aluminum Conc., mcg/L
Calcium gluconate (0.465 mEq/L)	APP Pharmaceuticals	10	9400
Elcys (50 mg/mL)	Excela Pharma Science	10	120
Magnesium sulfate (4.06 mEq/mL)	Fresenius Kabi USA (APP)	50	300
Potassium acetate (2 mEq/mL)	Hospira	50	200
Potassium chloride (2 mEq/mL)	Hospira	20	100
Potassium phosphate (3 mmol/mL)	Fresenius Kabi USA	50	32,800
Sodium acetate (2 mEq/mL)	Hospira	20	200
Sodium chloride (4 mEq/mL)	APP Pharmaceuticals	30	200
Sodium phosphate (3 mmol/mL)	Fresenius Kabi USA	5	16,300
Infuvite Pediatric	Baxter	50	30
Multitrace-4 Pediatric	American Regent	3	6250

[a]For comparative purposes only. Aluminum concentrations vary depending on manufacturer and vial size.

References

1. Bhatia J. Fluid and electrolyte management in the very low birth weight neonate. *J Perinatol.* 2006;26(suppl 1):S19–S21.
2. Chawla D, Agarwal R, Deorari AK, Paul VK. Fluid and electrolyte management in term and preterm neonates. *Indian J Pediatr.* 2008;75(3):255–259.
3. O'Brien F, Walker IA. Fluid homeostasis in the neonate. *Paediatr Anaesth.* 2014;24(1): 49–59.
4. Holliday MA, Segar WE. The maintenance need for water in parenteral fluid therapy. *Pediatrics.* 1957;19(5):823–832.
5. Choong K, Bohn D. Maintenance parenteral fluids in the critically ill child. *J Pediatr (Rio J).* 2007;83(2 suppl):S3–S10.
6. Meyers RS. Pediatric fluid and electrolyte therapy. *J Pediatr Pharmacol Ther.* 2009;14(4):204–211.
7. Roberts KB. Fluid and electrolytes: parenteral fluid therapy. *Pediatr Rev.* 2001;22(11): 380–387.
8. Guarino A, Vecchio AL, Dias JA, et al. Universal recommendations for management of acute diarrhea in nonmalnourished children. *JPGN.* 2018;67(5):586–593
9. Adrogue HJ, Madias NE. Hypernatremia. *N Engl J Med.* 2000;342(20):1493–1499.
10. Lorenz JM. Assessing fluid and electrolyte status in the newborn. National Academy of Clinical Biochemistry. *Clin Chem.* 1997;43(1):205–210.
11. Taylor SN, Kiger J, Finch C, Bizal D. Fluid, electrolytes, and nutrition: minutes matter. *Adv Neonatal Care.* 2010;10(5):248–255.

12. Eliason BC, Lewan RB. Gastroenteritis in children: principles of diagnosis and treatment. *Am Fam Physician*. 1998;58(8):1769–1776.

13. Foster BJ, McCauley L, Mak RH. Nutrition in infants and very young children with chronic kidney disease. *Pediatr Nephrol*. 2012;27(9):1427–1439.

14. Schmidt GL. Fluids and electrolytes. In: Corkins MR, ed. *The A.S.P.E.N. Pediatric Nutrition Support Core Curriculum*. 2nd ed. Silver Spring, MD: American Society for Parenteral and Enteral Nutrition; 2015:107–128.

15. Tzamaloukas AH, Malhotra D, Rosen BH, Raj DS, Murata GH, Shapiro JI. Principles of management of severe hyponatremia. *J Am Heart Assoc*. 2013;2(1):e005199.

16. Arcara KM. Blood chemistries and body fluids. In: Tschudy MM, Arcara KM, eds. *The Harriet Lane Handbook*. 19th ed. Philadelphia, PA: Elsevier Mosby; 2012:639–650.

17. Marcialis MA, Dessi A, Pintus MC, Irmesi R, Fanos V. Neonatal hyponatremia: differential diagnosis and treatment. *J Matern Fetal Neonatal Med*. 2011;24(supp 1):75–79.

18. Taketomo C, Hodding J, Kraus D, eds. Magnesium sulfate. In: *Pediatric and Neonatal Dosage Handbook*. 20th ed. Hudson, OH: Lexicomp; 2013:1176–1178.

19. Hines EQ. Fluids and electrolytes. In: Tschudy MM, Arcara KM, eds. *The Harriet Lane Handbook*. 19th ed. Philadelphia, PA: Elsevier Mosby; 2012:271–292.

20. Freeman BK, Hampsey J. Nutrition and growth. In: Tschudy MM, Arcara KM, eds. *The Harriet Lane Handbook*. 19th ed. Philadelphia, PA: Elsevier Mosby; 2012:524–563.

21. Giapros VI, Papaloukas AL, Andronikou SK. Urinary mineral excretion in preterm neonates during the first month of life. *Neonatology*. 2007;91(3):180–185.

22. Aladangady N, Coen PG, White MP, Rae MD, Beattie TJ. Urinary excretion of calcium and phosphate in preterm infants. *Pediatr Nephrol*. 2004;19(11):1225–1231.

23. Rigo J, Pieltain C, Salle B, Senterre J. Enteral calcium, phosphate and vitamin D requirements and bone mineralization in preterm infants. *Acta Paediatr*. 2007;96(7): 969–974.

24. Iacobelli S, Bonsante F, Vintejoux A, Gouyon JB. Standardized parenteral nutrition in preterm infants: early impact on fluid and electrolyte balance. *Neonatology*. 2010;98(1):84–90.

25. Berg CS, Barnette AR, Myers BJ, Shimony MK, Barton AW, Inder TE. Sodium bicarbonate administration and outcome in preterm infants. *J Pediatr*. 2010;157(4): 684–687.

26. Nesargi SV, Bhat SR, Rao PNS, Iyengar A. Hypercalcemia in extremely low birth weight neonates. *Indian J Pediatr*. 2012;79(1):124–126.

27. Taketomo C, Hodding J, Kraus D, eds. Calcium chloride. In: *Pediatric and Neonatal Dosage Handbook*. 20th ed. Hudson, OH: Lexicomp; 2013:316–318.

28. Taketomo C, Hodding J, Kraus D, eds. Calcium gluconate. In: *Pediatric and Neonatal Dosage Handbook*. 20th ed. Hudson, OH: Lexicomp; 2013:320–324.

29. Taketomo C, Hodding J, Kraus D, eds. Potassium acetate. In: *Pediatric and Neonatal Dosage Handbook*. 20th ed. Hudson, OH: Lexicomp; 2013:1542–1543.

30. Taketomo C, Hodding J, Kraus D, eds. Potassium chloride. In: *Pediatric and Neonatal Dosage Handbook*. 20th ed. Hudson, OH: Lexicomp; 2013:1544–1546.

31. Taketomo C, Hodding J, Kraus D, eds. Potassium phosphate. In: *Pediatric and Neonatal Dosage Handbook*. 20th ed. Hudson, OH: Lexicomp; 2013:1551–1553.

32. Taketomo C, Hodding J, Kraus D, eds. Sodium phosphate. In: *Pediatric and Neonatal Dosage Handbook*. 20th ed. Hudson, OH: Lexicomp; 2013:1734–1738.

33. Kalhoff H, Manz F. Nutrition, acid-base status and growth in early childhood. *Eur J Nutr*. 2001;40(5):221–230.

34. Cuzzolin L, Fanos V, Pinna B, et al. Postnatal renal function in preterm newborns: a role of diseases, drugs and therapeutic interventions. *Pediatr Nephrol.* 2006;21(7):931–938.

35. Kalhoff H, Manz F, Kiwull P, Kiwull-Schone H. Food mineral composition and acid-base balance in preterm infants. *Eur J Nutr.* 2007;46(4):188–195.

36. Manz F, Kalhoff H, Remer T. Renal acid excretion in early infancy. *Pediatr Nephrol.* 1997;11(2):231–243.

37. Lawn CJ, Weir FJ, McGuire W. Base administration or fluid bolus for preventing morbidity and mortality in preterm infants with metabolic acidosis. *Cochrane Database Syst Rev.* 2005;(2):CD003215.

38. Drukker A, Guignard JP. Renal aspects of the term and preterm infant: a selective update. *Curr Opin Pediatr.* 2002;14(2):175–182.

39. De Curtis M, Rigo J. Nutrition and kidney in preterm infant. *J Matern Fetal Neonatal Med.* 2012;25(suppl 1):55–59.

40. Kermorvant-Duchemin E, Iacobelli S, Eleni-Dit-Trolli S, et al. Early chloride intake does not parallel that of sodium in extremely-low-birth-weight infants and may impair neonatal outcomes. *J Pediatr Gastroenterol Nutr.* 2012;54(5):613–619.

41. Peters O, Ryan S, Matthew L, Cheng K, Lunn J. Randomised controlled trial of acetate in preterm neonates receiving parenteral nutrition. *Arch Dis Child Fetal Neonatal Ed.* 1997;77(1):F12–F15.

42. Aschner JL, Poland RL. Sodium bicarbonate: basically useless therapy. *Pediatrics.* 2008;122(4):831–835.

43. Sugiura S, Inagaki K, Noda Y, Nagai T, Nabeshima T. Acid load during total parenteral nutrition: comparison of hydrochloric acid and acetic acid on plasma acid-base balance. *Nutrition.* 2000;16(4):260–263.

44. Subramanian S, Agarwal R, Deorari AK, Paul VK, Bagga A. Acute renal failure in neonates. *Indian J Pediatr.* 2008;75(4):385–391.

45. Mirtallo JM. Aluminum contamination of parenteral nutrition. *JPEN J Parenter Enteral Nutr.* 2010;34(3):346–347.

Index

D

E

F

H

J

K

L

M

P

S

T